For Don
a fellow Traveler - Reader
for your colleagueship
[signature]

HEALTH CARE REFORM IN SWEDEN, 1980–1994

HEALTH CARE REFORM IN SWEDEN, 1980–1994

Andrew C. Twaddle

AUBURN HOUSE
Westport, Connecticut • London

Library of Congress Cataloging-in-Publication Data

Twaddle, Andrew C., 1938–
Health care reform in Sweden, 1980–1994 / Andrew C. Twaddle.
p. cm.
Includes bibliographical references and index.
ISBN 0-86569-289-0 (alk. paper)
1. Health care reform—Sweden 2. Medical care—Government policy—Sweden. 3. Public health—Political aspects—Sweden.
I. Title.
RA517.T86 1999
362.1'09485'09048—dc21 99-12565

British Library Cataloguing in Publication Data is available.

Library of Congress Catalog Card Number: 99-12565
ISBN: 0-86569-289-0

First published in 1999

Auburn House, 88 Post Road West, Westport, CT 06881
An imprint of Greenwood Publishing Group, Inc.
www.greenwood.com

Printed in the United States of America

The paper used in this book complies with the Permanent Paper Standard issued by the National Information Standards Organization (Z39.48-1984).

10 9 8 7 6 5 4 3 2 1

To the Memory of
Martin U. Martel
1929–1995
Professor of Sociology
Brown University
Master Teacher
Devoted Mentor
Respected Colleague
Beloved Friend

Contents

Figures and Tables

FIGURES

TABLES

Preface

As part of what has been called a "New World Order," the welfare systems of the developed world have come under substantial challenge. New transnational corporate development, new international trade agreements, and other instruments of a global economy are focused on increasing the profitability of business, which has meant scaling back programs that have raised the "cost of doing business": unemployment insurance, pensions, family benefits and—most costly of all—health benefits.

This development makes Sweden a place of special interest. With the post–World War II development of the welfare state throughout the Western world, Sweden had taken the lead. By the 1970s, Sweden was considered a model of the successful welfare state. It had a broader range of more elaborate programs providing more security to more people than could be found in any other country. It had the lowest infant mortality and the highest life expectancy of any country in the world (challenged only by the other Scandinavian states and, later, Japan).

Investigators from other countries, particularly the United States—which had the least developed welfare state, providing fewer programs to fewer people, and in the 1960s had the lowest life expectancy and the highest infant mortality of any developed nation in the world—flocked to Sweden to learn from its success. I was among the second generation of those investigators, looking at the ambulatory health services in Göteborg in 1978–1979.

Like most American researchers, I was most impressed with the number of problems that seemed to have been solved in Sweden while seeming to be beyond solution in my own country. I confess to becoming quite enamored of the Swedish model, even while publishing critical assessments of the substantial problems that remained in primary care. I returned to Sweden in 1980, 1983, and 1990. On that last visit, I detected what seemed to me to be a sudden shift in the health policy debates in Sweden.

Instead of speaking about the medical care system in terms of effectiveness, solidarity, and public planning, the discussions were focused on competition, markets, and privatization. There were serious proposals and programs to bring in the concept of diagnosis-related groups as a means of accounting for medical care costs and for generating a "market" where services could be "purchased" by public authorities from either public or private "sellers." To me it was like being at sea in the North Atlantic and finding my compass pointing south. The direction seemed to me to have turned 180 degrees. At a conference in Stockholm in 1990, I charged that Sweden was taking some of the most pernicious features of the U.S. health care system without adequate critical reflection. I was roundly criticized by a friend who is a physician and a Conservative politician for not appreciating that they understood that "the American medical care system is the worst in the world and nobody here would think of imitating it."

Nonetheless, Sweden seemed to be taking on more of the characteristics of the U.S. system, and focusing on shifting the public system into a more market-like mode of operation. On the one hand, I was, and remain, surprised and dismayed at how easily the Swedes seemed prepared to give up what still seemed to me to be a model for the rest of the world. On the other hand, my curiosity was aroused. How do you explain such a sudden shift in the direction of policy development? I raised the question and was provided with answers that seemed to me to be much too easy and unconvincing. I resolved to return to Sweden to take a closer look.

The opportunity was provided by Tema H of Linköpings Universitet. They expressed an interest in having me visit to pursue a very different agenda: to explore with philosophers a typology of health problems I had developed many years ago. Not only was that project interesting, but it would put me in place to take a closer look at the changes I was piecing together from fragments of information that filtered through to the United States. At Tema H, I found several colleagues and students who were willing to discuss issues that were of interest to me, to provide me with references, and to use their contacts to help me arrange interviews. I must especially acknowledge the help and guidance of Lennart Nordenfelt, Jan Sundin, Lars Söderström, Thomas Brante, Ulla Lundh, Bengt-Erik Eriksson, Per-Erik Liss, Bengt Richt, and a wonderful staff: Peter Berkesand, Yvonne Blixt, Lena Hector, and Monika Thörnell. I am forever indebted to them for guidance and support.

I was able to move for several months to the Institutionen för Socialmedicin at Akademiska Sjukhuset of Uppsalas Universitet, where I had the pleasure of association with Claes-Göran Westrin, Björn Smedby, Kerstin Carsjö, Mats Thorslund, Ragnar Berfenstam, and Eric Paulson. Ulla Sigeman was tireless in her secretarial support.

An old friend, Bengt Mollstedt, provided me with a much-needed introduction and orientation to the problems, mobilized his considerable contacts on my behalf, and offered a vital critical foil to my thinking throughout the project. In all my work in Sweden over the past twenty years, he has been my anchor. A new acquaintance whom I met when I interviewed him as a subject for this study, Bo Holmberg, then chair of the Parliamentary Committee on Health and Welfare and now governor of the Södermanland province, also helped me contact respondents. He has been a source of continuing support as well.

Lars Bergqvist, Professor of Economics at Tema H, very kindly read the entire manuscript and corrected my misspellings in Swedish. My colleague Richard Hessler spent two days with me in Stockholm to help with interviewing members of Parliament. My colleages Don Granberg and Ken Benson kept me appraised of developments in their areas of expertise, the Swedish political system and Swedish industrial policy, respectively. Sara E. Priddy of the Academic Support Center at the University of Missouri drew the figures.

To all of these people I express my gratitude for sharing knowledge, for sharing resources, for giving of their valuable time, for providing a home, for friendship, for support, and for criticism, all of which were needed more than they can appreciate. Needless to say, nothing accomplished here could have happened without them. Equally needless to say, they should be held harmless for any misunderstanding, error, or opinion expressed herein.

The people at Greenwood Press were extraordinarily helpful and pleasant. From my first contacts with Jane Garry, to the early editing under Marcia Goldstein, to the final copy editing and typesetting with John Beck's book producing firm, I experienced working with solid professionals who were determined to make this book as perfect as they could. They were a pleasure to work with, and I look forward to our next project together. The reader can safely assume that any remaining errors are the result of my inadequate response to their prompting. To all of them, my deep gratitude.

In the text there are passages translated from the Swedish. Unless otherwise noted, I am responsible for those translations. I regret that space limitations prohibited supplying the original Swedish in this publication.

While I was doing the work reported here, Sarah Wolcott, whom I am blessed to have as my wife, was doing a study of the teaching of reading in the Swedish public schools, which became her doctoral dissertation. We shared data, insights, observations, and interpretations. That sharing has enriched this study and penetrated it in ways I can no longer identify. And the sharing of our lives has made all these enterprises more joyful, enriching and meaningful. May she forever be a part of my life.

I now turn you over to the text in the hope that what I saw and heard and how I thought about it may help others in Sweden and elsewhere to better understand and cope with the new developments that shape all our worlds.

HEALTH CARE REFORM IN SWEDEN, 1980–1994

CHAPTER 1

To Market, to Market . . . : The New Politics of Medical Care in Sweden

To market, to market to buy a fat pig,
home again, home again, jiggity jig.
Nursery rhyme

If it ain't broke, don't fix it.
American folk saying

By the mid-1970s, Sweden had built the most comprehensive welfare state in modern times, at the centerpiece of which was the health care system. Judged by conventional standards of technical quality, availability, accessibility, and acceptability, it was at least as good as any other system ever devised. From the standpoint of providing very high-quality services to an entire national population, it was among the most successful, perhaps the most successful, in the world. It may have lacked in flexibility, but not to a degree seen as problematic by most Swedes. It was among the most expensive in the world, exceeded only by the system in the United States of America. This is to say the system was not without problems, only that the problems were "good" ones: those born of success.

The principles upon which the medical care system, and indeed the whole welfare state, was built were those developed and encoded—but not originated—by the *Sveriges Arbetares Socialdemokratiska Partiet* (Social Democratic Party: SAP). The groundwork had been laid by the state church, beginning in the sixteenth century, which established public education, health care, and social support for those in need, and by the popular movements of the late nineteenth century (Olsson, 1993). The system was solidly rooted in a centuries-old Swedish tradition of assuming public responsibility for those "not strong enough" to meet their own basic needs under the prevailing economic system, whatever the reason for their being "weak."

In the 1980s, Sweden began changing that medical care system. The reasons were not entirely clear, nor was the process or even the long-term direction of change. One strategy could have been to build on the successes of the system and to make it more effective or efficient. Indeed, some parts of that system—for example, child health and maternal health—were organized so as to produce high levels of professional satisfaction, the approval of clients, and important impacts on the level of health in the population. Professionals working in those sectors held up their system as a model for the world (Twaddle, 1987). However, rather than building on such successes by treating them as models for those parts of the system that have been more problematic, such as general medicine (Twaddle, 1986), the political direction was to substantially modify, if not abandon, the *principles* of a national health service and to introduce "market mechanisms" into the financing and organization of medical care. Instead of "quality," "effectiveness," "equality," and "solidarity" being the core rhetoric in talking about the medical care system—the dominant vocabulary heard in the late 1970s and early 1980s—one heard "efficiency," "productivity," "market mechanisms," "competition," and "privatization."

We submit that this is a drastic change. It is one not obviously driven by problems in medical care, either its technical quality or the quality of care it provides. Many reasons were advanced by those promoting the changes, most of which referred to alleged inefficiencies in the delivery of services: rapidly increasing costs, long waiting lists for elective surgery, delays in transfers from hospitals to nursing homes, and so on. These problems were certainly there, but, for reasons we will elaborate, seemed inadequate to explain the new political course.[1]

Other reasons advanced by the proponents of change in the early 1990s had to do with the new international economic environment in which Sweden found itself. Not just medical care but all of the welfare state must change, it was argued, to enable Sweden to compete in the modern world. The economy had become increasingly internationalized and the sector most exposed to international competition had increasingly found the "Swedish model" a handicap. The European Union, which Sweden joined (with the support of all parliamentary parties other than the Left Party) had regulations requiring modification of welfare-state structures. For purely economic reasons, it was argued, Sweden must change. While much more compelling, we think these arguments are still insufficient as explanations. Our reasons will be presented after we have established some groundwork.

We also submit that an analysis of the changes in Swedish medical care policy have implications other than those for medical care in Sweden or even the future of the Swedish welfare state. There was an international resurgence of "classical" or "neo-liberal" economic theory as a basis for social and economic policy. From a perspective focused on the development of public systems of social welfare to one focused on market, competition, and privatization, we had seen a resurgence of the right in Thatcher's Britain, Reagan's United States, and other countries as well. Sweden is the country that had gone furthest in developing a public welfare model and might be seen as the country best suited to resisting a rightist revival. That it felt and continues to feel those pressures is not surprising. How it handles them is of interest to all people facing the "market" as the organizing principle of political life.

This work is intended to explore in some detail the nature of the proposed changes in medical care, the context in which those changes were being proposed, and the steps that were taken to implement change. We will be providing a documented and data-supported argument leading to a conclusion that the current climate is fundamentally a political one. In so doing, we hope to provide a new bit of understanding relevant to the condition of the modern world.

In the remainder of this chapter, we will spell out in more detail a description of the Swedish medical care system at its zenith of comprehensiveness, the late 1970s and early 1980s. That description will show a strong system of medical care; one in need of modifications and adjustments, but one with fundamentally solid principles. We will then try to outline the changes in policy direction that were evident between 1980 and 1994.[2] That outline will show that the features that made the medical care system strong were the ones being modified, leading to a potential for a less-effective and less-efficient system. While far from showing that the system was weakened, it does show that the system was placed at risk.

Our broad question was this: *Why are the Swedes placing an exceptionally strong medical care system at risk by changing from principles of pubic responsibility and planning to those of the market?* This question is particularly interesting in light of the fact that the system, indeed the whole "Swedish model," was devised to protect certain centrally important activities *from* market forces. Indeed, it has long been held that one of the characteristics of professional activity, emphatically including medicine, is that it is not a business and must not be operated on market principles (e.g., Carr-Saunders and Wilson, 1933; Parsons, 1968; Abbott, 1988). After presenting the strengths and weaknesses of the medical care system as of 1980 and the policy directions during the 1980s and early 1990s, we will present a plan of analysis. This introduction should be sufficient to frame the problem of this work more sharply.

THE SWEDISH SYSTEM 1980

As of the early 1980s, the Swedish medical care system seemed to be largely a success story, albeit one with much room for further improvements, particularly with reference to primary care and cost control.[3] Its main features, as we saw them, were as follows:

- There was universal access to medical services. A system of financing through general taxation provided that everyone could get medical care when needed. There were no cost barriers. The criteria for service was medical need, leaving physicians free to exercise their best professional judgment unbound by patients' social circumstances. Needless to say, this was a spectacular achievement from the perspective of an observer from the United States!
- The medical surveillance of children was excellent. All children received screening examinations, immunizations, and care in a system that maximized the potential for early detection of problems from birth through the compulsory school years. Pediatricians worked simultaneously in a large teaching hospital and in ambulatory care. They had high morale, seeing their work as effective and interesting.
- Medical surveillance of pregnancy was almost universal, with most prenatal care being delivered by nurse midwives and all but high-risk births being attended by nurse midwives. Maternal health physicians were able to concentrate on the complicated cases. They also had high morale.
- Infant and maternal mortality was among the lowest in the world and life expectancy among the highest.
- The public saw public medical care as providing high technical quality (Zetterberg, 1979). Indeed, the capacity of Swedish medicine could match that of any other country. The physicians were as well trained as any and the infrastructure was as sophisticated. That capacity was available to anyone in need, making the average technical quality of care much higher than that of other, equally advanced medical care systems.
- There was a system for allocating technology and personnel. A system of regional (high technology, teaching) hospitals, county hospitals, and local hospitals, each with limits on the kinds of specialties and technologies they could have, had effectively controlled the duplication of services that had driven up costs in the United States. In the late 1970s, for example, there were the same number of CAT scanners in Columbia, Missouri (c. 60 thousand population) and in the country of Sweden (c. 8.3 million).
- The system was cost effective at a unit level. Indeed, the cost per unit of service, such as a day in the hospital, was among the lowest in the developed world. Hospitals and clinics were run more efficiently than in the United States. On such measures as the cost per (specific type of) surgical operation, cost per patient day, cost per clinic visit, and so forth, Sweden compared favorably with countries with much lower investments in medical care. Among the most sophisticated systems, they were among the cheapest at the point of delivery.

Yet, as noted, there was substantial room for improvement. Indeed, some aspects of the system seemed not to be working well at all, either with reference to the quality of care or the cost of medical services. The most important were the following:

- Swedish medicine was highly specialized, more than any other country in the world. Indeed, in 1978 only 9 percent of the physicians were in general practice and only 14 percent practiced in ambulatory care. Most were in highly specialized hospital positions.
- District medical care was overburdened and underdeveloped. Most primary care districts were very large relative to the personnel serving them. To manage the demand, almost all general practitioners "blockaded" their telephones twenty-three hours a day with answering machines, making it all but impossible to make contact in less than several days.[4] People sought care for emergent conditions in the hospital emergency rooms, as access to appropriate primary care was limited.
- By international comparisons, Sweden had the lowest number of ambulatory physician visits per capita of any developed country and the highest number of hospital days. In the United States, Kaiser Permanente, a pre-paid group plan with its own hospitals, had shown that medical care costs could be reduced by approximately 40 percent in the U.S. context by providing each unit of care in the cheapest appropriate setting. Sweden seemingly took the opposite approach, and delivered each unit in the most expensive possible setting.
- The medical care system in Sweden was among the most expensive in the world, exceeded only by the United States. Part of the cost was associated with the very high proportion of old people in Sweden, at that time nearly 15 percent. Even with that, however, a conservative estimate would be that Sweden could cut its per capita medical care costs by half with no reduction in quality simply by doing everything possible outside the hospitals consistent with good quality.
- There was a single, bureaucratically organized system of care. While it was organized differently in different sectors (e.g., child care, maternal care, primary care) it did not differ from place to place within sectors. A planning process that took diversity into account at every step seemed to produce a system with no diversity in organization. This was an increasing problem, as an efficient bureaucratic system that seemed to meet the needs of Swedes well was less acceptable to the growing numbers of immigrants, who found it "cold and impersonal."[5] It is not clear that all segments of the population were equally well served.

The problems, then, seemed to be at the macro level. What we, as outside observers, thought was needed was a shift of care from the hospitals to ambulatory care, an increase in the numbers of primary care physicians, and improvements in the accessibility of primary care. At the micro level, the level of service delivery to patients, the system worked more efficiently than almost any other in the world. Unit costs for services were low.

While there were things that could be handled more efficiently at lower levels of organization, such as some routine purchasing decisions, it seemed to be the case that keeping central control over the allocation of personnel and technology was cost effective and consistent with high-quality care (cf. Hollingsworth, Hage, and Hanneman, 1990). While some district physicians seemed to work a fairly relaxed schedule as compared with their American counterparts, it was not clear that they were slower than other workers in Sweden, nor was it clear that the slower Swedish pace was not responsible for gains in quality.[6]

The overall picture was one of a system that worked well but had some important "bugs" that indicated a need for further development. None of the problems seemed to be inherent in the nature of public organization of services or the "Swedish model." Indeed, the problems were in principle solvable because there was an organization that could respond to them. Given the rapid development of the system, problems were not surprising.

THE CHANGING DIRECTION OF NATIONAL MEDICAL CARE POLICY

Since 1980, a series of reforms has been introduced into medical care. In 1982, a new law governing all medical care nationally took effect, decentralizing responsibility for the medical care system to the twenty-six counties and three independent municipalities. In 1984, the so-called Dagmar reform capped the expansion of private practice and provided for greater control over state medical care expenditures. In 1992, the so-called Ädel Reform decentralized all responsibility for the care of the aged from the counties to the municipalities. Also in 1992, a Care Guarantee (*Vårdgaranti*) reform provided that patients with one of twelve diagnoses associated with long waiting times for treatment were "guaranteed" treatment within three months or referral to another clinic. Finally, a Family Physician (*husläkare*) reform took effect in early 1994, requiring every permanent resident of Sweden to sign up with a primary care physician, thus converting primary care from a system of district medicine to a point-of-service system.[7]

Here we will note the highlights of each reform with an emphasis on changes in the structural arrangements that seemed to have been responsible for the success of the system up until 1980.

Heath and Sickness Care Law of 1982

In 1975, a Commission of Inquiry (*Hälso- och sjukvårdsutredningen*) was appointed to revise the national laws governing medical care in the form of a *ramlag*. The Commission completed its work in 1979 (SOU 1979:78), and a proposition was made to the *Riksdag* in 1980 (Regeringens propositionen 1981/82:97). The new law effectively repealed an eighteen-year-old Medical Care law (*Sjukvårdslagen* 1962:242) and a proclamation providing additional regulations (*Sjukvårdskungörelse* 1972:676).

The earlier regulations had been quite detailed and increasingly obsolescent in the face of rapid changes in medicine (Twaddle and Hessler, 1986).[8] The directive establishing the Commission of Inquiry was intended to produce a national law that was less detailed, one that would allow more local decisions to be made, and one that had the flexibility to remain relevant in a period of great changes.

The Commission proposal would have decentralized all operational responsibility for medical care to the counties while retaining responsibility in the national government for the allocation of technology and personnel. The law as enacted, however, significantly weakened the national role in this regard.

The law consisted of four main sections.[9] The first defined health and sickness care as consisting of prevention, diagnosis, and treatment of disease and injury, removing monitoring and dental care from the Commission proposal. The second set general goals for medical care (quality, accessibility, safety, equality in terms of delivery) and standards for the provider–patient relationship (respect for independence and integrity, good relationships). The last, which embodied most of the important changes, empowered the national government to set special terms for medical care in time of war.

It placed responsibility for providing medical care with the county governments and provided for urgent care of persons visiting counties. It mandated hospitals and defined hospital and ambulatory care. It mandated an appropriate system for transportation of the sick. It called for planning medical services in a manner that takes account of population needs and non-county run organizations. The national government was empowered to create multicounty regions to facilitate cooperation among counties (3–9 §).

It also mandated that each county establish a board to administer health and sickness care services and empowered counties to establish other agencies under the board (10–12 §) and required counties to hire appropriate personnel, requiring a physician be responsible for medical care activities, and term limits for physicians in training. It authorized the national government to set qualifications for positions (13–16 §). It allowed counties to charge patients for services, provided all were treated alike; they limited hospital charges to pensioners, and they set a three-year limit on attempts to collect bad debts (17 §).

The national government retained the power to oversee the whole medical care system, including the right to conduct inspections (18 §) as well as the right to issue directives to protect individuals or direct work activities in general.

In brief, then, the law removed the national government from all direct delivery of health and medical care services and gave the counties authority to run their own systems under some broad guidelines. The national government retained the authority to set minimum qualifications for work in the system and to exercise oversight. A myriad of detailed regulations were superseded by a *ramlag*.

The Dagmar Reform of 1984

After 1980, private practice of medicine had expanded rapidly, as measured both by the number of mostly part-time physicians who joined the sickness insurance funds and by the numbers of claims on those funds. The Social Democratic response was to introduce "legislation aimed at controlling and containing spare-time private practitioners: the Dagmar Reform. This reform is also an instrument to redistribute a small proportion of the health care budget and to institute a system of prospective payment for that small proportion" (Rosenthal, 1989).

At that time, the financing of medical care was mostly from county council taxes (71%). Eight percent came from the national social insurance system, and 10 percent came from national government subsidies. Under the new legislation, the national moneys (insurance and subsidies) were combined and provided as a block grant based on population size. Private practitioners could no longer directly bill the national sickness funds, but had to work under negotiated contracts with the county council boards.

The reform was quite successful in reducing private practice. Calltorp (1989b) showed data from *Riksförsäkringverket* documenting a drop from well over 5 thousand physicians in the sickness insurance program in 1984 to just over 2 thousand in 1985. As he expressed it, "Through this reform relatively free opportunities for physicians to attach themselves to sickness insurance full or part time came to an end" (p. 63). Calltorp contended that the Dagmar Reform (Regeringens propositionen 1983/84:190) had it's most important impact in establishing block grants.

> The most important part of the Dagmar reform was the consolidation of a large part of the state's payment to the counties in a lump sum allocated according to a per-capita model. Earlier, an allocation according to performance had been in effect. . . . (p. 63)

> The construction of the Dagmar Reform created an important instrument enabling the state to institute resource control. The state's payments to the counties, including the compensation collected from employers for financing general health insurance, is divided in lump sums to the counties. (p. 70)

As a result of the reform, the state could predict and control its expenditures. Counties could control the numbers in private practice.

One immediate sequel to the Dagmar Reform was the development of three forms of private health insurance, and a large number of physicians—Rosenthal (1989) estimated 20 percent—signed on to at least one of them (Calltorp, 1989a). As shown by Olsson (1993), this was just one of many private initiatives in the late 1980s to open nongovernmental alternatives in welfare. While there had been some growth in private practice as a result, the numbers of physicians involved remained well below the 1984 peak a decade later.

Another sequel is that during the 1980s the percentage of GNP spent on medical care in Sweden actually declined. Sweden was one of the only nations in the world where that had happened as of 1996. While other factors were likely involved, the capping of state expenditures was certainly an important factor.

The Ädel Reform of 1992

The Ädel Reform takes its name from the *Äldredelegationen*, a commission created in 1988 to develop a better way of coping with the rapidly growing population of aged persons. Its primary directive was to look into the division of responsibility between the twenty-three counties, which, in addition to three freestanding municipalities, had total responsibility for medical care, and the 224 municipalities, which had responsibility for housing and social welfare needs.

The Commission proposed responsibility for the care of the aged be transferred from the counties to the municipalities.[10] For several years, commissions had been at work to find a way to integrate medical care and social care of the aged (e.g., SOU 1987:21). The reasoning was that parallel organizations with overlapping responsibilities were inefficient and coordination of care was unnecessarily complicated. Further, individuals had difficulty discovering who was politically responsible, old people were sometimes forced to change residence when their care needs changed, and the division of responsibility among persons caring for the aged followed administrative jurisdictions more than the logic of care needs (Edström-Fors, 1991).

The result was four laws—introduced in 1990, passed in 1991, and effective in January 1992 (SFS 1990: 1402; 1990:1403; 1990:1404; 1990:1405)—which decentralized responsibility for the care of the aged, including long-term medical care, from the counties to the municipalities. Some twelve other laws had to be substantially modified as part of the reform, including the health and sickness care law of 1982 (Hedin, 1991).

The main thrust of the legislation was to assign to the municipalities responsibility for nursing homes and other care facilities that provide long-term somatic medical care. In so doing, municipalities were empowered to create the necessary administrative structures and required to build appropriate facilities or to pay for facilities provided by others. The state funding of counties and municipalities was altered to accommodate the changes and a grant was made to ease the transition for the municipalities (Socialstyrelsen, 1993a).

One provision in the law on fiscal responsibility (SFS, 1990:1404) dealt with patients in hospitals whose medical treatment was completed but who occupied beds because there were no spaces in more appropriate facilities to house them. Such patients were known as "bed blockers" (Thorslund and Parker, 1992). Not only were they in a more expensive facility than they needed, they were preventing other patients in need of care from finding a place in the hospital. This was a factor in the waiting lists for elective surgery. A large number of beds were being blocked in the large cities. What the bill did was to provide that the municipalities would be responsible for the cost of the hospital bed one day after the hospital notified them that the patient was ready for discharge. The municipality was then faced with the alternative of finding an appropriate place for the patient to stay or paying for a very expensive acute care hospital bed. According to several informants in Sweden who monitored the medical care system carefully, this provision seemed to have been fruitful, as the number of patients blocking beds had been sharply reduced as of 1993 (Könberg and Petersson, 1993; Mollstedt, 1993; Eliasson, 1993; cf. Socialstyrelsen, 1993a).

Almost immediately, reports of a sharp decline in the quality of care for the aged surfaced (Johansson, 1993e). Those working in the municipalities with social services spoke of the "deskilling" of medical care when it was turned over to an organization with no experience managing medical services.[11] Several articles appeared in the national press pointing to evidence that the quality of care had deteriorated (Johansson, 1993c; 1993b; 1993d; 1993a). Even the editors of Dagens Nyheter, who seemed to be fully in accord with the ideologically neo-liberal Lindbeck Commission report (Ekonomikommissionen, 1993), wrote that the competence of care in nursing homes had become a real concern ("Ädel var en viktig reform," 1993). Indeed, the first-year audit of the program by Socialstyrelsen noted that quality of care was an issue that needed attention (Socialstyrelsen, 1993a).

From an economic and administrative point of view, the early reports suggest that the Ädel Reform was a success. An initial report from Socialstyrelsen, *Ädel i Stockholm*, said that the municipality was providing care cheaper than the county had done (Hernbäck, 1993). At the same time, there was evidence of price gouging severe enough for the Minister of Health to issue a warning that he would seek legislation to control municipalities that took "shameless" fees for beds in nursing homes (Karlsson, 1993).

Britta Olby (1991) writing just before the reforms took effect, noted that the goals of the reform were defined mostly from the perspectives of the administrators and politicians (efficiency and cost) and secondarily from the perspectives of care givers (technical quality and work environment). Patient perspectives (communication, continuity, information, quality of care) were ignored. That given, it is perhaps not surprising that the early results appeared as they did.

The *Vårdgaranti* Reform of 1992

Another important initiative in 1992 was a "care guarantee." This was accomplished not through legislation but through the annual "Dagmar negotiations" between the national government and the counties, based on a 1991 agreement between the state and *Landstingsförbundet* (Regeringens skrivelse 1990; Socialstyrelsen, 1991). "The guarantee aimed at increasing access for certain treatments that had a queue problem, to shorten waiting times and to contribute to a more equal distribution of medical care utilization over the nation" (Socialstyrelsen, 1993b).

For a list of conditions associated with long waiting times, mostly elective surgery, a "guarantee" was issued that if the patient were not treated within three months he or she could go to any other clinic for treatment and his or her home county would have to pay for it.[12] Within a few months, the waiting lines in Stockholm were shorter and the number of operations being done had gone up. By October 1993, surgical queues nationally had been reduced by 20 percent (Johansson, 1993f; Socialstyrelsen, 1993b). This legislation was repealed in 1994 when the Social Democrats returned to power. In 1998, the press was again reporting problems with excessive waiting for treatment in Stockholm.

The Point-of-Service Primary Care Reform of 1993

Proposals for the development of a *husläkare* had been a central mission of the Liberal Party (*Folkpartiet liberalerna*) since the mid-1970s.[13] In 1977, the government, a coalition of the Conservative (*Moderaterna Samlingspartiet*), Center, and Liberal parties formed a Commission of Inquiry (*utredning*) to propose means of countering the trend toward high technology and highly specialized hospital care by shifting the emphasis in development in medical care toward ambulatory care (*öppen vård*). That commission proposed that ambulatory care outside the hospitals be built up step by step to a point-of-service primary care physician system in accordance with the Commission's proposed models. The models included the development of care centers (*vårdcentraler*), expansion of training opportunities for general physicians, retraining programs for other specialists to change to general medicine, and studies directed at expanding primary care as a proportion of all care (SOU 1978:74).

Prior to that report, decisions had already been taken administratively to cap specialty training outside of general medicine, geriatrics, and psychiatry while expanding the size of medical school classes. The result was that a much larger proportion of medical students would be forced into general practice. In addition, the conversion from solo receptions to care centers combining general practice, district nursing, and other primary health care at single locations was already beginning. While no action was taken on the Commission proposal, those trends continued.

With the return of the Social Democrats in 1982, the family physician proposal went onto a back burner until the return of the Liberals to government in 1991, holding the Ministry of Health and Welfare and the Ministry of Health within it.

In May 1992, the government introduced a new proposal (Socialstyrelsen, 1992a) for a *husläkare*. It went out for *remiss*,[14] modifications were made as a result, and a proposal was made to the *riksdag* in the fall of 1992 (Regeringens propositionen 1992–93:160). In presenting the bill to the parliament, the Ministry of Health framed the goals "to guarantee the public a free choice of physician and physicians, with some restrictions, the right of free establishment. The law shall include publicly employed family physicians" (Socialstyrelsen, 1992b). The bill, as summarized in the report of the parliamentary committee on Health and Welfare, covered the following issues:

- It provided that family physicians came under the Health and Sickness care law (1§) and must be certified in general medicine, but they could be either public or private (2§).
- It (3–7 §) made provision for enrollment with a physician, assigned responsibility to the county to see that everyone had a family physician, and set a system for linking physicians and patients in county records.
- It provided that people could change family physicians (8 §) and specified the duties of the family physician to provide and coordinate care for listed patients and provided flexibility for negotiations between counties and physicians (9–11 §). It set upper and lower limits on the size of family practices (1 thousand to 3 thousand patients) and limited discretion of physicians in accepting or refusing patients (12–16 §).
- It provided for "free establishment" of private physicians as family physicians (17–19 §).
- It provided for compensation through (1) capitation allowances supplemented by (2) consultation fees for services provided and (3) patient fees.
- It provided flexibility for counties to reduce payments to physicians not performing up to standard with respect to productivity (20–25 §).
- It provided provisions for patient fees and travel costs (26–27 §).

What emerged was something quite different from the proposal of the late 1970s. Instead of just a development of general practice in the context of a system of district medicine, the 1993 law created a point-of-service system without a geographic base.[15] This was something quite similar to the system of general practice in the U.K.

It is difficult to say what effect the law had other than a sharp increase in the total cost of primary care. For one thing, it was in effect only one year when it was repealed by the incoming Social Democratic government. For another, the law was passed, in May 1993 after seventeen counties had already made decisions to establish a point-of-service primary care system (Socialutskottet, 1992/93). It is difficult to sort out which changes were taking place anyway and which were the result of the law.

Indeed, when interviewing opinion leaders in the spring of 1993, it was impressive how little interest there was in the proposed law (outside the Ministry of Health, of course). Labor leaders, left politicians, and the like did not have it high on their agendas, being much more concerned about neoliberal initiatives that threatened to undermine public education, labor laws, public services, and the democratic process. Even when pressed, they did not think there was much to be concerned about. When the opening to private practice was pointed out to them, they opined that Swedes would not tolerate the dismantling of the public system. Gösta Tibblin, the first Professor of General Medicine in Sweden, thought the reform would have had a major impact if introduced in 1978. In 1993, however, most of the problems with primary care had been solved, so he thought the reform was of little importance.[16]

Other Initiatives

The next initiatives came from the Committee on the Organization and Financing of Medical Care, (*Kommittén om hälso och sjukvårdens finansiering och organisation, HSU 2000*). That committee appointed two expert groups to frame discussion.[17] The first presented three models: a reformed county model, a model based on family physicians, and a model based on a national health insurance scheme (SOU, 1993:38). The second report—a committee on setting priorities under the chairmanship of oncologist Jerzy Einhorn, a Christian Democratic member of Parliament—released a report affirming the priority of medical ethics. That is, patients should get care according to their medical needs. Considerations of wealth, age, ethnicity, and so on are not legitimate grounds for allocating resources.[18]

Another potential source of reforms impacting medical services is in the Commission that is working on changes in the Social Insurance laws. This was the highest priority of the liberal Minister of Health in the 1991–1994 government. In 1994, it was too early to tell what would come out of that commission. One possible result was the dismantling of the health services and their replacement with a straight insurance scheme. Were this to happen, it could result in a more expensive care system, with those expenses passed through to the patients, greater inequalities in care, and much more uneven quality of care. Many on the left feared the direction would be toward the "2/3 society" they wished to avoid.[19]

REFORMS AT THE COUNTY LEVEL

As much reform activity as there was at the national level, especially after 1982, the activity of county governments was at least as important. Indeed, several counties had begun experiments in "reforming" medical care, some by incorporating one or more "market mechanisms" into their delivery systems and others by increasing the priority of cost savings in budgetary decisions.

Market-Model Counties

In the late 1980s and early 1990s, some counties introduced changes in their medical care delivery systems targeted at such things as the governance of the system, changing the allocation of resources, changing the relationships among various components of the system, increasing patient "freedom of choice," improving the work environment for those in health occupations, and so forth (Landstingsförbundet, 1991b).

Among the most central elements of most of these reforms was an attempt to follow the lead of the U.K. by dividing the "purchase" of medical care from the "sale" of services. In general, this meant that public authorities were to decide what services were needed and what the overall budget for medical care would be. They would then contract with medical care providers, who would themselves no longer be employees of public authorities but independent contractors (Landstingsförbundet, 1990; 1991a; 1993c; 1993b). It was thought—despite the experience of the U.K.—that medical care would be delivered in a more "efficient" manner without damaging the quality of services.[20] Politicians would be able to focus on their role as advocates of patients by no longer being in a position where they had to defend the system (Landstingsförbundet, 1990).

Among all of these reform efforts, three were taken to be special "models." In Bohus County on the west coast, Dala Country in north central Sweden, and Stockholm County, incorporating the capital city, there were more comprehensive plans for changing the medical care system. These model counties (Landstingsförbundet, 1995) are of special interest.

Bohus County

Beginning in 1989, Bohus County—the fastest growing county in Sweden, located on the west coast—took the first step in reforming the medical care system by creating a database of costs for treatment of specific diseases. In 1990, it restructured the political and administrative organization of medical care with the goal of capping the rise in costs while maintaining a high level of quality. The major thrust was to decentralize the governance of the system.

In place of the earlier hospital and primary care boards, the county was divided into fourteen health and medical care districts, each with a board responsible for the health of the population. The boards could "purchase" care from "individual physicians, care centers, care teams, cooperatives, private physicians, occupational health units, or hospitals" (Landstingsförbundet, 1991b, 12). At the district level, the role of politicians was changed to prioritize representation of patient interests.

The county authorities were owners of the medical care facilities. They financed services and took ultimate responsibility for health and medical care. At this level, politicians maintained a dual role as "producers" and "purchasers" of care. The main responsibility of the county was to allocate funds to the districts using a population-based model. Funds were allocated to the primary care sector, which in turn paid for specialty and hospital care. The districts were expected to "shop" for the best prices. Hospitals "sold" medical services from a "price list" based on a form of "diagnosis related groups" borrowed from the United States. Each diagnosis had a price, and hospitals collected money according to the case mix of diseases embodied in patients they admitted. Beginning in 1993, 95 percent of all hospital care was compensated according to this model (Lanstingsförbundet, 1993b). A special board was created to oversee the quality of care. It was entirely separate from medical care "production" and the county politicians.

The overall goal was to provide a more efficient system of medical care and to alter the political process to "focus increasingly on what should be done . . . and devote less time to deciding how [it] should be accomplished" (Landstingsförbundet, 1990, 21–22).

Dala County

In 1991, the County of Dalarna undertook an ambitious reform designed to allocate resources according to need, restrict politicians to a role as "purchasers" of medical care, and compensate hospitals and clinics according to the work they actually performed (Landstingsförbundet, 1995). The main change was in the method of financing medical services.

The main feature of interest was that all funds for medical care were given to the primary care sector, which then contracted with hospitals and clinics for specialty and inpatient services. The providers of medical care became independent contractors who negotiated contracts with the political authorities but were no longer governmental agencies themselves.

The county was divided into fifteen medical care districts, one for each municipality. In each district there was a politically elected commission with seven to eleven members. That district commission was responsible for making an overall plan for medical care in the district, seeing to it that there were one or more primary health care centers and that the work of the centers was coordinated with other entities, such as occupational health units. It was at this level that contracts were made with the primary health care centers. Primary care centers had three to five district physicians, each responsible for approximately 2 thousand patients. The plan was that the primary health care center would be able to document and follow the health of the population in the area. The planners held that this would improve public health surveillance as well as provide a more personalized service for individual patients (SIAR, 1990; Landstingsförbundet, 1991b).

The overall governance of the system remained with the county government, which set goals and coordinated the overall work of the system. Through an eleven-member politically appointed board, they allocated funds to the medical care districts based on population size and composition, the most important element of which was the age distribution of the population. The county Board of Health negotiated agreements with the hospitals and clinics, including which clinics would be part of the medical care system and what conditions and fees they would impose for providing care. Hospitals and clinics would no longer be on an annual budget, but would be "profit centers," compensated according to the services actually provided.

Patients in the system were normally assigned to the primary care center nearest them, but they could change centers and/or physicians as long as the change was recorded. In addition, patients could consult physicians other than their primary care provider, generalist or specialist, by paying a higher fee.

Stockholm County

Beginning in 1992, Stockholm County changed both its system for governing medical care and its system of financing services for the sick. The most important component of change was from a budget-driven, centrally governed system to one organized around a "purchase-sale" system.[21] Providers (physicians, clinics, hospitals) were paid according to the services delivered (SPRI, 1993).

The county was divided into nine medical care districts, in eight of which the acute general hospital was removed from the previously integrated system and made a freestanding unit, compensated by the volume and type of services delivered. A Board of Health oversaw the medical care for the county. The board continued to run the hospitals. Three standing committees were formed from the board. One was responsible for purchasing services for the county; one negotiated contracts with the hospitals, which were defined as "producers"; and one worked with issues involving the quality of services. The board also allocated funds to each of the districts according to population size and composition (with the greatest weight on age), and negotiated agreements between the primary care chiefs and the clinic chiefs.

Each district was governed by a district committee with the responsibility of seeing that the population's need for medical care was met. It was responsible for the operation of the primary care system, psychiatry, and geriatric care. It was primarily the purchaser of acute medical care (Landstingsförbundet, 1991b, 1993a; SPRI, 1993).

Budget Model Counties

Other counties maintained "traditional" politically centralized, budget-driven systems. Among these were Jönköping, Kronoberg, Värmland, and Älvsborg Counties. Smaller experiments could be found in a large number of other counties.

Jönköping County

In contrast to the market-model counties that all tried to introduce one or another form of market mechanisms into the organization and financing of medical care, Jönköping tried to improve the efficiency of the kind of system that had characterized the Swedish model. It was a country of approximately the same population size as Bohus County, but which had been losing population since the beginning of the 1980s. Its population tended to be somewhat older than in the market-model counties (Landstingsförbundet, 1993a).

In contrast to the market-model counties, Jönköping centralized political authority at the county level. The county authorities created a system of governance in which the emphasis was on setting goals and following them up. Beginning in 1994, all work in medical care was financed from revenues. Compensation was based on services provided in the service sector and in surgical specialties. Care centers were financed by a combination of capitation, fees per visit, and fees for defined services. The main changes from earlier forms of governance were an increased weight placed on specification of work activities to be performed by specific units and a much more aggressive monitoring of performance, particularly costs and demand. A DRG system was explicitly rejected (Landstingsförbundet, 1993a).

Kronoberg County

Kronoberg in southeastern Sweden worked to bring down the cost of medical care by a traditional hierarchical process. Rather than allocating resources based on emerging need, they devised a system for budgeting based on the results of the previous year. All service chiefs were assembled at a conference and given the task of reaching consensus on how to reduce the previous year's budget and allocate the next year's among the clinics. In essence, they let the clinics "own the problem" on the presumption that they would then support the solution (Landstingsförbundet, 1995). With the exception of microbiological laboratories, all medical care was financed by allotment.

With the commitment of the county authorities to reducing costs, the decentralization of the decision making to the clinic level, and the commitment of service chiefs, Kronoberg had the largest reduction in medical care costs of any county in Sweden between 1990 and 1994, with increasing savings in every year of that period (Landstingsförbundet, 1995).

Värmland County

Värmland County also had a system for funding medical care by allotment. Local hospitals and primary care were funded according to need while the allotment for the county hospital in Karlstad was paid directly to the central district. The county authorities decided how the budget was to be divided between the central hospital and the local hospitals. Clinic chiefs had a role in long-range planning of services, which strongly influenced the allocations. Budgeting was based on these discussions and decisions on the amount of savings that must be realized.

This system realized savings between 1990 and 1994 equal to that in Kronoberg County. This was accomplished, according to the Federation of County Council's report, by building a strong consensus on the need for budgeting according to need and the need for realizing a reduction in medical care costs. Clinic chiefs were able to reach some degree of consensus on ways to reallocate activities and funds toward primary care and local hospitals.

In 1994, the county began an experiment in using DRGs to audit costs and expenditures, creating, it was thought, a stronger basis for making political decisions (Landstingsförbundt, 1995, 16–18).

Älvsborg County

Älvsborg County had what was called "traditional hierarchical financing by allocation" (Landstingsförbundet, 1995, 18). It had organized its medical care system in a manner identical to Kronoberg and Värmland with the following exception: The county authorities allocated the money for primary care directly, rather than having that task done by more decentralized agencies (Landstingsförbundet, 1995). While not as successful as Kronoberg and Värmland in reducing costs, Älvsborg County was more successful than any of the market-model counties in that regard.

Other County Experiments

Smaller experiments could be found in a number of other counties. These tended to focus on changes in administration of medical care and on making working hours more flexible to make medical care a more attractive arena of employment.

Some counties—for example, Södermanland and Jämtland—took measures to strengthen the capacity of the central country authorities to direct medical care. Various commissions that had managed medical care were eliminated. In their place, the county council established a number of committees, increased their frequency of meeting, and assumed more responsibility for setting goals and making plans. While the County Council made the political decisions, implementation was more decentralized.

One feature was the division of control over the purchase and production of medical care. Specialized services were put on a negotiated fee for service basis. The claim was that the citizens would thus have more influence, resources would be used more effectively, political debate would be vitalized, and freedom of choice would be increased with reference to the location of care.

Gävleborg County established a population-based system of resource allocation with the purchase and sale of services outside the primary care districts. Blekinge County put some services on a fee-for-service basis, conceptualizing those service units as "profit centers." Skaraborg County decentralized its political structure so that seventeen primary care committees, consisting of municipal politicians, could better link medical and social services. More resources were given to primary care and the number of hospital beds was reduced.

The Counties of Södermanland, Östergötland, and Kristianstad all established programs in which working hours could be made more flexible, reducing the number of weekends worked by individual employees. One consideration was to increase the retention of medical care workers in the system. Several counties—including Jämtland, Kalmar, and Uppsala—started providing management training to employees, most often targeted at ward nurses, to increase the efficiency at the unit level. Jämtland provided this training for health care teams as a unit in order to improve cooperation on the job. Norbotten County instituted a program to get "ideas from the grassroots," having discovered that empowered workers are more productive and effective. Örebro County instituted a program to improve the physical fitness of health care workers and coupled that with a beefed up rehabilitation program to reduce sick leave and increase effectiveness.

Some of these reforms fit well within the Swedish model developed right after mid-century, while others suggested greater or lesser degrees of departure from that model. In general, the market-model counties were less successful in containing costs than were the more traditionally budget-driven counties. An analysis of these results, however, goes beyond the scope of this study.

THE TASK OF THIS REPORT

We can now be somewhat more specific about our research objective. We want to understand why there was an attempt to reform medical care in a manner that shifted the fundamental principles from those of central direction to decentralized direction, from a planned system to one organized by market principles, from public to private services. There seemed to be much to lose in this change and little evidence that it would produce gains in quality or efficiency. To answer this question, we will explore in much more detail the structure of the medical care system and the problems it was addressing. We will then explore in some detail the development of the economy—in part because the medical care system functions inexorably in an economic environment (although not exclusively so), and in part because many in Sweden saw the state of the economy as the driving force behind medical care reform. We will then look at the state of the Social Democratic Party, which took a leading role in developing medical care, especially after World War II, and the rise of the right-wing parties that opposed much of the direction taken by the Social Democrats over the past century. Against that background, we will assess the changes in medical care and the state of the Swedish model.

In Chapter 2, we introduce some theoretical considerations that have provided direction to our analysis. These include a model of how medical care systems developed in this century in all Western countries, three models for organizing medical care—professions, markets, and a democratic political process—and some thinking on the internationalization of economies. Taken together, these identify strains in medical care, options for change, and reasons why one kind of option is being preferred over the others.

In Chapter 3, we present our methods, the ways in which we collected and analyzed information about the system.

In Chapter 4, we look at the development of medical care in Sweden with a focus on how it met the problems common to all Western medical care systems and how it met the particular strains all such systems were addressing at the close of the twentieth century. Here we will review how key decision makers in Sweden saw the problems of medical care and we will present some data bearing on the issues they raised.

In Chapter 5, we turn to the economy. We describe the economic downturn of the 1980s, the pressures exerted by the European Union, and the impact of the 1991 Tax reform. We offer our thoughts about the nature and existence of an economic crisis and its implications for medical care.

In Chapter 6, we discuss the political arena. We examine the decline of the Social Democratic Party and the rise of more right-wing parties as a possible line of explanation. We will see that a core element of the Social Democrats, in addressing real economic problems, abandoned some central principles of the party, causing a loss of confidence among the electorate. At the same time, the right, led by the Conservative Party, exploited the SAP weakness and capitalized on a variety of propitious external facilitators to gain power and to put forward their program.

In Chapter 7, we bring these lines of analysis together to show how the economic climate facilitated, but did not cause, the change in policy direction. It was the exploitation of those economic events by the Conservatives at a point where the Social Democrats were at their weakest that enabled the changes. In short, we see them as more political than economic. We also step back from the arena of medical care and look at the Swedish model of which it is a part. It is challenged but far from certain that it will not prevail. We end by laying out some broader issues for medical care in other developed countries.

An afterword briefly reviews events in Sweden that have followed the period of this study and which could form the basis for a continuation of this work.

NOTES

1. We leave these assertions undocumented here, but return to them in Chapter 4.

2. We take as a benchmark the publication of the Hälso- och Sjukvårds Utredningen report in late 1979 (SOU 1979:78).

3. Richard Hessler first studied Swedish medical care by interviewing members of the Hälso- och Sjukvårds Utredningen in 1977–1978. Andrew Twaddle first studied Swedish medical care by interviewing primary care providers in Göteborg in 1978–1979. It is on the basis of that experience that this characterization is offered. See Hessler and Twaddle, 1982; 1986; Twaddle, 1986; 1987; 1988; 1989; Twaddle and Hessler, 1986 for more details and documentation.

4. This is an understatement. With two people trying to get through by phone during the "telephone hour," it took us an average of seven working days to reach district physicians by phone. They were generally booked for several weeks in advance for all but acute care, making them an inappropriate source of care for most emergent conditions.

5. There were broader complaints about treatment in hospitals. These were identical with views found in other societies, however. Hospital care is tied to routines that exclude the patient as an active participant. To a great degree this is inherent in the nature of hospital work. On patient alienation, see Twaddle, 1979.

6. Swedes take coffee breaks morning and afternoon where people in the work setting get together for informal discussion. This seems to result in better work relations, better capacity for informal problem solving, less subjective stress,

and higher morale than is found among their more "hard-driving" American counterparts. They also have more vacation time and opportunities to be off work to meet parental obligations. From an American perspective, their work pace seems quite relaxed. They do not, however, seem to be less productive, at least in the academic work settings we observed.

7. District medicine was organized so that physicians and others have responsibility for the health of a community, including primary care for the inhabitants as well as clinical epidemiological surveillance. A point-of-service system is one in which all care is coordinated by a primary care physician. Rather than have a health care team assigned to a district, individuals sign up with primary care practitioners. The point-of-service system is the core of the British national health service and is one of the options gaining popularity with insurers as a form of managed care in the United States.

8. The law covered political responsibility for services, supervision of the counties, organization of hospitals, administration of medical care, governance of hospitals, administrative responsibilities in hospitals, qualifications and division of responsibility among physicians, hiring of other personnel, admission procedures for patients, financing of services, and so on. The proclamation provided additional regulations for administration of medical care, and spelled out responsibilities and authority of chief district physicians, hospital directors, and clinic chiefs. They allocated medical positions, set qualifications for physicians, and divided responsibility among various medical groups (SOU 1979:78; cf. Hulstrand, 1982; Landstingsförbundet, 1982).

9. A translation of the law appears in Appendix A.

10. Sweden had the largest proportion of aged people of any nation. The numbers were growing rapidly. With aging goes an increasing chronic disease burden. Between 1960 and 1990, the number of beds providing care for the aged had doubled, but relative to need, the "demand for service and care was increasing faster than the input of new resources" (Thorslund, 1992).

11. From interviews see especially Pettersson in Twaddle (1994b).

12. This list included the following conditions: coronary artery tests, coronary artery operations, angioplasty (PCTA), cholecystetomy, inguinal hernia repair, hip arthroplasty, knee arthroplasty, surgery for benign enlargement of the prostate, surgery for female incontinence, surgery for prolapsed uterus, cataract surgery, and hearing tests.

13. "Point of Service Primary Care Physician" is my translation of the Swedish *husläkare*. Official Swedish translations use the term "Family Physician," but the actual change legislated is more akin to the point-of-service primary care form of managed care being imposed on U.S. citizens by the insurance industry or the British general practice system. It does not carry the connotation that all members of a family will be treated by the same physician.

14. This is a formal process in which the proposal was widely circulated for commentary, with a specified deadline. Interested organizations and individuals respond to the whole proposal or to discrete parts of the proposal. Those commentaries are published, often with the bill the government presents to the *Riksdag*. In this instance, the commentary was published in Socialstyrelsen, 1992b.

15. Point of service is one form of what is called "managed care" in the United States. It is a system in which each patient is listed with a primary care physician

who then coordinates all care. Referrals to a specialist can be made only through the primary care physician. On international comparisons, those systems built around general practice and in which the general practitioner can screen referrals to specialists are the ones consuming the smallest proportions of their respective national resources.

16. We should also note that in April 1994, the *Riksdag* took actions to repeal the *husläkarlag* (Dahlin, 1994). The New Democrats, who had supported the passage of the law in 1993, voted to repeal it in 1994. Together with the Social Democrats and the Left Party, they objected to the system of compensation, the listing of patients, and the free establishment of physicians. They held that the law diminished freedom of choice for patients.

17. Expert groups were preferred in the Conservative-dominated government (1991–1994) to Commissions of Inquiry. Members were hand picked and represented bodies of expert opinion rather than a forum for negotiating interests. Indeed, "special interests" (which under the 1991–94 goverment included professions and labor, but not corporations) were to be excluded from the decision-making process.

18. In the spring of 1994, the Social Democrats resigned from the HSU 2000 committee in protest over the government's proposal for a *Vårdnadbidrag* to replace child and family allowances with a single child-support payment. The remaining members of the committee stated they would not try to issue a report before the next election (Medicinsk Ekonomi + Teknik, 1994). The final report was not issued until 1996.

19. This is a pointed reference to the United States, where it is held that two-thirds of the population has improved living levels and one-third is experiencing sharply reduced levels of living. In fact, the situation in the United States has proved to be much more difficult. Eighty percent of the population experienced declines in real income during the 1980s. Only the top 10 percent experienced improvement, and only the top 1 percent substantial improvement.

20. On the U.K., see, for examples, Bion, 1994; Chaston, 1994; Light, 1991; 1992d; Söderlund, 1994; Tierney, Sladden, Andersson, King, Lapsley, & Llewellyn, 1994.

21. Officials noted specifically that a system for separating the purchase of medical care from the sale of services had earlier been introduced in Great Britian. The idea there was that public authorities would be responsible for deciding what kinds of services they wanted and for arranging contracts with providers to deliver the service. They, the public authorities, would have no role in the organization of services, which would be offered by professionals in the private sector. The U.K. was clearly a model for some of the reforms in Sweden. See note 20.

Chapter 2

Factors Underlying Recent Changes in the Swedish Medical Care System: Theoretical Considerations

In trying to get an understanding of the changes that took place in the Swedish medical care system between 1982 and 1994, a first step is to organize some ideas about what might lie behind them. In this regard, some earlier work attempted to develop a model of changes in medical care organization that characterized economically advanced countries over this century (Twaddle, 1979; 1982; Twaddle and Hessler, 1977; 1987). That model shows how attempts to solve a problem of poorly trained practitioners in the early part of the century led to a new set of problems focused on the financing of the system and its ability to relate to patients in a humane way. It provides a framework for placing the Swedish experience in a larger social context.

A second set of ideas has to do with ways in which medical care can be organized: as a collective responsibility in a democratic context, as a professional service, or as a market commodity. Ideal types of these models are described along with some thoughts about how they fit some existing medical care systems and how we might think about changes over time, particularly recent time.

A third set of ideas has to do with the socioeconomic developments of the past that have varyingly been called "postmodern," "postindustrial," or "post-Fordist." What these refer to, in part, is the progressive internationalization of economies in ways that make economic activity more independent of the state, thus weakening the capacity of the state to manage its own economic affairs.

Taken together, these models (1) describe master trends in medical care, (2) present options for medical care organization, and (3) suggest reasons why the trends are toward the strengthening of one option over the others. Together, they are used to define more clearly the research question for this study.

INTERNATIONAL TRENDS IN MEDICAL CARE ORGANIZATION

At the turn of the twentieth century in the United States, there were a large number of poorly trained physicians. The nineteenth century had been a time of great ferment, in which a number of occupations developed to challenge the mainstream medical profession (Twaddle and Hessler, 1987).[1] Those physicians who were trained in universities, a distinct minority, were seeking a way to set some minimal educational standards for medicine based on the germ theory of disease.[2] At the same time, moneyed interests were seeking ways to dampen growing demands for redistributive social changes, partly buttressed by social epidemiological linkages between disease and the conditions of poverty. By focusing on the germ theory of disease, which saw health problems as internal to patients, it could diffuse reform efforts (Brown, 1979).

Both sides found common ground and arranged for the Carnegie Foundation to commission Abraham Flexner to visit every medical school in the United States and Canada. He issued his report in 1910. In it, he noted that only a handful of schools provided both solid scientific training and well-supervised clinical training. His report set the standard for contemporary medical education, and hence the modern medical school.[3]

By creating an institution in which physician training was combined with research into the causes and treatment of diseases, the medical school has been associated with a "knowledge explosion" that has continued at an accelerating pace throughout this century (see Figure 2.1).[4] It came at a time of increasing need for medical care as the population was entering a period of rapid aging. Both of these factors created an increase in demand. Diagnosis and treatment became more complex, requiring more effort in each case. At the same time, the number of physicians declined as substandard medical schools were closed. The result was an increase of work pressure on the individual physician.

Medicine responded as any other system under stress. First, it increased the scale of organization by moving work out of the homes of patients and into clinics and hospitals. This trend was reinforced by the need to share technologies developed with the new knowledge and sought as a means of saving labor. In contrast to industry, mechanization made medicine more labor intensive. Second, physicians began to specialize in small subareas of medicine. From the patient perspective, this constitutes fragmentation of service, as the patient often needed to see several physicians to treat different problems. Medicine became less well coordinated and it required more sophistication on the part of patients if they were to use it

Figure 2.1
Trends in Medicine Affecting the Physician–Patient Relationship

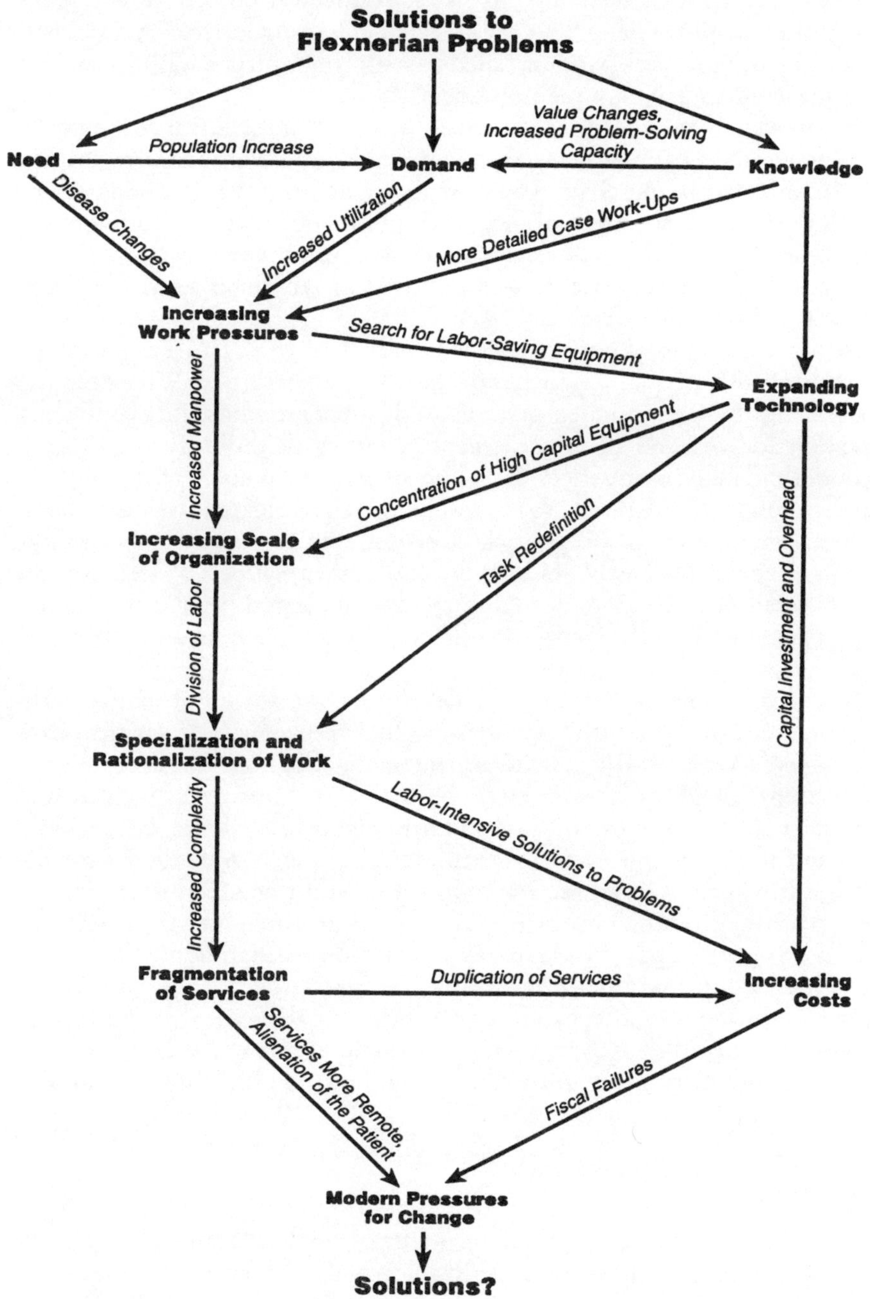

Source: Andrew Twaddle, *Sickness Behavior and the Sick Role* (Boston: G. K. Hall, 1979).

effectively. The increased use of high technology, the greater labor intensiveness of medicine as a result of bureaucratization and technological elaboration, the increased unit costs of specialized as compared with generally trained physicians, and the inefficiencies introduced by inappropriate consultations as patients failed to match symptoms with specialists all combined to drive up medical costs.

What started as an attempt to solve a problem in technical competence thus generated new problems associated with organization of a complex system and escalating costs. The new issues became the financing of the medical care system and its ability to respond appropriately to the needs of individual patients. As physicians gained autonomy in the professional–patient relationship, patients lost control. In technical terms, patients became alienated (cf. Twaddle, 1979, Ch. 8).

In other developed countries, the specifics of the historical development have differed in detail from one place to another. Whatever the differences, modern medical schools with substantially similar curricula developed at the end of the nineteenth century or the beginning of the twentieth. The consequences were the same everywhere, with substantial differences in degree as, for example, the U.K. elected to build a large general-practice sector by political decision, while Sweden allowed physicians to specialize freely. As a result, the degree to which problems were experienced differed from one country to another and the timing of a felt need to respond to the problems differed by as much as a decade. The trends, however, were identical.

At the time this model was first developed, we were noting the early development of a potential problem, in that the growth of medical care costs was faster than the growth of the overall economy in every European country and the developed non-European countries as well. It was clear that such a state of affairs could not continue for long. There was a limit to the percentage of GNP that could be spent on medical care, although it was not clear precisely where that limit was. Somewhat more clear was the growing expression of hostility to the medical profession, which was only in part associated with the antiestablishment ethic of the late 1960s. People complained more about inconsiderate and sometimes abusive treatment at the hands of an impersonal medical bureaucracy. Voices were heard demanding a more humane system of care.

We can now say a bit more about the new "crises," both fiscal and interpersonal.[5]

The Fiscal "Crisis"

Over the past two decades, the growth of medical care costs accelerated. Much of that growth was technologically driven in that new, sophisticated, and expensive methods of treatment were added to the options within medicine. Much was a result of the ways in which medical care had been organized, an example of cultural lag.

The technological development is well known and does not require additional documentation. Suffice it to say that new interventions were developed at both ends of the life cycle. It was during this period that transplantation technology, which had begun on a small scale earlier, flowered into a standard means of treatment for people *in extremis*. CAT scanners became commonplace. NMR machines were developed. In vitro fertilization, genetic diagnosis, and neonatal intensive care were developed and disseminated.

These technologies added to costs in several ways. At the most basic and obvious level, they cost millions of dollars to manufacture and more millions to buy. There was a marked increase in the direct capital cost of creating and maintaining a medical care facility as a result. Second, these new technologies reinforced the pressures toward bureaucratization and specialization and they increased the labor intensiveness of medical care. Technology thus created a "feedback loop" that continuously drove up costs. While the strength of this loop was strongest in countries with less political control over medical care, as in the United States, it was still significant in countries that politically rationed the distribution of new and established technologies, as in Sweden prior to 1982.[6]

In most countries, physicians were granted control over clinical decision making. They were either in complete charge of the purchase and use of technology (as in the United States), or a powerful interest group that had the major voice in selecting and using technology. Since new technology is always more interesting than old established practices, and since it provides new capabilities that might be of use to patients, there was a "technological imperative" in medical care that placed a bias toward using the more complex, expensive, and challenging tools in diagnosis and treatment. The result was that there was a tendency to use the more expensive options more often than their effectiveness would warrant and for conditions that could be managed as well or better with cheaper tools. In the United States, where, until very recently, each unit in the medical care system had to meet its own costs and there was no organization at any level that could make allocative decisions for technology, there was a greater use of expensive tools than in countries with regional or national agencies that could enforce rationing.

What we have described here might be considered the long-term development of an impending crisis. During a period of economic expansion, as characterized most Western economies for most of the post–World War II era, the increases in costs were manageable. The additional expense was "covered" by growth in the economy. During the 1980s, however, Western economies entered a period of depression (negative growth) or stagnation. The ability of societies to absorb medical care cost increases was compromised, making it seem mandatory that some way be found to bring the growth of medical care costs under control. The notation in sociological work in the 1960s that medical care threatened to bankrupt the societies it served seemed to have come to fruition.

In the United States, where most of the cost of medical care was borne by employer-sponsored private insurance, corporations found that health insurance was the fastest rising part of their labor costs. Even more important, the cost of health insurance commitments already made to retired workers posed threats of bankruptcy in the very near future. In an honored tradition of "lemon socialism" (Carnoy and Shearer, 1980), the corporations took an interest in promoting national health insurance, making it appear more likely that the United States would soon join the rest of the civilized world in providing universal access to medical care for all of its citizens.

In those countries where a national system of health insurance already existed or where there was a national health system, it might be expected that there would be renewed interest in cost containment, more effective use of resources, and rationing of care. Indeed, that seemed to be the case in Sweden, where there was renewed talk along these lines and a marked increase of activity in policy-making circles showing an intent to make substantial changes in the medical care system. The nature of those proposals, the identification of interests promoting them, and some assessment of the quality of the various arguments is the core of the present study.

In the United States, the only developed country with neither a national health insurance nor national health system, the thrust of health care reform was more directed toward reducing medical care expenditures and increasing the profits of those financing medical care—the corporations and the insurance industry—sometimes at the expense of the quality of care and equity.[7]

The "Crisis" of Alienation

The other crisis noted in the model is that of the alienation of the public, particularly as they become patients. Here we use the term "alienation" in its technical meaning: a loss of control over important resources. It has been argued that the development of the patient–physician relationship (and perhaps all public–professional relationships) was characterized by a growing autonomy of the professionals *in that relationship* coupled with a growing alienation of patients, again *in that relationship* (Twaddle, 1976; 1979; 1982).[8] Further, that autonomy–alienation relationship can be seen as having at least four dimensions: clinical, organizational, economic, and interactional.

Clinical

If we go back to the early part of this century, we encounter a situation in which the knowledge base of medicine was not much more sophisticated than the knowledge of the average patient. In that circumstance, the patient was in a position to make a greater contribution to the mutual understanding of his or her disease and in the selection of treatment. While the physician had more experience with diseases, and hence was a valued advisor, it was not the case that patients were expected to defer to the physician's judgment in every instance. Indeed, several physicians wrote books intended to provide the corpus of medical knowledge so that patients could handle their own conditions (e.g., Pierce, 1895).

As medical knowledge grew, it grew apart from "common sense." The expertise needed for effective diagnosis and treatment became more esoteric and arcane. Physicians became more autonomous in making the decisions that set diagnoses and selected treatments. Patients had to defer more to expert knowledge and hence became more alienated.[9]

Organizational

Early in this century, most contacts with physicians took place in the homes of the patients. Physicians spent most of their time making house calls. Medical care took place on the "turf" of the patient, which meant that physicians were guests of their patients, constrained to follow the rules of the household. As medical care moved out of the patients' homes and into the clinic and hospital, medical care was at the same time shifting to the turf of the profession. The imbalance of power in the professional–patient relationship that had earlier been partly redressed by the guest–host relationship was now intensified by that same relationship. In addition to having to defer to the physician's expert knowledge (and monopoly of resources) the patient now had to defer as well to the "house rules" of the medical institution. Hospital routines are designed to ensure technical quality and to facilitate the work of the staff, often at the inconvenience of patients.[10] The increased control of physicians was matched by a loss of control by patients.

Economic

Early in the century, medical care was delivered in a democratic context wherein the physician provided care to anyone who needed it, irrespective of ability to pay. The patient then paid the physician for the services, with money if he or she had it, with goods or services if he or she didn't. The option of bartering for services was common. It was part of the medical tradition that paying patients were charged more to offset the cost of delivering care to the poor.

The bartering option and the cost-shifting practices came to an end during the 1970s in the United States. All medical services became based on a cash economy, in which physicians set fees, determined the number and kind of services each patient needed, and issued a bill. The patient was forced to pay, either out-of-pocket or through insurance, or do without. In part this was a result of the enactment of Medicare and Medicaid, which provided insurance coverage for a substantial sector of the poor population. Even more, it was the emergence of investor-owned, for-profit providers who shifted the bottom line from service to earnings.[11] Again, as physicians gained autonomy, patients gained alienation.

Interactional

One consequence of these developments is that physicians increasingly lived in a different world from their patients. On the one hand, they lived more of their lives in a medical culture, where the modes of thinking, the kinds of decisions taken, and the assessment of people from "outside" are "common sense" within a culture that is increasingly removed from "common sense" in other cultural contexts (cf. Bloom, 1963). On the other hand, especially in the United States, physicians became enormously wealthy as compared with the average patient. In the United States, the average income of physicians grew from 2.5 times the industrial wage in the 1930s to 40 times the industrial wage in the 1980s (Twaddle, 1979).

Both these developments made communication between physicians and patients more problematic. The language used by physicians was remote from the language of their patients. Their assumptions about priorities and their assessments of the abilities of patients to follow advice, either because of their understanding or their command of resources, became increasingly unrealistic. In short, physicians and patients became alienated from each other.

Implications

This analysis suggests that public expressions of disaffection with medical care might be expected to increase over time. It has been suggested that the increases in malpractice litigation in the United States (Press, 1984; Twaddle and Hessler, 1987) were such an expression. The growth of complaints to the Medical Responsibility Board in Sweden and the General Medical Council in the U.K. (Rosenthal, 1988) could be seen in a substantially similar light. One would also expect that increasing complaints of cold, impersonal treatment, or "being a disease and not a person" would be more common.

It would also suggest that alternatives to medical care might become more attractive, particularly as these hold a promise of more "holistic" and humane treatment. Groups competing with medicine that had previously been dismissed by professionals as "quacks" became more popular with the public and exerted a claim for official recognition and legitimacy. Chiropractors, faith healers, diet promoters, and the like not only saw greater patronage but also recognition as licensed professionals.[12]

In the context of these large-scale trends in medical care organization, there are differences in the ways in which such services can be constructed, each having implications for the operation of the system and its ability to meet public expectations and needs. We turn now to that question.

MODELS FOR MEDICAL CARE: DEMOCRATIC, PROFESSIONAL, AND MARKET

It is a basic assumption for this study that the activities of any society that are aimed at minimizing disease and illness and identifying and healing the sick are social activities.[13] That is, they are patterned in ways that reflect the decisions of the members of the society, either those directly shaping "medical care" or those that indirectly constrain "medical care."[14] The central point is that any system is a matter of decision. There is no "natural" way of organizing such that any one form of organization is *a priori* superior to any other. At the same time, it is fair to speak of advantages and disadvantages of any form of organization so long as one is clear about the criteria for making such judgments.

Another basic assumption about the ways in which the social response to health problems is organized can be described in terms of different modalities of organization. Toward that end, this section describes three *ideal types*[15] that together are thought to encompass the range of organization found in the sphere of Europe (including North America) and areas under the influence of Europe with respect to health care activity. No historical example of health care organization, of course, corresponds exactly to any one of these ideal types. In reality, health care systems contain a mixture of elements from all of these types. At the same time, most systems contain more elements from one of these types than from the others. Development of ideal types is a way of gaining conceptual clarity about the elements and dimensions of a more empirical analysis. They are ways in which people think about health care systems and hence may have some import in understanding decisions made about those systems (see Table 2.1).

The first is activity organized by the community as a whole.[16] People sharing a geographical space can and do make collective decisions, even while the range of such decisions can vary greatly in scope and content. Any system for constructing health care activity by collective decision making, directly or indirectly, will be called a *democratic mode of organization.*

The second ideal type is activity organized by specially chosen experts.[17] While all societies have people who have special powers or capacities for identifying and responding to health problems, it is only in the more eco-

Table 2.1
Models for Medical Care

Facet	Democratic	Professional	Market
Definition	Decision-making by citizens or representatives accountable to the citizenry	Decision-making by experts with special training and credentials based on abstract knowledge.	Decision making by consumers under conditions where there are a large number of providers acting independently and perfect knowledge of price and quality.
Dominant Actors	Political parties, politicians, civil servants	Professionals	Business interests
Dominant Value	Equity/Equality	Effectiveness/Quality	Efficiency
Dominant Goals	Preservation and extension of democracy; influence in decision-making	Enhancement of knowledge, improvement of technique and capacity, application to problems within domain of expertise	Profit
Mode of Regulation or Control	Elections, opposition parties	Socialization, ethical standards, informal sanctions, formal sanctions imposed by colleagues	Competition
Enhancing Factors	Tradition of democracy; equality of power; constitutional limits	Public trust; absence of exploitation	Newness of market, absence of hegemony, trust busting
Undermining Factors	Concentration of power, wealth and control	Overextension of claims. professional threats to democracy. market incursions into professional sphere	Concentration of economic power; strength of professional ideologies; strength of democracy.

nomically advanced societies that these people separate their health role from other areas of activity or make their livelihood from their health care activities. In such cases, the claim to being a health care provider is that they have knowledge which is difficult to acquire and which is not shared by others in the community. It is sometimes the case that such professionals are allowed to organize health care activity among themselves. In those cases, we can speak of a *professional mode of organization*.

The third ideal type is activity organized by economic purchasing power. For this to happen, health care must be seen as a commodity that can be traded as any other good or service. The terms of trade are set in a commercial context; that is, services are offered for a price and are purchased by those who see themselves in need. To the extent that anyone is free to offer services and the only qualification for purchasing them is the ability and willingness to pay, we can speak of a *market mode of organization*.

Clearly, no society has organized in a way that can be represented cleanly by one of these models. Nevertheless, the ideal types can be useful benchmarks for discussion.

In a less systematic way, each of the ideal types has already been discussed with reference to medical care organization. In the discussion of medical care, for example, Talcott Parsons (1968; cf. 1951; 1964; 1975) argued that the market was unsuitable for medical care organization. Given the importance of medicine for individuals and the vulnerability of the sick to exploitation, only a professional mode of organization that makes the patient's needs central would be appropriate. Other observers have discussed medicine as a market activity, with special emphasis on its putative superiority to democratic and professional modes of organization in providing a more efficient and cost-effective service (e.g., Lane, 1991; cf. Enthoven, 1980; 1986; Enthoven and Kronick, 1989; Hirschman, 1992; Jönsson and Rhenberg, 1985; Saltman and von Otter, 1987; 1989; 1992; Saltman, 1992). Several observers have framed the discussion of medical care changes in terms of a conflict between professional and market modes of organization, seeing the growing strengths of market modes of organization as a threat to professional modes (e.g., McKinlay, 1976; Esping-Anderson, 1985; 1990; Relman, 1980; 1983; Kassirer, 1995; Tambour, 1997; Sherrill, 1995; Ginsberg, 1996).

All of this would suggest that these dimensions might be both relevant and fruitful for clarifying discussion of medical care organization, particularly the role of interests in modes of organization and political agendas for changes. The first step, of course, is to attempt to gain greater clarity on the definition of each type. Only then can we discuss empirical cases that mix elements of all these modes, albeit in very different ways. Our first task, then, is to present a set of definitions that clearly distinguishes the three models in order to have the conceptual clarity needed to classify observed systems. That is to say, the first step is to construct some ideal types.

For each of the three modes we will attempt to identify (1) a formal definition of the mode of organization in what can be conceived as its pure form as well as main types of variants, (2) the kinds of actors who will be dominant, (3) the kinds of social values it emphasizes, (4) the kinds of goals it sets for the population it organizes, (5) the main modes of social control or regulation, and (6) factors that enhance and diminish that mode vis à vis others (that is, that enhance or undermine its dominance).

Democratic Organization

Definition

A democratically organized system is an institutionalized means for people to make and administer collective decisions. In its ideal form, it is a way of decision making in which every member of the community participates. It is a way of organizing collective activity that is characteristic of many tribally organized societies, particularly before contact with Europeans, and some small towns.[18]

In all but the smallest population units, at least some of the decision-making authority is delegated to people who are in some way chosen to make decisions on behalf of the collectivity. These representatives generally set policy on behalf of the larger community. They decide what goals the community will have and what means will be employed to reach those goals. To be legitimate, they must represent the "will of the people." When representatives work at such tasks as an occupation they are politicians. To the extent that they are collectively accountable to the larger population, we can meaningfully speak of a democratic system. To the extent that some people are excluded from participating in the decision-making process, democracy is compromised.

As a pure type, a democratic mode of organization can hardly be said to exist in the developed world, particularly in the arena of health care. In most countries considered democracies, in which there is a strong representative element in government where legislation is done by parliaments or other bodies elected by the general public, the democratic mode is at least approximated.[19]

Dominant Actors

In a democracy, political parties are most often the means for organizing democratic activity by serving as a forum for goal setting. Political parties tend to represent constituencies with particular interests. They frame political agendas designed to further those interests. In parliamentary systems, it is in the arena of negotiation among the parties that political planning takes place. In nonparliamentary systems, it is more often the case that individual politicians negotiate goals and parties become a vehicle for election only. In either case, the dominant actors will be successful politicians: legislators and elected executives. Civil servants tend to exercise a restraining force. They set and administer routines for implementing legislation and they resist changes, thus mediating against sudden alterations in political direction or pace.

Dominant Values

The core value of democracy is *equity*. Only the participation in decision making by equals allows for a democratic process. Inequality creates coercion. A "company of equals" allows for colleagueship, open sharing, and free and independent decision making. It is only under such conditions that everyone's interests can be taken into account and final decisions can have full legitimacy.

Dominant Goals

The dominant goal of any democratic model of decision-making is the preservation and extension of democracy. Ensuring that there is a process by which everyone can participate in decision making is of primary importance. In the making of decisions, the main issue is control over the mechanisms for public decision making—in most societies, the legislative bodies and the units that give political direction to administrative units. In a democratic system, these decisions are generally made to distribute resources in a manner so as to meet conditions democratically defined as "fair."[20] The democratic mode promotes universal access to those resources defined as basic and places limits on inequity in the distribution of others.

Mode of Regulation/Social Control

In any but the smallest societies there is a diversity of interests, making it likely that any group of politicians will represent not the whole community but the portion that was able to mobilize a majority (or plurality, depending on the system) in the last election. To continue in power, politicians must be able also to mobilize a majority (or plurality) in the next election as well. Elections and opposition parties, then, are the main means of social control in a democracy.

In some systems in which there is a fundamental governing document which regulates the decision-making process (for example, a constitution), there may be other agencies that regulate conflicts or constrain interests that are counter to democratic principles. Such agencies may be administrative units (as in most parliamentary systems) or judicial units (as in the United States). In either case, there are some attempts at legislation or administration that fall outside permissible bounds. The body in question has the power to invalidate such decisions, to redress grievances, and to set limits on the concentration of power.

Factors Enhancing Democratic Organization

The main factor enhancing the democratic mode of organization is a strong tradition of democracy with rough equality of power distributed throughout the community. It is essential that each person in the community be free to express views, make proposals, and have a voice in decision making. This means there must be protections against intimidation and exclusion. Strong institutions designed to protect the right of participation are an asset, especially if they have the authority and power to constrain any who would set limits on the rights of others. In a representative system, free elections with full participation of the electorate under conditions where all points of view can be heard and taken into account in decision making are factors enhancing democratic modes of organization.

Factors Undermining Democratic Organization

There are four major limiting considerations in discussing democratic modes of decision making. The first is the atrophy of the model when a powerful group of people or interests captures the decision-making and implementation apparatus. In extreme and highly visible form, we can talk of any dictatorship as an abrogation of democratic decision making, even when that dictatorship is popular (e.g., the Third Reich in Germany, the Peronista regime in Argentina, or the early Soviet regime in the USSR). In less extreme and less visible form, we can still talk about an abrogation of the democratic model when only one side of the political spectrum can participate in decision making or parts of the population are not permitted to have a voice in decisions (as in apartheid South Africa or, to a lesser degree, the repression of working-class parties in the United States). Indeed, the most fundamental threat to democratic decision making is any concentration of power.

The second limiting consideration is in the development of an administrative apparatus. In larger political units, the administration of goal-directed activities is usually delegated to a full-time paid staff. Civil servants typically are not fully accountable to representatives or directly to the people. In most societies, they are provided protection from arbitrary dismissal, which also insulates them from full accountability. Such administrative units are often resistant to political direction and have an inertia which can impede or frustrate changes in goals or means (cf. Myrdal, 1982).

The third limiting consideration is the development of a system in which organized groups gain special access to community decision makers and distort the decision-making process for private gain. This can take the form of petty corruption, in which bills are passed, rules interpreted, or influence wielded in a way to generate advantages for individuals in exchange for special compensation for the public figures involved. Unless widespread, this behavior can discredit individuals without necessarily discrediting the institutions. It can also take the form of a more fundamental corruption in which organized private interests become the dominant source of influence on the legislative and/or administrative process, as when lobbying distorts or replaces political debate and policy making.

In general, the more any individual or group of individuals has a disproportionate share of resources (wealth, power) of the community, and the more they can mobilize resources, the more they can use force or fraud to further their ends, the less effectively the political system can represent collective decisions. When government becomes more responsive to factions than to the common good, argued James Madison (1961), representative government ceases to serve either liberty or justice.

Professional Organization

Definition

In most developed societies there are some people who make claims to be able to make decisions on behalf of others on the basis of their expert knowledge. The professional bases that claim on his or her formal training in a field that requires abstract knowledge that is useful to others and which requires that those without such training defer to the professional (Abbott, 1988; Brante, 1992). Some theorists (e.g., Freidson, 1970) have added that professionals are people who have been granted autonomy in the conduct of their occupational activities (Simpson, 1971, 261). Others have contended that the professional has formal technical training that has been validated with some provision to assure that the knowledge and skills are put to "socially responsible uses" (Parsons, 1964; cf. Freidson and Lorber, 1972). As Denzin (1968) observed, it is not enough for individuals to have these characteristics. To be a profession, they must organize on that basis to have a claim to license and mandate for the exclusive practice of the occupation. In this regard, medicine is a prototypical profession.

As an occupation based on expert knowledge, then, professionals have some special body of knowledge that is abstract, a mission to apply that knowledge in the interest of clients, and a claim to the trust of clients in the performance of their work. In effect, that means that they enjoy high status and of necessity a large degree of autonomy in defining, performing, and evaluating their work.

To organize around professional activity means that only experts will define the content of that activity. They have a mandate to develop requisite skills and to apply those skills solely in the interests of people in need of them. They will be given the exclusive right to set and maintain standards of practice on the condition that they enforce performance ethically.

When an activity is organized around professionals rather than a democratic process in the community, that sphere of activity is removed from democratic decision making. Instead, a small group of people is given license to make those decisions. To the degree that professionals are prepared to use that license to enhance their own positions and exclude others from participation in decision making, and/or others in the community grant that license, professional organization is not only undemocratic, it is antidemocratic. To the extent that a population has a commitment to democracy it will limit and constrain professional organization.

Dominant Actors

If an activity is to be organized by experts, professionals will be the dominant groups. That dominance is typically not generalized; it is limited to the problems the professional knowledge is supposed to solve. There are certainly national differences, however, in the perceived scope of those problems.[21] Taken to an extreme, it might be held that only persons with certain credentials should be allowed to participate in any decision-making process.[22]

Dominant Value

The dominant value of the professions is effectiveness, generally expressed as quality. Professions are generally oriented to increasing their knowledge, refining their skills, and applying both in the most effective manner to solving the problems of clients or patients.

Dominant Goals

To the degree that professionals take their expertise seriously and to the degree that they feel a need to maintain the trust of clients or potential clients, their goals will include enhancement of knowledge, improvement of technique and capacity, and application to problems within the domain of expertise. Aside from that, the goal of the professional will be to maintain, enhance, and defend their domain of dominance. Professional associations assert the exclusive right of decision making for their experts, try to discredit any attempt by others (including other professional groups) to gain access to decision making within that domain, and work to enhance the rewards (both status and compensation) for their members.

Mode of Regulation/Social Control

Given that professional organization is premised on expert knowledge, a public perception of the usefulness of that knowledge, and client trust, it follows that there are severe limits on the ability of "outside" groups to regulate professional activity or to control any but the most obvious and egregious violations of conduct norms. To a degree not found in other forms of organization or with reference to other kinds of occupational groups, one element of public trust is that the professionals will regulate themselves.

The dominant mode of regulation is socialization. A long, arduous, and rigorous training period with frequent quality checks and a process of certification allows the development of technical expertise and the internalization of a value system that includes core ethical precepts in a culture that places heavy emphasis on putting the needs of "cases" first, even before those of the practitioner.[23] When problems emerge, informal means of resolution are typical, such as "talking to" the violator, boycotting the practice (refusing referrals), and, under extreme circumstance, seeking to revoke the license to practice (Freidson, 1970, Ch. 7). If the state is required to intervene, it is dependent upon the testimony of other professionals to make its case.

Factors Enhancing Professional Organization

Professional activity is enhanced when the public is convinced that the activity is important to its welfare, the professionals have provided effective screening for ethical standards, and the professionals are socialized to a primary value putting the welfare of clients first. Of core importance is public confidence in the "dedication," and "self-sacrificing" nature of the professionals and confidence that exploitation is not an issue. Of secondary importance (as long as a minority of the population is adversely affected) is restraint in fees, keeping professional services affordable, an ethic of charity care, and/or some means of financing care that ensures that ability to pay does not dictate services. These lead to professionals being granted, or maintaining, the freedom to organize their own activities. Implied in this is that professionals are insulated from markets. Services will be provided to those in need irrespective of their power or wealth. Resource mobilization must not depend primarily upon the selling of services. The provision of professional services must be provided by other means, such as public contributions through taxes or voluntary contributions. Investment in technology, education, and infrastructure would seem to be essential and only partly an activity of the professionals themselves.

Factors Undermining Professional Organization

If other aspects of decision making are in the realm of democratic organization, professional autonomy must be constrained. Four things may undermine professional organization: (1) a perception that professional claims have expanded into domains that the community wishes to preserve for democratic decision making, (2) professionals themselves becoming a threat to democratic decision making outside the perceived sphere of professional competence, (3) the work of the profession absorbing an inordinate portion of the resources of the population, or (4) a move on the part of market organizations to capture professionals in the interests of profits.

In the first instance, the tendency of professionals to expand their sphere of influence may lead to democratic movements to constrain professional activity. Restrictions on the authority of the church in most Western societies may serve as an example. The movements to restrict involuntary mental-hospital commitments may be another. As any concentration of wealth or power may threaten democratic organization, professional organization may be perceived as a threat when professionals become wealthy from practice income, leading to feelings of exploitation.

As much as the activity of the experts may be seen as needed and valued, there are other things valued as well. Should, for example, the cost of medical care continue to increase at the current pace, it will in only a few years interfere with the ability to allocate resources to other goods and activities that are necessary for good health (i.e., food, clothing, recreation) or to achieve other goals (e.g., education, collective security). We are now at a point where it is recognized that the unchecked growth of medicine threatens to bankrupt societies.

In many societies, the growing strength of market modes of organization may undermine professional organization as well. Increasingly, business interests are finding opportunities for nonprofessional groups to enhance profits by coopting professionals.

Market Organization

Definition

A perfect market must meet three conditions. First, the largest unit in the arena must have a trifling amount of the total economic activity. There must be a large number of units. Second, each unit must act independently. Economic competition must be impersonal. "The essence of perfect competition, therefore, is not strong rivalry, but rather the utter dispersion of power to influence market behavior" (Stigler, 1968, 181). Third, participants in the market must have perfect knowledge of (proposed) transactions. In the empirical case, perfect markets are an abstraction; in Weber's terms, an "ideal type." They do not exist, but under rare circumstances may be approximated. Among business interests, and among neoliberal economists, markets are often assumed, even when all of the stipulated conditions have been violated.

In a market, activity is organized around people who see needs that might be filled by providing goods and services for others to purchase. The only requirement for participation as a provider is that a person have something to put up for sale. The only requirement for a purchaser is to have the means to execute a transaction (i.e. money or some equivalent medium of exchange).

Dominant Actors

Business interests dominate markets. Markets consist of those who create (or have) goods and services to sell. Indeed, it is the action of buying and selling that defines markets. If the actor is the creator of the goods and services and seeks to develop a demand for the product to increase production or the like, we can speak of an entrepreneur. The conception of an individual who by his or her own creative efforts takes personal financial risks and builds a new enterprise is internalized by nearly every businessperson and is put forth in debate to suggest that the market generates creativity and energy.

With the advent of the limited-liability corporation owned by stockholders and controlled by a board of directors, the reality became quite different for most people in business. The major actors work for a salary. In the sense that managers sell their labor and do not control the means of production, management can be thought of as "proletarianized." To the extent that they take financial risks, it is with other people's money, for which they are not personally responsible. Such people act as representatives of the organization, and to that extent might be considered professionals. Neither of these images should be pushed too far, but they do suggest that the actor as entrepreneur is not characteristic of many firms in the market.

Dominant Value

The core value of the market is efficiency, generally expressed as a ratio of costs and profits. The lower the cost of inputs consistent with earning a profit, the more efficient the system is seen as being.

Dominant Goals

Actors in the marketplace are motivated by the potential for profits. Unlike the professional expert who limits his or her occupational activity to a particular body of knowledge and set of skills, they are indifferent to the nature of the product being marketed. Indeed, it is considered not only permissible, but "smart" to change product lines with shifts in demand.

While the profit motive was conceived as a factor explaining the behavior of individuals, each of whom constituted his or her own firm, it has been applied not only to the entrepreneur but to the corporate firm. Even though salaried managers are compensated by a contractual agreement, they supposedly are judged according to the degree to which the firm shows a profit. Entrepreneurs are directly rewarded with higher incomes if their investments "pay off." There is a substantial difference between entrepreneurs and managers in the degree to which they assume personal risks in starting and building their businesses. The entrepreneur puts his or her own capital at risk. If the business succeeds, he or she earns a profit. If it fails, he or she loses the investment. Managers never put their own resources at risk and do not face the prospect of personal loss of wealth if the business fails.[24] Nevertheless, the theory of the market treats profit as the motive for economic behavior.

Mode of Regulation/Social Control

Competition among a myriad of units with approximately equal power in the economy will force each of them to provide goods and services on equivalent terms if the quality of information to consumers is good. A market is thus self-regulating, as firms are forced to lower prices if their product is provided more cheaply by another firm. The mechanism of regulation is generally expressed by supply and demand curves. As supplies increase relative to demand, prices will fall. As demand increases relative to supply, prices will rise. As prices increase, the supply will increase. The market keeps a balance between supply and demand by the price mechanism.

As a market is self-regulating and prices will always be at the lowest point consistent with supply and demand, any other form of internal social control is seen as irrelevant. Indeed, the ideology of those who work in markets is one that sees external regulation, particularly democratic, as not only unnecessary, but harmful, creating artificial imbalances between supply and demand and/or reducing the connection between supply, demand, and price (cf. Carniero, 1967; Sumner, 1883).

The state has a limited function of creating the climate for market activity, most importantly by enforcing private agreements as expressed in contracts.

Factors Enhancing Market Activity

A new product which quickly generates a myriad of small companies leads to a situation where the conditions of a pure market are most closely approximated. Under pure market conditions, it is likely that the theory of the market works.

It might be accepted by some adherents of market theory—but by no means all—that to the extent that the conditions of the pure market are violated (for example, by concentration of economic power), aggressive political activity on the part of the state (e.g., trust busting) enhances market activity. Many of those same people would endorse the use of the state to provide an infrastructure (e.g., roads) that facilitates price equalization over a sufficiently large territory to ensure a myriad of suppliers and minimization of transportation costs.

Factors Undermining Market Activity

Any concentration of economic power either in the reduction of the number of units or in the increasing share of the market enjoyed by any one of them violates the assumptions of market theory. Such developments distort the market by allowing for (1) the manipulation of supply, demand, and price independently of one another, (2) the direct control of some firms by others, and (3) a rapid reduction in the number of competing firms as smaller and weaker ones are absorbed into or destroyed by the larger and stronger ones. Indeed, this kind of "Social Darwinism" has been raised by some into an ideology that sees the "survival of the fittest" as a desirable outcome that ensures that only the best firms and the best products are retained. Social Darwinism, however, is a distortion of market theory. While it was a predicted outcome of market activity by some theorists supporting democratic development (Marx, 1973; 1974), the concentration of economic power destroys markets. To the extent that markets do tend toward a smaller number of larger units over time and to the extent that concentrated power constrains decision making, markets are self-destroying.

Market activity is weakened to the extent that professional activity is strong. Allocation of goods and/or services by occupational monopolies (e.g., licensed professions, guilds) that operate under exclusive societal mandates limits the freedom to provide goods or services on the one hand and limits freedom of choice by clients on the other. When such a monopoly can be used to "control quality" by restricting supply, a situation is created in which prices can be set by agreement among the providers. When such a monopoly controls a set of services that are thought to be of such importance that "cost is no object" (Montiero, 1973), the link between price and demand is nonexistent.

Market activity is also weakened to the extent that democratic decision making is established and decisions about the production, distribution, and pricing of services are made by collective decision making (e.g., the state). The conditions here are similar in their market effects to those of professional activity, except here the center of decision making is distributed to the whole citizenship, which will generally delegate that authority to a representative body.

Mixes of Models: Toward Reality

It is nowhere the case that a society is organized around one of these models, and only under the most ideological conditions that a group dominating a society seriously attempts to establish one of these models in its pure form.

Near-pure democratic activity might be best approximated in some small, tribally organized societies (e.g., the Lenape at the time of the first European contacts). Some populist movements, such as the New Left movement in the United States during the 1960s and the current U.S. anarchist movement, have seriously attempted to establish "participatory democracy" as a mode of operation for the society. In modern times, these movements have generally been small and marginal to the larger society.

While there have been some statements endorsing professional activity as a mode of organization for whole societies (e.g., Plato's philosopher king, Compte's sociology queen), it has been the historical case that professional activity has been seen as appropriate for some activities (most notably medical care) and not at all for others. The empirical case has been that the part of human activity that is cordoned off and limited to professionals has been larger or smaller at different times and places. As a model for societies, professional activity has not been even approximated anywhere.[25]

There have been more serious attempts to establish the market as the mode of organization for societies. It could be argued that the notion of limited government in the establishment of the United States could be seen as an attempt to establish a market-driven society, were it not for the fact that the concept of market had not yet appeared and the society was based on subsistence agriculture. Nevertheless, from time to time the market has been reified as the answer to all problems, as in Reagan–Bush's United States, Thatcher's U.K., and Bildt's Sweden. In all of these instances, democratic and professional institutions were seen as so strong that there was no real chance that the market could take everything over.[26] Most of the supporters of these movements were people who wanted some adjustment in the direction of the market, but who would not support a totally market economy should that become a serious possibility.

The reality for modern societies, then, is that there is a mix of democratic, professional, and market activity. The issues that arise among these modes of organization are ones of balance, whether one mode is too strong, or needs to be strengthened. Could we achieve a more effective result if the professionals had a larger voice? Could we achieve a more efficient result if we allowed the market to "free up" decision making by providing more choice and allowing activity to follow demand? Could we achieve a more equal distribution of activity if we allowed the community to come to a consensus about how resources could best be allocated for the common good?

We want to briefly address the extent to which different models may be characteristic of different spheres of activity within medical care organizations before turning to the next section, in which we will address the extent to which there may be a historical shift taking place from one mode of organization to another.

Spheres of Medical Organization

Production, Distribution, and Cost

Medical care organization consists of different spheres of activity that can, in principle, be combined in different ways to constitute a total system (see Table 2.2). On the one hand there are a number of activities that together constitute the production of medical activity. These include such things as selecting people who will learn medicine, the selecting of the kinds of things they will be expected to learn, creating standards for testing whether they indeed know what they should know to be credentialled as physicians, allocating opportunities for specialized training, certification of specialists, producing technological solutions, managing the division of labor between medicine and related fields, and the discipline of practitioners whose behavior does not meet the standards of acceptable behaviors (technical, moral, or otherwise).

On the other hand there are a number of activities that together constitute the distribution of medical activity to a population that has needs for medical services. Included here is the system of financing care (for the general public, in some societies only for those who cannot afford to purchase care themselves, or for those with special needs), and the system of allocating personnel and technologies.

A third sphere consists of control over the cost of medical activity and focuses on who makes the decisions that result in expenditures. We can look at those in the contexts of clinical decisions to make use of resources in individual cases, infrastructure decisions in the provision of technologies, and the control of the cost of professional personnel.

Not only is it likely that each sphere of activity can be organized in a different way within any given society, but there may be differences among societies as well. In Table 2.2, three societies with which we have some

Table 2.2
Modes of Medical Care Organization by Sphere of Activity in Three Selected Countries

Type of Activity	U.S.	U.K.	Sweden
Production of Services			
Selection of Students	Professional	Professional	Professional
Curriculum of Medical Schools	Professional	Professional	Professional
Standards for Credentialling/Licensing	Professional	Professional	Professional
Allocation of Specialty Training	Professional/ Market	Democratic	Democratic
Certification of Specialists	Market/ Professional	Professional	Professional
Discipline of Malpractice			
informal	Professional	Professional	Professional
formal	Professional/ Democratic	Professional	Democratic
appeals	Democratic	Democratic	Democratic
Allocation			
Distribution of Physicians	Market	Democratic/ Market	Democratic
Financing of Care for General Public	Market	Democratic	Democratic
Financing of Care for Indigent Patients	Democratic	NA	NA
Financing of Care for Special Populations	Market/ Democratic	NA	NA
Distribution of Technology	Professional/ Market	Democratic	Democratic
Distribution of Hospital Beds	Market/ Democratic	Democratic	Democratic
Distribution of Ambulatory Care Sites	Market	Democratic	Democratic
Costs			
Of Case Management	Professional	Professional	Professional
Of Technology	Market	Market	Market
Of Professionals	Professional	Democratic	Democratic

familiarity have been selected to represent a range of modalities of organization at the macro systemic level. The United States (up to 1960) represented a system organized around a fee-for-service payment system with very limited public regulation, the closest approximation to medicine in a market system in the developed world. Sweden (in the period between 1970 and 1990) represented a decentralized public system in which counties provided services under a set of guidelines from the national government, which established minimal standards. The United Kingdom (from 1945 to 1975) represented a centralized national system of publicly provided medical care.

In all the cases under consideration, the production of medical care organization, particularly the practitioners, was left in the hands of the professionals. Nonprofessional organizations entered only in the arena of discipline across the three societies. In the sphere of discipline, the early, informal procedures were left to the professionals. Others entered only when the professionals were unable to resolve the problems themselves. In the United States, the judicial system is sometimes the first formal mechanism used. In that case, the judiciary may be called into play more to provide compensation for injury than to discipline the profession.[27] In Sweden, there is an administrative agency (*hälso- och sjukvårdsansvarsnämden;* HSAN) that consists of jurists, politicians, union representatives, and professionals. That body relies heavily on the physician representative for judgments. While it is nominally political, it generally leaves control in professional hands (Rosenthal, 1988).

Only in the United States can specialization can take place by declaration. Physicians can specialize without formal specialty training or certification. This might be considered a market organization of specialty allocation. At the same time, there is a system of graduate training with certification procedures, a professional system.

It is in the allocative sphere that substantial variations can be found. Here there is a tendency for the United States to opt for market solutions and for the U.K. and Sweden to opt for democratic solutions. By and large, it is not the case in any of these countries that professionals make deliberate decisions on the allocation of personnel or technology for any geographic area. Instead, U.S. physicians make individual decisions based on the kind of livelihood they see possible in localities they individually see as desirable. U.K. hospital physicians locate where there are positions available and community physicians locate in areas that are not closed based on desirability and compensation differentials. Swedish physicians apply for vacant positions.

The control of costs varies by the kind of cost. In all three societies, professionals control the costs of case management. By this we mean the resources spent on each case. The patient's decision is limited to seeking care. All other costs are generated by professional decisions. Technology costs are dictated by the market in all three societies, with professionals making decisions on the purchase of major equipment within a market context. Professional compensation is set by the professionals themselves, although more frequently in negotiation with insurance companies in the United States and by physicians negotiating with politicians in the U.K. and Sweden.

It would thus seem to be the case that different models could apply in different spheres of activity within a system of medical care.

Organization of Medical Spheres

The United States is more representative of the market approach than either the U.K. or Sweden. It is also the only country in which nonprofessionals are encroaching on clinical decision making. The introduction of diagnostic related groups (DRGs) as a means of funding medicare in the early 1980s provided hospital administrators a means to influence discharge decisions. They calculated the number of days and/or procedures that bring each case to the cost that was compensated by Medicare and told the physician the government required them to discharge their patients on that day.[28]

Sweden is a more democratically organized country with broader participation of health occupations in clinical care and more political decision making relative to allocative decisions. Physicians have felt more constrained in their incomes and freedom to locate where they wish. The distribution of services has been more equitable.

INTERNATIONALIZATION OF THE SOCIOECONOMIC SPHERE

A final set of ideas behind this project has to do with developments in the macrosocioeconomic sphere, specifically with respect to the internationalization of the economy and, by implication, of society as well. It is no longer the case that nation states can be the arena in which macroeconomic decisions are made and implemented. Indeed, there is much speculation about whether the economic models that have been credited with successful management of national economies in this century are still relevant. Work on transnational social organization, however, is new to the social sciences and we do not yet have models that provide a fully satisfactory basis for analysis. As expressed by Gøsta Esping-Anderson (1990, 222), "Ours is an epoch in which it is almost universally agreed that a profound realignment, if not revolution, is underway in our economy and society. The proliferation of labels . . . often substitutes for analysis. But it mirrors the recognition that we are leaving behind us a social order that was pretty much understood, and entering another the contours of which can be only dimly recognized."

Economic Internationalization

Most analysts would agree that there has been a large and important change in the organization of economic activity.[29] The following list identifies some of the main characteristics of the change as identified by global post-Fordist theorists. Particularly good summaries can be found in Bonanno and Constance (1997).

	FORDISM	GLOBAL POST-FORDISM
Nature of "Regime"	• National economies based on domestic mass production and consumption regulated by welfare states • National and multinational corporations • Rigidity	• International economic relations based on flexible accumulation (decentralization of production, "information" of labor), global sourcing, and transformation of the nation state • Flexibility
Goals	• Growth of national internal market • Extraction of low-cost resources and labor from Third World by First-World multinational corporations • Matching domestic production with domestic consumption • Development of international trade	• Avoid higher cost of doing business in First-World states • Bypass regulations (e.g., environmental) and welfare-state arrangements • Deindustrialize First World • Deregulation of global finance, capital flight to newly industrialized and Third-World states
Mode of Regulation	• Strong local, regional, and national controls • Breton Woods Agreement • Stable, neocorporatist labor–capital arrangements mediated and enforced by welfare state (social security, unemployment) • Keynesian economic policies; state as bearer of monetary constraint, consumer credit • National relations • Collective bargaining, corporatist "class compromise" • International relations	• Absence of local, regional, and national controls • GATT, EC/EU, NAFTA, IMF, World Bank • Internationalization of capital • Transnational corporations • Globalization of economy

Characteristics

- Centralized production, strong unions
- Full-time employees with job security, benefits, step increases on ladder
- Corporations identified with nations
- Financial and research capacity located in First World
- Development of welfare state

- Decentralized production, weak unions
- Part-time and temporary employees with no security, benefits, or career ladders
- Corporations independent of nation state
- Financial and research capacity remains in First World
- Rollback of welfare state

Consequences

- National sovereignty
- Social norm of consumption
- Growth of service sector
- Homogenization
- Strong worker bargaining power
- Improved working conditions, wages, and job security
- Political decision making in democratic process
- Steady or reduced class differences
- Growth of middle class
- Facilitation of worker association, communication, and organization; workers identify with job and class

- Separation of sphere of influence of the state from sphere of influence of capital
- State fiscal crisis
- Segmentation
- Weak worker bargaining power
- Poorer working conditions, lower wages, and loss of job security
- Political decision making removed from democratic process
- Increased class polarization
- Decline of middle class
- Fragmentation of workforce; workers identify with residence, ethnicity, nationality, and consumption patterns

In the industrial, modern, or "Fordist" era, mass-production economies were organized around firms that were geographically based in a single country, even when they had substantial international activity. Production was organized in plants which centralized labor activity. Labor unions were organized and legitimated. A welfare state provided support for workers who were subjected to new pressures of cyclical unemployment.

In the postindustrial, postmodern, or global post-Fordist era, a more "flexible" and decentralized economy is organized around firms that have no national home. Production is decentralized, with workers scattered in different places around the globe, and "globally sourced," in that each component can be gotten from any of a variety of places. Nonunion and part-time labor replace full-time union workers. Collective bargaining is delegitimated and labor unions weakened or abolished. The state loses power to regulate environmental impacts and welfare-state provisions are scaled back and weakened to reduce taxes and the costs of benefits.

To underline the facts that seem to have particular importance, the nation state becomes incapable of economic or social regulation, and the working class, including most of what was earlier the middle class, is pushed into a new condition of powerlessness in the absence of any internationally organized labor movement. Until a real international law with real enforcement powers can be created, it seems likely that we will experience growing unregulated capitalist development and growing social anarchy.

The most immediate manifestations of the pressures of internationalization for the Swedish economy are tied to the development of the European Union and Sweden's decision to seek admission. The internationalization of the European economies has taken place in a framework constructed by and in the interest of the international business community. The regulations developed in the European Community and passed on to the European Union are premised on neoliberal economic theory.[30] They are antiunion, pro–free market, and opposed to restrictions that promote social policies. Meeting the conditions of those regulations is a requirement for gaining admission to the European Union.

A decision to join the European Union was taken by the political leaders of all the parliamentary parties, with the exception of the Left Party, in 1990. At that level there was a near consensus across the political spectrum that Sweden should join the EU. On the basis of that consensus, then Prime Minister Ingvar Carlsson formally applied for admission to the European Community in 1991 (Johansson, 1994), and the Swedish parliament formally decided to apply for admission to the European Economic Community in 1992 (R&D Tema, 1993). After a time of negotiation with the EU on conditions of membership, with the most important issues being the impact of membership on Swedish democracy, the implications of a common defense policy on Swedish neutrality, the amount of the annual dues Sweden would pay, and the amount of regional support the less-developed parts of Sweden would get, Sweden joined the EU in 1994.

Swedish business did not wait for the referendum, however. They moved rapidly with the support of the center–right government to meet the conditions of membership. They made a rhetoric of competition, markets, and privatization the center of a new ideological debate in place of the liberty, equality, and brotherhood approach that seemed only a few years before to be a solid core of Swedish values.

Implications for the Welfare State

These tendencies were strongly reinforced by an economic downturn in the 1970s and 1980s. The welfare state, which was built during a long period of economic expansion, made economic demands that were difficult to sustain during a long period of economic stagnation and recession. One consequence of this shift has been that the Swedish model came under attack. That model consisted of a corporatist mode of decision making, a policy of wage solidarity, public provision of basic social services on equal terms to all residents of the country, and special support for the "weakest" members of the society. The objective was to provide for a leveling of social and economic opportunity and outcomes, not in any absolute sense, but certainly more than found elsewhere in the developed world (Duffy, 1989; Immergut, 1989; Hicks and Kenworthy, 1998). Sweden had built by far the most comprehensive system of social insurance in the world, providing for income protection (unemployment insurance, sickness insurance, job retraining and placement, early pensions, etc.) and social services (education, health and medical care, home help, etc.). These programs were publicly financed by the national, county, and local governments.

One manifestation of the economic downturn and the pressures of internationalization was increased pressure from industry, particularly that exposed to international trade, to reduce taxes and regulation in order to make business more competitive. Marginal income tax rates were cut in the early 1980s and a major tax reform was passed in 1990 (Åsbrink, 1990). A series of measures were taken to deregulate finance and business during the 1980s. The results that everyone can agree upon were (1) a financial crisis for the state as an enormous budget deficit grew rapidly, and (2) a bank crisis following rapid investment in European real estate by Swedish banks at a time when real estate values were inflated, leaving massive unsecured debt when the market dropped. Beyond that, agreement evaporates.

One side, consisting of the Swedish Employers Federation (*Svenska Arbetsgivareföreningen*; SAF) and neoliberal economists (e.g., Ekonomikommissionen, 1993), has argued that the cause of the crisis is the growth of the welfare state itself. By expanding services beyond the ability to finance them, Sweden had been "living beyond its means" and must sharply scale back the provision of social services to balance the state budget. Indeed, SAF has been sounding that theme since the 1970s (Edgren, 1973; Strender, 1974; SAF 1975). In seeking models for their scenario, they settled on ancient Athens and Uruguay (Langby, 1983).

Their case rested on the contention that Sweden was falling behind the rest of the developed world in economic development. Those promoting this view pointed to the declining profitability of Swedish industry, inefficiency in the public sector, an overextended welfare state, and the difficulty of democratic decision making when technical expertise is needed to make intelligent decisions. They sought to reduce taxes, deregulate finance and business, and introduce "market mechanisms" into the public sector by separating purchasers and sellers for services. Further, they sought to reduce the arena of democratic decision making by replacing the corporatist structure with expert groups and restricting the domain of parliamentary decision making (Ekonomikommissionen, 1993).

While the neoliberal perspective gained hegemony in the Swedish political debate, it was criticized for its one-sided presentation of facts. Walter Korpi (1992) led this charge by looking at the long-term development of the Swedish economy in comparison with other European and Organization for Economic Co-operation and Development (OECD) states and a group of states most like Sweden. He found no evidence that Sweden was falling behind, only that the growth rate in wealthy countries tends to be lower than that in countries with weak economies. Labor economists noted that transfer payments were in balance, indicating that the financial problem was not with the core welfare programs. Indeed, the main foreign debt was private, not governmental. At the same time, labor held that Sweden had come to a point where the thrust of welfare policy must change. Instead of expanding the scope and size of the system, attention must turn to the most effective use of resources. For the system to work however, the emphasis must be on full employment, leveling of incomes, and equal access for everybody. This required public democratic solutions to problems (LO, 1986).

As noted, on the political spectrum the shift to neoliberal thinking was not limited to the right-wing *Moderaterna Samlingspartiet*. It was found in all of the so-called "bourgeois parties" and even in the Social Democratic party (Feldt, 1991; cf. Andersson, 1993). The result was that many Social Democrats felt abandoned by their party and wondered what it meant to call it a "socialist" party (Augustsson and Hansén, 1991; cf. Wickbom, 1989).

These issues will be reviewed in more detail in later chapters. Suffice it to say here that the climate of debate changed drastically. Instead of being the framework within which issues were discussed, the Swedish model became the focus of the discussion (e.g., Bergström, 1993; Gröning, Korpi, Nilsson, Ström, Wibe, Arvidsson, Bäck, Pinheiro, Åmark, 1993; Lovén, 1992).

Measured by the percentage of gross national product devoted to welfare services, then, the era of the growth of the welfare state seemed to have come to an end. The issues under discussion were the extent to which the achievements of the past several decades could be protected, the means for protecting them, and the best structure of services that could be attained versus the extent to which the whole idea of a welfare state was a mistake and the welfare of the country required that it be dismantled as quickly as possible.

Implications for Medical Care Organization

The core activity of medicine has been both more international and more local than other welfare activities. On the one hand, medicine as a body of knowledge and practices has been international since at least the eighteenth century. The content of medicine and the standards for medical care have been shared throughout the developed world and widely diffused to the less developed world in this century. A hospital and the nature of medical work do not differ substantially from one country to another. Medical training is quite similar in all medical schools, regardless of location, as are standards for treatment. On the other hand, medicine is a local activity. Except for the most esoteric treatments, people do not tend to travel long distances to get medical care. Indeed, unless unavailable locally, people seldom leave town for primary care.

What this means is that trends toward internationalization of economies will probably have little special significance for medicine. That is, one would expect the pressures on medical care activity to be grossly similar to those on the welfare system in general. It would be under pressure to privatize and introduce competition into the public sector. The main caveat is that medicine may be in a stronger position to resist change than are other welfare activities. It is treated as a special category of service that requires a licensed monopoly to maintain standards. In its core activities, it has been relatively immune to external controls. Indeed, that is at the core of what it means for medicine to be a profession. To the degree that physicians see the preservation of their organization as a profession as important and threatened by pressures to behave more in a market mode of organization, they may be able to withstand pressures to become more like businesses.

THE RESEARCH QUESTION

Given (1) that Sweden is undergoing the same pressures as in the rest of the developed world, having to deal with both financing the rapidly increasing costs of medical care and the increasing alienation of patients; (2) that professional, democratic, and market means of organization can be distinguished and used to describe different spheres of medical care activity; and (3) that there is an important intensification of market modes of organization in the developed world, it seems reasonable to raise the question of the degree to which the professional/democratic organization of Swedish medical care might be attenuated and taken over by a market. If that is the case, it would be important to try and understand the implications of such a development for health and medical care.

The first question must be to see to what extent the recent sociohistorical development of medicine fits the model described in the first section of this chapter. Has the development of the modern medical school resulted in the same changes as found in the United States? That is, has practice become more bureaucratized and specialized? Has care become more fragmented and costly? Are the main problems encountered in the medical care arena those of financing and alienation? If so, how have these features been manifest? Have they taken similar or different forms from those found in other countries? How has the national and cultural climate modified or specified these developments?

A second question is how one can describe Swedish medical care in terms of the models provided in the second section of this chapter. To what extent is medicine a profession as opposed to a market or a democratically organized activity? Which activities are organized as a market and which democratically? How much autonomy do physicians have in what areas? How are the activities of related occupations, such as nursing, physical therapy, and laboratory technicians organized? How do they relate to medicine?

The third major set of questions has to do with the current pressures for change in medical care activities. What changes are being promoted for medical care and who is promoting them? What are the issues that need resolution in debating the changes? What groups are resisting change and on what grounds do they resist? How well grounded in research are the arguments for and against change? To what degree are pragmatic and ideological forces driving changes?

A fourth set of questions involves the projected consequences of changes. What are the likely outcomes for medical care organization? What are the likely consequences of alternative outcomes?

NOTES

1. Starr (1982) provided an excellent analysis of the emergence of medicine as a profession in the nineteenth century. It would be fair to say that medicine was not a profession before the end of the century, so the term is used very loosely at this point. We will provide a more precise definition in the next section.

2. The germ theory, developed in the 1870s, became the first scientific basis for clinical medicine. It posited that microorganisms caused disease, that every disease had a specific microorganic cause, and that cures could be affected by discovering a chemical substance that could kill the microorganism without simultaneously killing its host. As Dubos (1959) showed, the germ theory contained an implicit promise that, one by one, all diseases could be eliminated and, by extension, death could be overcome. He suggested that the germ theory constituted an ideology.

3. And, not coincidentally, "socialistic" public-health-oriented solutions became "second-class medicine." The move to improve health through social reform was effectively slowed and brought under the control of the establishment. During this same period the socialist labor movements in the United States were repressed by military force. That these movements were allowed more freedom to develop in most European countries partly accounts for the different development of medical care in the United States.

4. This model was initially developed in collaboration with John Stoeckle and elaboated in a number of contexts (e.g., Twaddle and Hessler, 1977; 1987; Twaddle, 1979; 1989).

5. In the current political climate, it seems to be the case that economic analysis has dominated the discussion, indicating a recognition of the fiscal crisis but not the interpersonal one. To the extent that economists offer the only line of analysis (and we don't here suggest that what they contribute isn't valuable), it is likely that the interpersonal crisis will be ignored. There is a danger that it might even be aggravated. If there are linkages between the two, as we suggest here, a failure to deal with the interpersonal crisis could make solution of the fiscal crisis impossible in the moderately long run, especially, as seems to be the case, when economic theory takes no account of the linkages. It could also lead to a crisis in the legitimacy of the political system in the slightly longer run.

6. A description of changes in the Swedish system from 1982 on appears in Chapter 4.

7. There was considerable momentum behind the idea of universal health insurance in the 1992 election, much of it coming from initiatives of the Washington Business Group on Health, representing the largest corporations in the United States. When the proposal failed to take the cost of health insurance off corporate budgets, the coporations withdrew their support. An analysis of the failure of health insurance reform in 1994 goes beyond the scope of this book. See, for example, Navarro (1989) and Starr (1982).

8. In other contexts, physicians may have lost autonomy. McKinlay (1976), for example, argues that physicians, as they become salaried employees, become "proletarianized."

9. In recent years, partly in reaction to the perceived overdominance of the medical profession, but probably more motivated by a desire to reduce the use of medical facilities, an ideology has developed that an individual's health is their own responsibility (read "fault"). With better health education, improved dietary choices, and "fitness" programs, individuals could stay healthy and avoid the need for medical care. Indeed, the medical profession has been portrayed as overtreating patients, particularly in the end stages of life, requiring that patients have legally empowered advocates to oppose medical recommendations and decisions. On the one hand, this is a response to the clinical bias first discussed by Freidson (1970). On the other, it illustrates the power of the Social Darwinist revival of the 1980s in the United States, the U.K. and other countries.

10. This was a good part of the concept of medicine as a system of social control (Parsons, 1951; 1975; Zola, 1975). Hospitalization, as much as anything, is a means of ensuring that medical treatment regimens are followed by placing all initiatives in the hands of providers.

11. In a television documentary on the refusal of investor-owned for-profit hospitals in Dallas to stabilize indigent patients in their emergency rooms, one physician made the memorable statement that medical ethics were in conflict with corporate policy.

12. Indeed, there does seem to be a growth in the number of chiropractors in the United States and in their patronage. They have grown from a marginal occupation in the 1950s (Wardwell, 1952; 1980; 1992) to a position more in the mainstream today. They have successfully sued organized medicine to rescind the ban on cooperation between medicine and chiropractic.

13. In this, we follow the distinctions among disease, illness, and sickness made in earlier work (e.g., Twaddle, 1980; Twaddle and Nordenfelt, 1994).

14. The quotes are to indicate recognition that medicine and medical care are not the only way to organize such activities. Indeed, the institution of modern Western medicine is only one option, although one that is so powerful in the current world that using this language has become the only viable way to discuss this generic type of activity without lengthy explanations of what one is intending to take as a topic. A direct decision is one directed to the sphere of activity, such as one to license some people who have met certain criteria as exclusive practitioners or decision makers in that sphere. An indirect decision may be one that is either more general or directed to a different sphere of activity and which nevertheless shapes or constrains the one under consideration. An example might be a decision to let the food supply be allocated by ability to pay, which can result in some people lacking means to purchase adequate nutrition, in turn resulting in increased disease, thus affecting medical care. Another might be the decision to allocate healers by a central plan based on population numbers, leaving populations that have greater need with inadequate resources while others with little need have a surplus.

15. In the same meaning as ascribed by Weber (1947); cf. Miller (1963).

16. By community, we mean any geographically based collectivity that constitutes a population. People in any area can function at some level as a collectivity. Discussion of decision making in such a context is, of course, more complex the larger the population under consideration. Much of what is here referred to as "community" is called the "state" in other literature. While I intend community to encompass the state, I do not wish to limit the definition to units that meet conditions of sovereignty, and I do want to include smaller units of organization, such as provinces, cities, villages, and so on. There is another definition of community as a "natural" order based on tradition and including family, neighborhood, and kinship, what Habermas called the life sphere (Brante, unpublished manuscript). That is not the meaning intended here.

17. In this type, I have been much influenced by discussions with Thomas Brante and Yvonne Villanueva-Russell.

18. The New England town meeting most closely approximates this kind of pure community decision making in the modern world.

19. The limit here is that in most if not all such countries there are some parts of the population whose views are excluded from the decision-making process (either prohibited or discouraged), while other groups to a greater or lesser extent dominate decision making. Scandinavian parliamentary systems in this regard are more open to a wider spectrum of the society and are more democratic than, say, the United States, where two centrist–right parties monopolize the legislative and administrative systems and no party represents workers or the nonwealthy (persons with net worths of zero or less).

20. It is to be expected that neither the concept of fairness nor the criteria for judging what is fair in any instance will be uniform throughout any but the smallest and most homogeneous communities. Indeed, different standards in this regard are characteristic of different social classes and ethnic groups.

21. There is another dominance issue, that of the authority of different experts in the professional arena. There may be different disciplines with different bodies of expert knowledge and some real ambiguity regarding which might be most beneficial at a given time and place under given circumstances (Abbott, 1988). It is the former, and not the latter, that most concerns us in this instance.

22. An aristocracy, oligarchy, or totalitarian state could in that way be seen as an instance of expert dominance. That, however, substantially perverts the concept of a profession with legitimate claims to expertise.

23. This is not a statement or claim that experts or professionals are more ethical (i.e., better people, more worthy, etc.) than others. It is a statement that there are fewer opportunities for other forms of regulation given the difficulty of lay judgment and that the society is more dependent upon ethical self-regulation than is the case for other kinds of occupations. There is a level at which it is true that only experts can judge whether a practice is knowledgeable or skillful. It may be true, however, that clients can to some degree judge when the practice is useful or profitable. What this implies is that other forms of regulation, such as the market (because of the vulnerability of patients to exploitation) and the law (because of technical incompetence of nonexperts in making judgments seen as technical in their essence) have been ruled out of consideration in any but the most peripheral conditions. Self-regulation, by placing more emphasis on ethical constraints, is one of the main avenues left. It is likely that ethical principles, at least as a set of agreed-upon rules of thumb, will be discussed more under those circumstances and even be more effective as a regulator than for other occupational groups in community and certainly in market modes of organization.

24. Indeed, the linkage has been broken entirely among higher managers in some of the large corporations, who get enormous raises in salary as their firms show signs of failing. There is reason to suggest that high-level managers of large corporations have become a closed, self-perpetuating group that has the capacity to reward themselves irrespective of performance. There are signs that as these abuses of power become more and more public the demand for democratic control of corporate behavior is growing.

25. There are totalitarian societies in which it is not obvious that any of the three models dominates. Physicians have at times been under the sway of a totalitarian ideology and worked in the service of a state that is in no way a democracy. Nor were market forces allowed to work. Nazi Germany is a prototype of special interest here. While physicians were instrumental in the creation of Nazi ideology, particularly with respect to genocide, it could not be said that they had professional autonomy (Lifton, 1988). The typology we present is therefore not exhaustive.

26. There are some indications that the strength of market forces has been stronger than anticipated by some people who "played along" with the neoliberal (right-wing, Social Darwinist) governments. There seems to be more cautionary commentary indicating limits to market mechanisms in the U.K. and Sweden, for example. In the 1992 U.S. election, the voters elected a government opposed to continued neoliberal politics. Swedish voters returned the Social Democrats to government in 1994.

27. Since the patients or their insurance carriers must pay for all medical care, it is often necessary to recover the costs of treatment. Since the society uniquely lacks any mechanism for income replacement when people are disabled as a result of disease or injury, suits are instituted to ensure a livelihood. The United States is also unique in not having a general welfare system or administrative means of resolving conflicts. The judicial system becomes, under these circum-

stances, a substitute for conflict-resolution agencies and for a welfare system. For the workings of the U.K. and Swedish systems, see Rosenthal (1988).

28. This is not the intent of the legislation, which provided for reimbursement of average costs on the understanding that hospitals would be paid more than their costs half the time and less half the time. Instead, the hospital administrators have taken the DRG reimbursement as the maximum amount the patient would be allowed to cost before requiring the discharge. In the year after DRGs took effect, hospital administrators in Columbia, Missouri, reported in interviews that their collections from Medicare had increased by two to eight times. It should be kept in mind that DRGs were introduced as a cost containment measure.

29. Antonio and Bonanno, unpublished manuscript; Antonio and Kellner, 1992; Bonanno, 1994; Borrego, 1981; Clarke, 1990; Constance and Heffernan, 1991; Friedland, 1991; Gramsci, 1971; Harrison and Bluestone, 1988; Harvy, 1990; Hicks and Misra, 1993; Huber, Ragin, and Stephens, 1993; Jameson, 1991; Lambert, 1991; Lipietz, 1992; Picciotto, 1991; Pitelis, 1991; Sassen, 1993.

30. The basic conditions of participation in the EU are the "four freedoms": free movement of goods, services, labor, and capital (Johansson, 1994). The contrast with the "four freedoms" proposed by Franklin Roosevelt in 1941 (freedom of speech and expression, freedom of worship, freedom from want, and freedom from fear) may be an indicator of the magnitude of the shift in focus the "new world order" is asking.

CHAPTER 3

The Nature and Scope of This Study

> Give a small boy a hammer, and he will find that everything he encounters needs pounding.
>
> Abraham Kaplan (1964, 28)

The general problem for this study, outlined in Chapter 1, was to understand the reasons for the sudden shift in the political debate on medical care policy in Sweden from principles of solidarity, equality, and central planning to principles of competition, markets, and privatization. This shift apparently took place in a very short time.[1] The reason for any shift was not immediately obvious, particularly one that entailed such a drastic change in direction. It seemed interesting and important to study the change.

As outlined in Chapter 2, there are some theoretical models, based for the most part on research on other topics, that suggested important leads in framing this problem. Trends in the organization of medical care that seemingly transcend specific national systems were noted, leading to increased problems on two fronts: the capacity of societies to fund increasingly expensive systems of medicine, and the increased alienation of the public from medicine at the clinical level. Different models (democratic, professional, and market) were developed for the organization of medical and other services. Each had implications for the quality of care. More important for the present, they provide benchmarks from which directions of change can be noted. Finally, models of trends toward economic globalization would predict a trend from professional and/or democratic forms of organization toward a market form. This would be especially the case when conservative forces gained the ability to make the market a hegemonic project (Jessop, 1991).

Against this background, it is now possible to offer a more precise statement of the research problem. First, we state more specific research questions, not as precise as hypotheses, for reasons we will elaborate upon, but sufficient to provide clear criteria of relevance for data collection and analysis. Second, we offer a statement of our research methods: the kinds of data we gathered, the methods of analysis employed, and the form of presentation.

THE RESEARCH QUESTIONS

As with any other human activity, medical care may be seen as a discrete entity, a set of actions circumscribed around a core focus and having some independence from other social concerns. To take such an approach has value, insofar as it can highlight special features of the activities that set it apart from other concerns. Some of those may entail features that would otherwise be overlooked and which can contribute to our understanding. At the same time, sociologists have increasingly come to appreciate that to focus only on a set of activities seen in isolation from others leads to a partial and often distorted view. It is at least important to see medical care, or any other institutionalized activity, in a larger context. All human actions are embedded in larger social patterns and cannot be fully understood apart from them.

With this in mind, this study will focus on three broad strategic questions. The first, which looks at medical care as an entity unto itself, can be stated as follows: *Are there trends in medical care in Sweden which have generated internal contradictions or other problems of a magnitude sufficient to require a basic shift in the underlying principles of organization of medical services?* As presented in Chapter 2, we want to review trends with respect to bureaucratization, specialization, technology development, fragmentation of services, and cost. Given the nature of the reforms at issue, we are especially interested in the resource demands of the medical care system—whether the system has become, or threatens to become shortly, unaffordable to the society. In other words, does medical care in Sweden threaten to bankrupt the society in the absence of radical reforms?

We also want to explore the extent to which there is a serious problem of alienation that differentiates Sweden from other Western countries. The key focus here is whether the conditions under which care is provided had deteriorated or otherwise become so intolerable that the public demanded better treatment (i.e., more humane, more responsive to their nonmedical needs, etc.). Keeping in mind W. I. Thomas's famous dictum, "When men [*sic*] define situations as real they are real in their consequences," it may be less the objective situation that is controlling, than the perceptions and beliefs of persons who make decisions about medical care organization.

The second question follows from the nature of the reform effort. As recalled from Chapter 1 proponents of market reforms argued that changing from a publicly run system based on central planning, assurances of equity with respect to quality and access, and solidarity to one that is more competitive, market driven, and privatized would be better in some substantial way. One key position they took was that weak economic growth, caused by the overextension of the welfare state, made the public medical care system unaffordable. Therefore, we ask the following question: *Has the development of the Swedish economy led to problems of financing public services sufficiently important as to make the medical care system unaffordable or the cost of that system a threat to the growth and development of the larger society?* Here, we want to review major events in the recent economic history of Sweden as these affect revenues, expenditures, and costs of services, particularly those in the public sector.

It is particularly important to focus on three facets of the economy: growth in the gross domestic or national product, the growth of revenues in the public sector, and the growth of public services, particularly medical care. This suggests it would be fruitful to search for both general trends and moments of change that would alter the balance between the demands of those services on the economy and the carrying capacity of the economy. Again, we want to be careful to focus on the perceptions of those who made decisions affecting medical care, as these can be more important in understanding policy than are the objective realities.

Our third general question comes from the recognition that whatever the case with reference to the internal condition of the medical care system and the general economy, decisions about reform of medical care and other social services are essentially political, if only in the narrowest sense that they will be made by politicians. Our position, however, is not that narrow, and we want to look more broadly at the issue of public policy making as it affects medical care. This leads us to the third of our general questions: *Has there been a shift in the political balance of power sufficient to account for a basic change in public policy?* Here we want to look at the balance of power among key interest groups in the society, their linkages to political parties, and their ability to influence social policy. Aside from problems in the organization of medical care and the economy in general, has something happened that has enabled political forces hostile to the welfare state to gain power at the expense of those in favor of strong public services?

More specifically, it is crucial to look for trends and/or moments of change in the relative power of interest groups with central roles in the economy: labor and large employers. As political parties are the vehicles through which programs are proposed and enacted, and parties are at least on occasion closely aligned with particular interests, it is important to look at the positions taken by specific parties over time and the relative strength of those parties with the electorate.

Put another way, we ask three general questions that are the subject of the following three chapters: (1) Is there a crisis in medical care, (2) is there an economic crisis, and (3) is there a political crisis? that can account for the sudden and dramatic apparent shift in medical care policy evident in Sweden between 1989 and 1993?

The Crisis of Medical Care

The questions to be raised in analyzing the possibility of a crisis in medical care organization follow closely upon the schema proposed in Chapter 2 under the heading "International Trends in Medical Care Organization." There we argued that following the establishment of modern scientific medicine in a medical school curriculum providing training in the basic sciences followed by supervised clinical training, there was an explosion of new well-grounded knowledge at a time of increasing need and demand for medical care. A scenario was constructed that called particular attention to the following elements (Twaddle, 1982):

- increased productivity of medical personnel as care moved from the home of the patient to more centralized settings.
- increased rates of technological development and more rapid introduction of new technologies.
- increased bureaucratization of services as technologies and personnel were centralized in hospitals.
- increased specialization of services as physicians sought to master knowledge and technique, gain access to technology, and respond to the bureaucratic imperative to rationalize work.
- increased fragmentation of services from a patient perspective as individuals received care for different problems from different specialists.
- increased costs of care resulting from increased labor intensiveness of medical service (particularly in the hospitals), capital and operating costs of new technologies, and lack of coordination among specialists.

According to the model, by the mid-twentieth century the core problems facing medical care were twofold. On the one hand, the growth in medical care costs were rising more rapidly than the economies of most First World countries, making the financing of care a core issue. On the other hand, the growing impersonality of medical care delivery and the growing gap between professional and lay knowledge had created a problem of alienation between the system and its clients.

Most of these trends were established well before mid-century and problems became apparent shortly after mid-century in most countries, but before the full growth of the welfare state, which is largely a post–World War II phenomenon. In Sweden, while the process of development can be traced to the 1940s, it was not until the 1970s that we can make the case that medical care became predominantly a public activity. For our purposes, it is especially important to review trends since 1970 with respect to control of technology, bureaucratization, specialization, fragmentation, costs, the financing of medical care, and patient alienation. In that way we will focus on the problems of the public system and the response to them.

The Economic Crisis

By the middle of the 1970s, Sweden had a system of social welfare that was more comprehensive than in any other country, both with respect to the scope of services provided and the inclusiveness of population coverage. It was a universal system of entitlement that required a large public sector. Indeed, by the late 1970s, the average Swede paid more than 50 percent of their income in taxes, receiving almost all of it back in services and/or transfer payments. Medical care and education were virtually free of charges, as were a variety of support services provided as needed. It could be argued that if any country had created a public sector that could threaten the overall economy, it would have to be Sweden. Further, the survival of the system would be more dependent on a well-functioning economy in Sweden than would be the case in other countries which had made lesser investments in public services.

To explore the robustness of the economy as a foundation for the welfare state, it is important to look for trends in the following facets:

- growth (or lack of growth) in the gross domestic product and/or the gross national product.
- factors that may underlie economic growth, such as productivity and levels of employment.
- growth in revenues at the state, county, and municipal level, as all of these had a role in financing medical care and other welfare services.
- factors such as tax policies and levels of employment underlying the revenue production of governments.
- growth of expenditures at various government levels, particularly those on welfare-state programs.
- budget surpluses and/or deficits resulting from the balance of revenues and expenditures, with special emphasis on transfer payments.

Given that there is evidence that national economies are becoming increasingly integrated with others, it is increasingly important to take note of economic features external to nations that affect their national economic performance. With this in mind, it is important to include the following in any analysis of an economic crisis:

- the cost of basic resources and materials purchased outside the nation, with particular emphasis on fuels and raw materials.
- the organizational ties of economic entities with entities outside the nation (such as subsidiaries or parent companies).
- the nature of economic cooperation at the state level (membership in transnational economic organizations, trade treaties, import/export restrictions, etc.).

Even with a good summary of all these items, it is difficult to settle on criteria that would help decide when a level of economic performance is insufficient to sustain a particular level of public welfare. It is important to explore the degree to which expert opinion was in agreement on the issues and to note the reasons for disagreements found. As with other policy areas, perceptions may override realities.

The Political Crisis

This is a bit more difficult to map in advance. There are a myriad of ways in which political perceptions and/or power can shift. In the Swedish case, however, we can advance some preliminary ideas. First, rightly or wrongly, the creation and development of the welfare state is seen as a product of the labor unions and the Social Democratic Party, which were in close alliance over most of this century. The Social Democratic Party was in government, either alone or in alliance with one of the middle parties (Center or Liberal) from 1932 to 1976. In 1976, a coalition of the Liberal, Center, and Conservative parties assumed control of the government in various combinations until 1982, when the Social Democrats were returned to power. A Social Democratic government was in control from 1982 until 1991, when a coalition of Conservative, Christian Democratic, Center, and Liberal parties assumed control of government.

This suggests three topics that would be worth closer attention. First, it is important to look more closely at the policies of the Social Democrats. What were they? How were they changing over time? What internal discussion were they having about the welfare state? To what extent were they indeed creating and defending the Swedish model? Second, what was the relationship between the Social Democratic Party and the labor movement? Did the party function as a political representative of labor during this period, or were there differences that may have weakened their ties? Did any of this affect the political position of the left in Swedish politics? What was the agenda of the nonsocialist parties with reference to the welfare state during their first (1976–1982) period in government and their second (1991–1994) period? To what degree were they in opposition to the Swedish model? Had their position changed? If so, why? What were the interests and policies of corporate and business organizations during the period? What were their ties to "bourgeois" parties? How did they participate in the policy-formation process?

RESEARCH METHODS

The research questions, while pointing to some kinds of evidence that should be collected, are not hypotheses, which would allow a much closer specification of that evidence. Instead, they indicate areas of inquiry for which many kinds of evidence may be relevant, some of which could not be identified in advance of the research, but had to be discovered as part of the research process.

The first requirement, then, was that the research frame a process within which the kinds of relevant evidence could be identified as an ongoing activity. That is, we needed an exploratory design, the end result of which might allow us to reach some conclusions but, more importantly, would allow us to formulate better questions, perhaps ones that lend themselves to hypothesis testing. Such a process requires

- a plan for data collection that would reasonably assure that the range of options for answering any of the research questions would be captured.
- openness to data sources and/or forms that may not have been anticipated.
- inclusion of information not only on medical care but on the social systems within which medical care is located.
- a format that would allow for interpretation.
- flexibility in seeking ways to piece together information so as to reach well-grounded conclusions.

The plan was to build a research design around a program of interviews with people who represented different organized interests in the Swedish debate on medical care policy. This included politicians, who made the legislative decisions; physicians and nurses, who were obviously affected by any changes in their work environs; other professional and highly skilled health workers;[2] and blue collar workers in health care.[3] In addition, we would seek interviews with researchers who study health policy and persons with an active role in implementing policy. At the time of the interviews with representatives of organized interests, we collected documents on health policy or related issues prepared by the organization represented by the respondent, including such things as the organization's analyses of policy changes and their effects on the organization, communications with members to mobilize a response, and documents prepared for public consumption on policy options.

We reviewed recent scholarly literature on Swedish health policy to learn what was known about the nature of the changes and the dynamics behind them. We actively sought not only published, but unpublished work or work in progress, in conjunction with interviews with researchers.

Simultaneously with the interviews but separate from them, we sought out reports by official agencies, such as *Statistiska Centralbyrån* (the Bureau of Statistics) and *Socialstyrelsen* (the Board of Health) on trends and problems in medical care organization and financing. We also undertook a daily review of a major national newspaper as well as occasional issues of other papers in order to capture public debate. Especially important was news coverage of the medical care system, with emphasis on reform efforts and political positions of various groups.

Data Collection

Prior to the field work for this study, there had been an opportunity to review documents analyzing the medical care system prepared by the Ministry of Health, the Federation of County Councils, the Swedish Medical Association (SMA), the Swedish Nurses Association (SNA), the Union of Municipal Employees (SKAF), and the editor of *Dagens Nyheter*. An analysis of those documents showed that what the County Councils, SMA, and Ministry of Health had presented at a conference at Emory University in 1992 as a "broad consensus" on the need for market reforms in medical care had been opposed or treated skeptically by the SNA and the SKAF (Twaddle, 1992).

Immediately upon our arrival in Sweden in January 1993, interviews were conducted with the presidents of the Federation of County Councils and the Swedish Nurses' Association, the Minister of Health, and the secretary general of the Swedish Medical Association, all of whom were acquaintances from earlier contacts. New contacts were made with the federation of blue collar labor unions (LO), the federation of white collar unions (TCO), the Health and Welfare Committee of Parliament, members of the Östergötland County Council in Linköping, and several academics who had published work on the medical care system. This constituted the sampling frame for the study. These interviews were supplemented by Richard Hessler's ongoing contacts with persons in the Western Region Planning Office in Göteborg. Others interviewed were either referred by these sources or were chance encounters.[4] At each interview we requested, and in each instance received, all documents prepared by the respondent's organization that included analyses and/or positions regarding the organization and financing of medical care in Sweden. Those documents were reviewed and analyzed for descriptions of the organizational perspective on the issues raised in Chapter 1.

Several visits were made to the Central Bureau of Statistics to review and purchase data being generated on medical care by the national government. Several visits were made to bookstores run by a variety of politically active organizations to collect materials on medical care they handled. These organizations were mostly in the Liberal–Social Democratic–Left part of the political spectrum and most of these materials were in opposition to the program of the four-party government in power at the time. As it was this part of the spectrum that was absent from the materials provided by official agencies, they were used mostly to assure a counterbalance to the government–SMA–County Council stance and to identify counterarguments and data for a more balanced analysis. It should be noted that books were collected representing a wide range of opinions and views, including extreme right-wing and left-wing positions.

The weekly report of the Parliament, *Från Riksdag och Department*, was monitored for the actions of government agencies and ministries as well as the *Riksdag* itself. This provided a comprehensive inventory of directives, commission of inquiry reports, committee actions, propositions, and legislation along with the main points raised in debates within those units. Visits were made approximately monthly to Fritzes in Stockholm, the official outlet for government publications and documents. There it was possible to collect the directives, propositions, commission of inquiry reports, propositions, parliamentary committee reports, and legislation identified in *Från Riksdag och Department*, as well as academic and other publications on public policy.

The national daily newspaper, *Dagens Nyheter*, was reviewed daily and other papers were read occasionally. All articles dealing with the economy, political positions, the development of Swedish involvement in international organizations and agreements affecting the economy or medical care, and the organization of medical care (with emphasis on the debates on the political direction) were indexed on computer files with brief summaries, allowing accurate retrieval. Entries covered news, editorials, *debatt* articles, and letters to the editor. These provided a relatively complete inventory of the kinds of issues and the range of arguments that were in the public discourse in 1993.

While many of our sources had known biases, taken together they represented as close to a comprehensive inventory of positions and opinions and information as we could devise. We actively sought viewpoints we may have missed and have found none. It is our belief that the information we collected provides an adequate base on which to proceed with assurance that we have at our disposal the full range of materials required to capture the issues and debates affecting our subject. Further, the process of data collection allowed for the kind of flexibility we needed to identify data sources and issues as an ongoing process. Given that we could not specify the substance of the research in advance, the procedures allowed for it to be defined as a component of the research while at the same time maintaining the rigor needed to provide a base of information on which well-grounded conclusions could be drawn. In short, it met the criteria of openness to new data sources, flexibility, range, and enabling interpretation.

Data Analysis

The analysis plan was to explore the major components of changes affecting Swedish medical care and then use that analysis to reflect on the theoretical issues posed in Chapter 2. The next three chapters take up structural changes in the medical care system, the economy, and political arrangements, exploring in each instance whether a credible case can be built that those changes required a sharp change in public policy affecting the financing and organization of medical care. Specifically, we wanted to explore whether the public system had failed and needed to be replaced with a market system. In those three chapters we attempt to provide the following information, not serially, but in an integrated form: (1) a chronology of the major events and/or junctures that have altered in some substantial way the structures and patterns of the respective system, (2) identification of issues debated at the time of each event as well as the most important groups in the society participating in the debates, (3) an assessment of the evidence bearing on those issues, and (4) a conclusion about whether those changes provide necessary or sufficient causes for a change in the orientation of public policy *vis à vis* medical care. This analysis will be offered in narrative form.

The final chapter addresses more explicitly the broad trends and provides an interpretation of the findings. It summarizes the previous chapters and links the findings to the theoretical issues presented in Chapter 2. We connect the findings to pan-national issues in the development of medical care in Western developed countries, to alternative models for organizing medical care, to models for discussing the internationalization of economies, and to selected issues in the theory of the state.

An Afterword summarizes major developments in Sweden following the study period and speculates on their implications for this analysis.

NOTES

1. At a conference in Stockholm in 1990, I heard discussion of markets, competition, and privatization for the first time. I did not hear those terms used anywhere in 1989.
2. Organized in unions affiliated with TCO, the largest being SKTF, *Svenska Kommunal Tjänstemannens Förbundet*, the Swedish Association of Professional Municipal Workers.
3. Organized in unions affiliated with LO, the largest being SKAF, *Svenska Kommunal Arbetares Förbundet*, the Swedish Union of Municipal Workers.
4. A listing of the individuals interviewed in each organization can be found in Appendix B. In each instance, interviews were tape recorded and transcribed. With minor editing, most were published in Sweden as a contribution to the ongoing debates (Twaddle, 1994b).

Chapter 4

The Medical Care Crisis: What It Is, If It Is

The first question is whether there is an internal crisis in medical care, as internal contractions of the system itself could be grounds for holding that a reform was necessary. We would accept as a crisis any state of affairs in which the medical care system would be unable to continue offering the level of service it had been providing or one in which it could not extend that level of service to segments of the population that were not yet receiving it. We would not accept as a crisis a situation in which problems could be identified but those problems could be solved by the working of the existing system. The questions for this chapter become the following: (1) Were there trends or structural contradictions evident that meant the medical care system was inherently doomed in its capacity to continue providing its best services to all those who had historically received them, and (2) Was the system incapable of further development to meet emergent needs of the population?

In seeking to answer these questions, we first return to the model of international trends in medical care organization presented at the beginning of Chapter 2. We provide a thumbnail sketch of the development of the Swedish medical care system with special emphasis on need, demand, knowledge, work pressures, technology, bureaucratization, specialization, fragmentation, and cost. We then turn to the issues that have most concerned Western medical care systems in economically advanced countries: financing and alienation. In the first instance, we explore whether the cost of the system had increased to a level where the nation could no longer afford to provide state-of-the-art services to all those who may have historically received them (i.e., who met the criteria of need and would have been provided the service at some time in the past had it been available). We especially want to look at trends in demand and need that might affect the capacity of the system to respond adequately. In the second instance, we explore whether the public has become less capable of participating in clinical decisions or decisions involving organizational arrangements, economic terms of delivery, or establishing a personal relationship with providers than had been the case in the past. Again, we will want to look at trends that indicate emergent problems. Against this background, we review the medical care reforms described in Chapter 1 to see what effect they had on financing and alienation.

Once we have a reasonable picture of the state of Swedish medical care as of the late 1980s, we turn to the political debate, reviewing selected opinions expressed in documents and interviews to see whether there is a claim that a crisis in medical care exists and, if so, who makes that claim. We identify the issues in medical care delivery that were being discussed in 1993 and link them to particular interest groups. Especially important is a delineation of the political agendas of the various interest groups, political parties, and others who were in the debate over medical care reform. Our key question at this point is, "Who wanted what in shaping the medical care system?"

In the final section of this chapter we review the evidence and draw conclusions about the following questions:

1. Is there a crisis in the organization and/or operation of the Swedish medical care system?
2. What problems does the Swedish medical care system face and how well is it organized to solve them?
3. What are the competing political agendas for changing or defending the Swedish medical care system?
4. Is there any reason to fundamentally change the nature of the organization of Swedish medical care in order to solve problems internal to the medical care system?

THE DEVELOPMENT OF THE SWEDISH MEDICAL CARE SYSTEM

No comprehensive history of Swedish medical care organization has been written,[1] although several people, all of whom were addressing issues in parts of that system, have noted important benchmarks in the development of the system (Heidenheimer and Elvander, 1980; Ibo, 1980; Garpenby, 1989; Calltorp, 1989a; Immergut, 1989; Olsson, 1993; Twaddle, 1994b) . A compilation of those benchmarks appears in Table 4.1.

As can be seen from the table, the fundamental principles of the modern Swedish medical care system were well developed by 1900. Sweden by that time had established public hospitals (1533), founded medical schools (early 1600s), developed scientific and professional organizations of physicians (1633, 1808), provided for public ambulatory care (middle 1600s), established a public health authority (1698), created acute general hospitals (1752), established the responsibility of the state for primary medical care (1773), created health insurance (c. 1870), and created income maintenance funds for the sick (1891). Clearly, the principle that medical care was a public responsibility to be provided through, if not always by, public authorities was firmly established in Sweden at an early date.

In this century, developments with respect to medical care have been to reinforce these basic principles and to build upon them:

- Swedish physicians organized a labor union in 1903 to represent their interests with the state. The SMA, *Läkarförbundet*, began as a voluntary association, but was reorganized in 1942 to require all physicians to join a local organization and a national organization that was a part of the SMA. The SMA is composed of organizations of physicians in different specialties and/or working arrangements (e.g., hospital officers, district physicians). While there are not infrequently different interests among the constituent groups, the SMA attempts to represent all physicians with state, county, and, recently, municipal authorities.
- Health insurance was expanded and made a public responsibility. In 1931, a national law established obligatory benefits and set fees for medical services, making health insurance universal in principle. A voluntary system of health insurance was made compulsory in 1947 and a state responsibility in 1955, at which point health insurance became universal in fact.
- The national government gained the authority to allocate technology and personnel. Following the Medical Care Law of 1962 (*Sjukvårdslagen 1962:676*), Sweden developed a system of rationing based on a hierarchy of hospitals. At the top, regional hospitals had the most esoteric and advanced technology. County hospitals were high technology, but at a lower level, and local hospitals were relatively low technology. There were regulations on the types of specialties that could practice at each level. Some—internal medicine, obstetrics and gynecology, and psychiatry—could be found in local hospitals. Cardiology, gasteroenterology, and the like were in county hospitals, and subspecialties such as pediatric endocrinology were found only at the regional hospitals. This system checked duplication of services, and provided a structure, making cost containment possible (Hollingsworth, Hage, and Hanneman, 1990).
- A Seven Crowns Reform in 1970 drew a line between public and private medicine, abolished fee-for-service as a means of reimbursing hospital ambulatory care, establish a maximum out-of-pocket cost to patients for medical services, and placed public medical care providers on salary.

This was the framework that was the basis for our characterization of the strengths and weaknesses of the system as of 1980, presented in Chapter 1. It was a system that provided comprehensive medical care to everyone resident in the country with very little out-of-pocket cost at the

Table 4.1
Landmarks in the Development of the Medical Care System in Sweden (up to 1994)

Date	Event	Meaning
1200s	Hospitalen and Helgeandshusen established	to deal with (1) leprosy and (2) the poor; shows public responsibility for indigent
1533	Act of 1533	Hospitals taken from religious authorities and placed under public control
Early 1600s	First medical school at Uppsala	Establishment of modern medicine
1633	Collegium Medicum founded	First organization of physicians
Middle 1600s	Stockholm, Göteborg, and Norrköping have Town Medical Officers	First use of medicine as agent of the political entity
1698	Collegium Medicum made cornerstone of public health	First organized public health authority
1736	Public Health Commission founded	
1752	Serafimer Hospital founded	First Acute hospital
1766	Public Health Commission dissolved	
1773	Central government took responsibility for whole of district medicine	First use of medicine as agent of the state
1807-1808	Swedish Medical Society (Läkarsällskapet) founded	Medicine organizing as profession
1813	Collegium Medicum became Public Health Board	
1817	Local Hospital Boards established	
1862	County Councils established	Political unit that later became responsible for all medical care
after 1870	Voluntary Sickness Funds established	First health insurance system; initially urban; 13% coverage by 1925
1877	Public Health Board became National Board of Health	
Late 1800s	Consultants appointed to public hospitals	
1891	Sickness Funds Law	First nationally sponsored sickness fund (income maintenance)

Table 4.1 (*continued*)

Date	Event	Meaning
1903	Swedish Medical Association (Läkarförbundet) founded	First trade union association in medicine
1931	Sickness Funds Law and Tariff Law	First obligatory medical benefits; set fees for services
1942	SMA reorganization	All physicians required to join a local organization and at least one national federation
1947	National Health Insurance Law	Transition from voluntary to compulsory health insurance
1955	National Health Insurance begins	Based on 1948 Höjer Commission report
1959	Hospital Act	
1970	Seven Crowns Reform	Abolished fee for service for ambulatory care delivered by hospital physicians
1983	Health and Sickness Care Law (1982:763)	Gave total responsibility for medical care to counties; placed total control of medical care in medical profession
1984	Dagmar Reform	Established block grants to counties and ended fee-for-service billing by private physicians
1987	Sickness Insurance Reform	No benefit day abolished; benefits paid on hourly rather than daily basis; employer administration of short-term sick leave
1990	Ädel Reform	Decentralized care of the aged from the counties to the municipalities
1993	Husläkare Reform	Established a point-of-service primary care system in place of district medicine.

Sources: Arnold Heidenhimer and Nils Elvander, *The Shaping of the Swedish Health System* (New York: St. Martins, 1980); Hirobumi Ibo, "Health Insurance and Medical Services in Sweden and Denmark 1850–1950," in ibid.; Peter Garpenby, *The State and the Medical Profession: A Cross-National Comparison of the Health Policy Arena in the United Kingdom and Sweden* (Linköping: Linköpings Universitet, 1989); Johan Calltorp (1989a), Ellen Immergut, "Procedures for Conciliation: The Institutional Basis of Swedish National Health Insurance, 1930–70," *Scandinavian Studies* 61:146–68; Sven Olsson, *Social Policy and Welfare State in Sweden* (Lund: Arkiv, 1993); Andrew Twaddle (1994a). ©1984 Andrew C. Twaddle.

point of delivery. At the point of service, it was well organized from the perspective of providers other than district physicians. District physicians in 1980 were mostly in community solo practices isolated from colleagues and the hospitals.[2] Other ambulatory care physicians had hospital appointments and worked in groups.

The main problem with the system was that general medicine was underdeveloped. There were too few general practitioners and there was too little incentive for physicians to choose general practice. The result was that districts, particularly in the large cities, were too large to be managed, patient access to services was limited, and inappropriate use of specialist services, especially hospital emergency rooms, was common.

The Western Pattern and the Development of Swedish Medical Care

Turning now to the model describing international developments in medical care, we see Sweden as very much part of the same pattern as described for other modern, Western industrialized countries.

First, the need for medical care increased. This is partly a function of population growth, which has been rapid since the early 1800s (see Figure 4.1). As presented in Chapter 2, need for medical care in a population is largely a function of age. An older population has more chronic disease and a younger one more acute disease. The latter requires more medical care per capita. With industrialization, which came very late to Sweden by comparison with other European and North American societies, there was the beginning of an increase in the proportion of aged persons in the society. Indeed, by the 1970s, Sweden had the population with the highest proportion of elderly persons in the world. In 1990, 17.7 percent of all Swedes were over the age of sixty-five and 8.02 percent were over seventy-five (Statistiska Centralbyrån, 1993).

Second, the development of medical knowledge was at least as rapid in Sweden as it was in other Western countries. While Sweden developed its first medical school in the early 1600s, it cannot be claimed that there was a firm scientific basis for medical practice before the latter part of the 1800s. Epidemiological knowledge developed earlier, of course, and was of value in recognition of disease patterns and, in some instances, for public health interventions. It was not until the germ theory of disease was framed around 1870, however, that we can meaningfully talk about a scientific basis for clinical practice. While a study of the development of Swedish medicine is lacking,[3] we may presume that knowledge spread among Swedish physicians as rapidly as it did among the British and much faster than it did among the Americans.[4]

Third, we have no information on the demand for medical care for the late 1800s and early 1900s in Sweden. It can be safely presumed, how-

Figure 4.1
Population Growth in Sweden (in Millions)

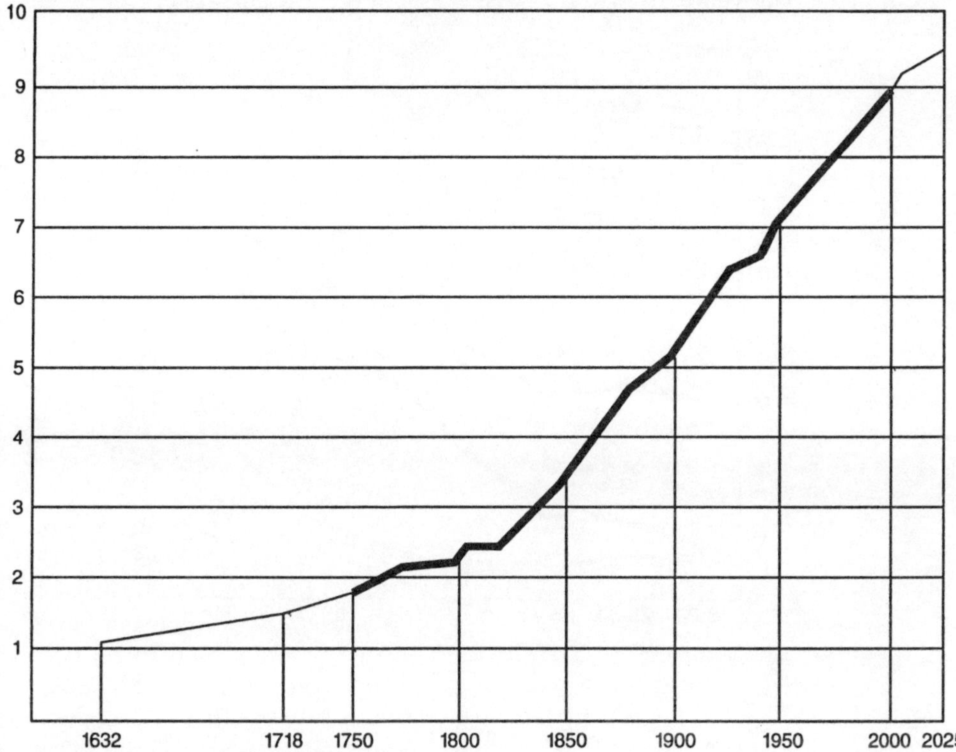

Source: Statistiska Centralbyrån, *Statistiska Årbok' 93 för Sverige* (Stockholm: SCB, 1993).

ever, that in the absence of strong competition from alternative healing traditions it increased rapidly during the early part of this century.[5] Certainly by mid-century demand was high, although with a distinctive pattern. Sweden had the lowest number of ambulatory care visits per capita of any European or North American country and the highest number of hospital days. This was less a function of demand than the peculiar development of medical services concentrated in hospitals with an underdeveloped primary care sector. In any event, in 1988–1989, 57 percent of all women and 43 percent of all men consulted an ambulatory care physician, an increase from 1980–1981. Almost 9 percent had consulted district nurses, also an increase over 1980–1981 (Figure 4.2). At the same time, an audit of the medical care system in 1990 concluded that primary care was still underdeveloped and needed to be "powerfully strengthened" at the expense of the hospital system (Järnebeck and Laxhed, 1990).

Figure 4.2
Contacts with Ambulatory Care by Age: 1980–1981 and 1988–1989

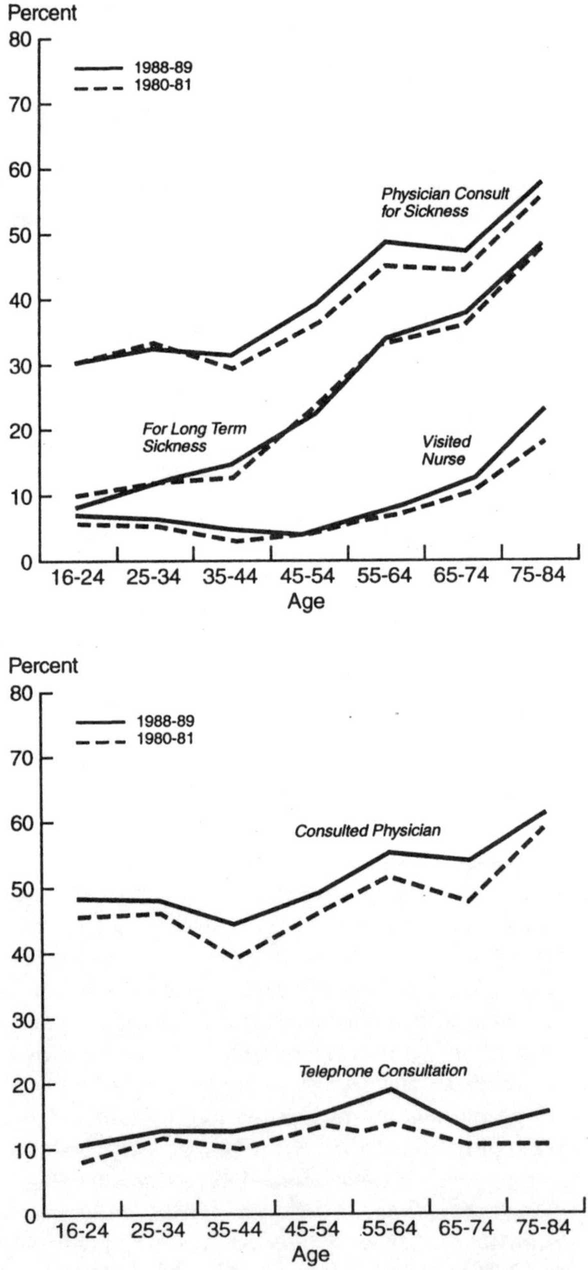

Source: Statistiska Centralbyån, 1990.

Fourth, work pressures on medical practitioners certainly increased during this century. It is unlikely that there was a sudden shift, as occurred in the United States after the Flexner Report, where increased demand was coupled with a sharp reduction in the physician supply.[6] Nevertheless, there is evidence of a steadily increasing demand for medical services in the continuing increase in physician visits and hospital days.[7]

Fifth, Sweden has certainly developed into a country with state-of-the-art technology from one that at the turn of the century could be regarded as economically and technologically backward. This applies as much, perhaps more, to medicine as to any other sphere of activity. Indeed, Sweden's medical care is focused on high technology, tertiary care treatment. Further, Sweden has taken a role far beyond its size in developing new technology. Some centers, such as the *Akademiska Sjukhuset* in Uppsala, *Karolinska Institutonen* in Stockholm, *Salgrenska Sjukhuset* in Göteborg, and the University Hospital at Lund are among the leading medical research institutions in the world.

Sixth, as in the rest of the developed world, the combination of a need for increased efficiency and the need for centralization of expensive technologies resulted in increased bureaucratization, specialization, and rationalization of services. In the 1940s, a decision was taken to build the medical care system around hospitals and specialists. Financing was focused on the development of state-of-the-art medical centers, to the relative neglect of primary care. Medical specialists so dominated the system that by 1978 only 9 percent of all physicians were in primary care and only 14 percent were in ambulatory care.[8] In the mid 1970s, the size of medical school classes was increased sharply and residency training opportunities in specialties other than general medicine, pediatrics, psychiatry, and geriatrics were capped. The result was an increase of primary care physicians to over 23 percent of all active physicians (Table 4.2). In addition, a myriad of new technical occupations were developed.

Last, fragmentation of services in principle was limited by having a system of district medicine. In 1970, Sweden was divided into small geographic units for the purpose of providing primary care. In each unit, there was a position for a general medicine specialist who was responsible for all the people in his or her district. That meant that everyone had a specific primary care physician who, presumably, would know them and provide a personal level of service. In practice, this system worked well in the rural areas and small towns. In the cities it was a far from realized ideal. There, many positions were vacant,[9] the districts were often too large for a general practitioner to service well,[10] patients went to emergency rooms for emergent and acute conditions because they could not get to see a primary care physician, and practice was taken up with the routine surveillance of chronic conditions.[11] Relative to need or demand, primary care was seriously underdeveloped as of 1980. The result

Table 4.2
Physicians in Active Service: Sweden, 1990

Physicians	Public	Private	Total	Percent of Total
General Medicine	3909	347	4256	17.41
Anesthesiology	1144	40	1184	4.84
Pediatrics	1234	86	1320	5.40
Dermatology	357	71	428	1.75
Internal Medicine	2629	407	3036	12.42
Endocrinology	136		136	0.56
Cardiology	454		454	1.86
Infectious Disease	375		375	1.53
Pulmonary Medicine	264		264	1.08
Gastroenterology	122		122	0.50
Nephrology	143		143	0.58
Rheumatology	189		189	0.77
Gerontology	487		487	1.99
Occupational Health	69		69	0.28
Social Medicine	51		51	0.21
ENT	54		54	0.22
Voice	18		18	0.07
Physical Medicine and Rehabilitation	113		113	0.46
Neurology	256		256	1.05
General Psychiatry	1315	249	1564	6.40
Child Psychiatry	296		296	1.21
Forensic Psychiatry	43		43	0.18
General Surgery	1855	429	2284	9.34
Pediatric Surgery	110		110	0.45
Hand Surgery	70		70	0.29
Neurosurgery	97		97	0.40
Orthopedic Surgery	931		931	3.81
Plastic Surgery	118		118	0.48
Thoracic Surgery	99		99	0.40
Urology	278		278	1.14
OB/Gyn	1329	253	1582	6.47
General Oncology	261	10	271	1.11
Gyn Oncology	51		51	0.21
Ophthalmology	642	105	747	3.06
ENT	661	192	853	3.49
Radiology	989		989	4.05
Pathology	958		958	3.92
No Specialty		123	123	0.50
Other Specialty		26	26	0.11
Total	**22107**	**2338**	**24445**	**100.00**
All Primary Care Specialties				**23.30**

was that for urban populations care was fragmented, being provided in specialty clinics, with different family members seeing different physicians and individuals seeing different physicians for different problems.

All these factors (expanding technology, increasing scale of organization, specialization, fragmentation) served to increase the costs of medical care, particularly after the middle of this century. Medical services increased from somewhat over 7 percent of gross national product in 1970 to nearly 10 percent in 1982, then declined to about 9 percent in 1987 and 8 percent in 1992 (Figure 4.3), while the absolute costs continued to increase (Figure 4.4).[12] As the proportion of aged increases toward 20 percent of the population and the proportion of the population out of work because of sickness continues to increase, the financial burden of health problems should continue to increase.

One way to look at these developments is to note that the changes in Swedish medical care are, at this level, absolutely characteristic of the Western world in general. There is nothing special in the patterns, although the specifics are unique. Here, as in many other instances, the devil is in the details.

For one thing, the magnitude of the burden of health problems is greater than for any other country, if one discounts epidemic- and famine-related events that are more characteristic of developing countries. Sweden has the highest proportion of aged people of any country, which generates an enormous upward pressure on medical services. The unit cost of delivering medical care grows geometrically with the age of the patient. In addition, Sweden faces this problem with a high-technology system built around tertiary care. This is the most expensive way to organize medical care. It means that the settings in which much care is delivered are overcapitalized and less capable of responding to personal needs than lower technology and less bureaucratic settings would be. This is not to take an antibureaucratic or antitechnology stance, but only to suggest that the balance between high- and low-technology settings needs to be explored.[13]

These points need to be held in mind as we turn to the core problems facing Western medical care systems: financing and alienation.

Financing

Four points should be clearly made with respect to the cost of medical care in Sweden. First, as in the rest of the developed world, the cost of providing medical services in Sweden has risen rapidly, more rapidly than the gross national product or any other part of the economy (Figure 4.5). The growth of medical care costs has paralleled that of other OECD countries (see Figure 4.3), and as of the middle 1980s was second highest among OECD countries, a position it had held at least as far back as 1960 (Figure 4.6, Table 4.3). Sweden thus shared in the interest all developed countries had in finding ways to cap the rise in the cost of medical care.

Second, OECD data show a trend after 1982 toward a reduction in the proportion of the Swedish GNP devoted to medical care. While most

Figure 4.3
Growth in Cost of Medical Care, 1970–1987, as Percentage of GNP for Sweden, Great Britain, the United States, and the Average of OECD Countries

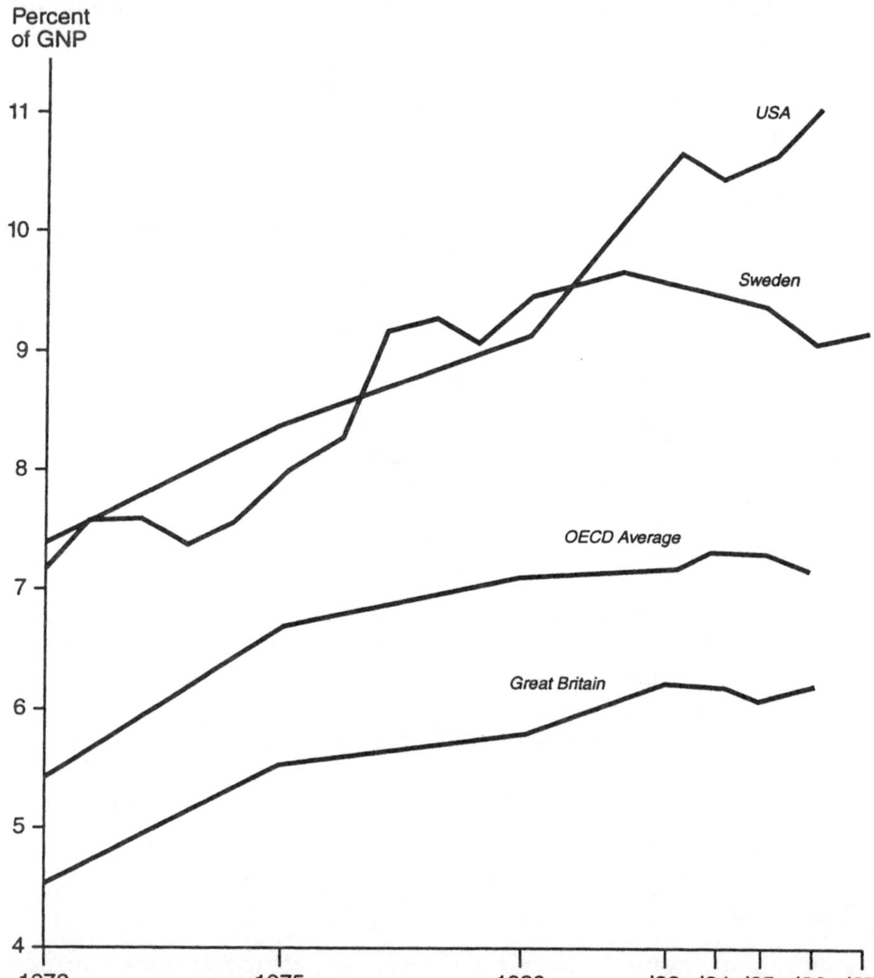

Source: OECD, *Financing and Delivering Health Care: A Comparative Analysis of OECD Countries* (Paris: OECD, 1987); Statistiska Centralbyrån, *Nationalräkenskaperna* (Stockholm: SCB, 1988): Johan Calltorp, 1989a, *Prioritering och beslutsprocess i sjukvårdsfrågor* (Uppsala: Institutionen för Socialmedicin), 13.

other countries experienced a leveling of the relative cost of medical care, partly as a result of strong economic growth, Sweden was the only OECD country to post an actual decline (see Figure 4.3).[14]

Third, even though it was never fully exploited, Sweden entered the 1980s with a system of allocating technology and personnel that pro-

Figure 4.4
Financing of Social Welfare Expenditures 1975–1991 in 1980 Prices

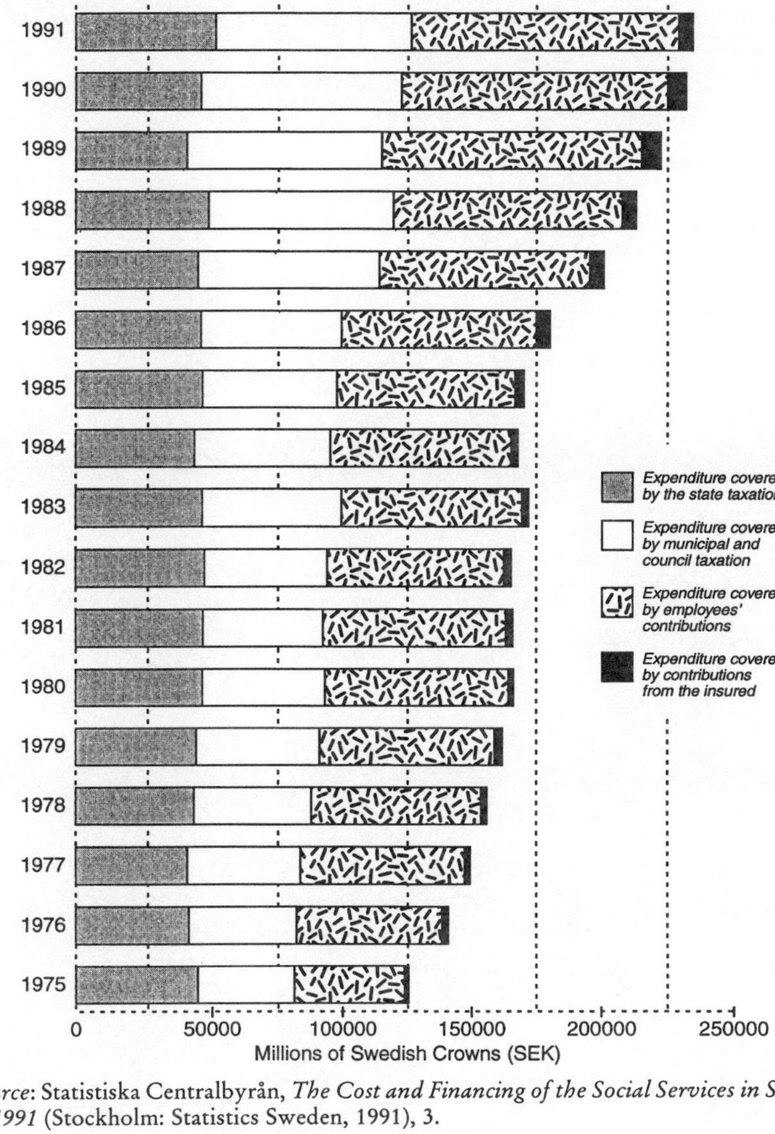

Source: Statistiska Centralbyrån, *The Cost and Financing of the Social Services in Sweden in 1991* (Stockholm: Statistics Sweden, 1991), 3.

vided a structure for effective cost containment. In fact, the system was used to allocate technology and medical specialties by level of hospital. That undoubtedly prevented the cost of the Swedish system from being much higher than it was. It was never used, as it could have been, to allocate resources between hospital and primary care. Had it been so used, the cost of the Swedish system might have been more modest.

Figure 4.5
Consumption within Selected Sectors Along with GNP, Controlling for Inflation, 1970–1986

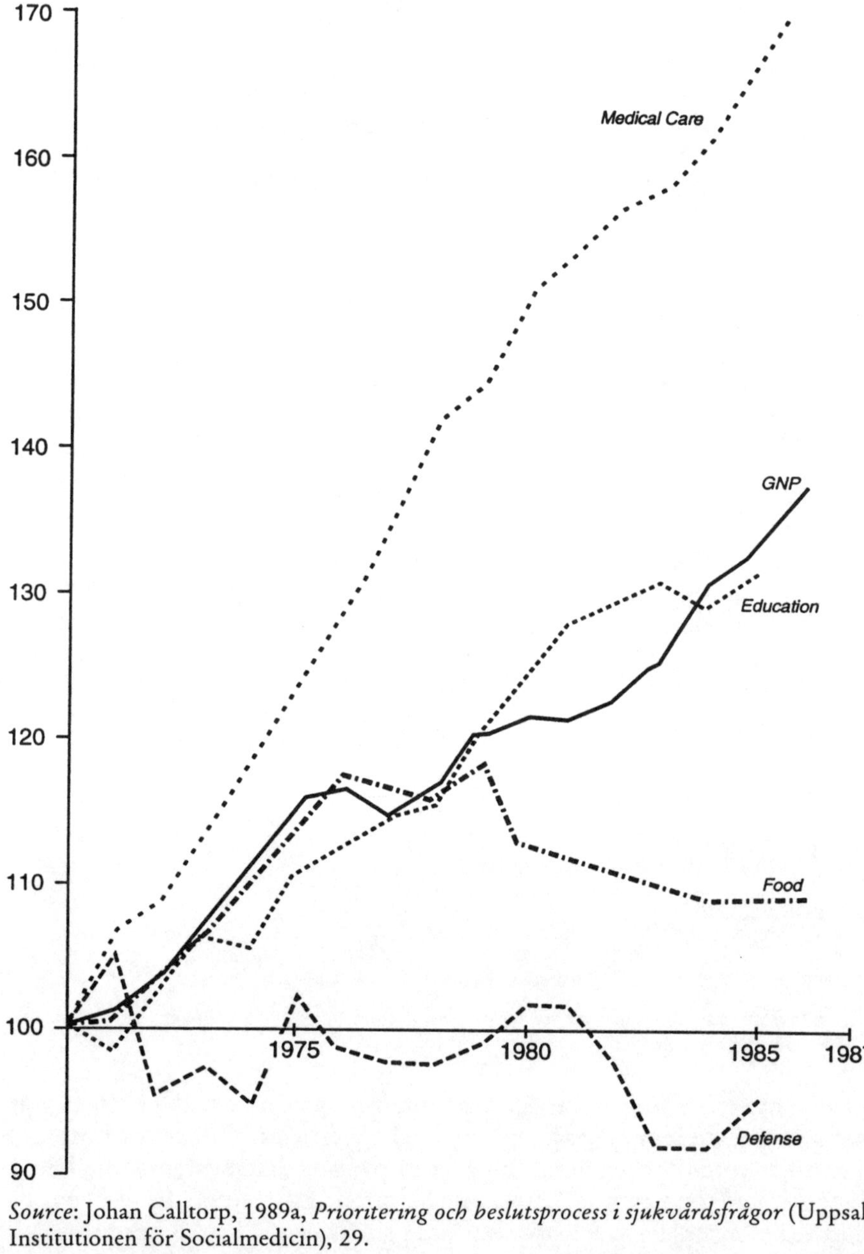

Source: Johan Calltorp, 1989a, *Prioritering och beslutsprocess i sjukvårdsfrågor* (Uppsala: Institutionen för Socialmedicin), 29.

Figure 4.6
Association of Health and Medical Care Costs and per Capita GNP in OECD Countries (Local currencies converted to U.S. dollars based on parity of purchasing power)

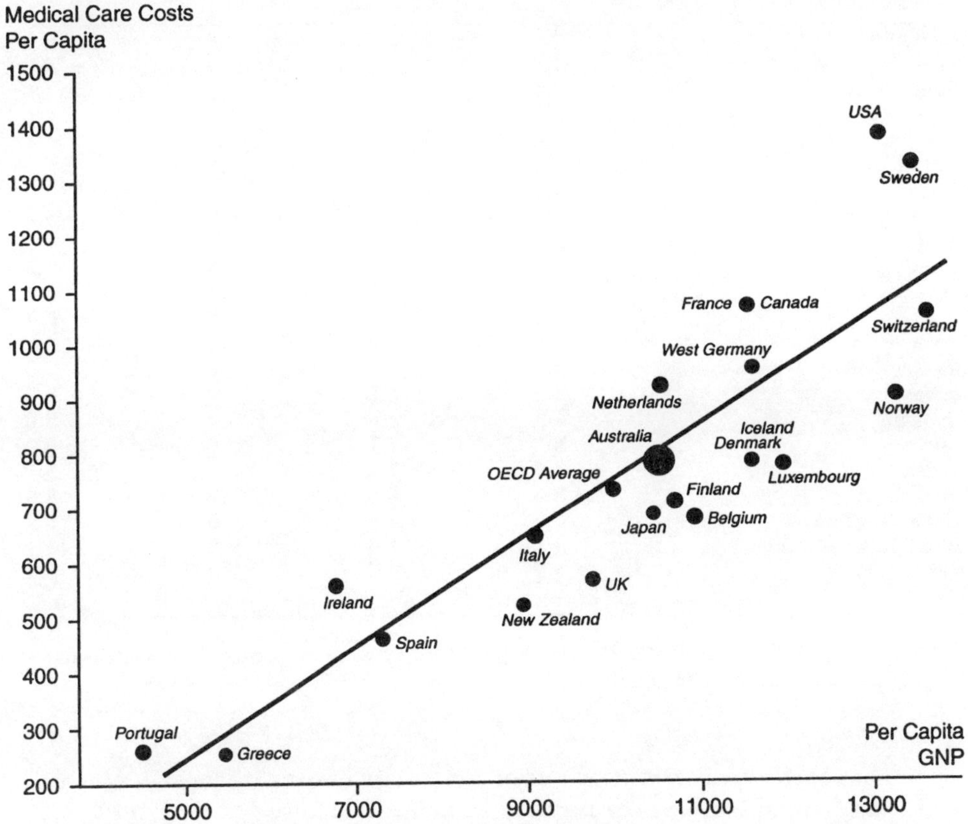

Source: OECD, *Financing and Delivering Healthcare: A Comparitive Analysis of OECD Countries* (Paris: OECD, 1987); Johan Calltorp, 1989a, *Prioritering och beslutsprocess i sjukvårdsfrågor* (Uppsala: Institutionen för Socialmedicin), 29.

Fourth, at the level of the discrete units in which medical care was delivered, the system was among the most efficient in the world. Hospital wards had fewer employees per bed and had lower costs than their counterparts in other countries, ambulatory care receptions were lower in cost, and expensive technology was monitored to see that it was used appropriately and efficiently shared. The high cost of the total system was not because the components of that system were inefficient. It was because there was a bias in the use of that system toward the use of its most expensive components.

Table 4.3
Health and Medical Care Costs as Percentage of GNP in OECD Countries

Country	1960	1970	1980	1986
Australia	4.6	5.0	6.6	6.8
Austria	4.6	5.4	7.9	8.0
Belgium	3.4	4.0	6.0	7.1
Canada	5.5	7.2	7.4	8.5
Denmark	3.6	6.1	6.8	6.1
Finland	4.2	5.6	6.3	7.5
France	4.2	5.6	7.4	8.5
Greece	2.9	4.0	4.2	3.9
Iceland	5.9	8.7	6.9	7.5
Ireland	4.0	5.6	8.5	7.9
Italy	3.3	4.8	6.8	6.7
Japan	3.0	4.6	6.6	6.7
Netherlands	3.9	6.0	8.2	8.3
New Zealand	4.4	5.1	7.2	6.9
Norway	3.3	5.0	6.6	6.8
Portugal	-	-	5.9	5.6
Spain	2.3	4.1	5.9	6.0
Sweden	4.7	7.2	9.5	9.1
Switzerland	3.3	5.2	7.2	8.0
United Kingdom	3.9	4.5	5.8	6.2
United States of America	5.2	7.4	9.2	11.1
West Germany	4.7	5.5	7.9	8.1

Source: Johan Calltorp, 1989a, *Prioritering och beslutsprocess i sjukvårdsfrågor* (Uppsala: Institutionen för Socialmedicin), 23.

That costs were seemingly out of control in Sweden, then, was not, as in the United States, because they lacked a structure for cost containment but, because that structure was never fully exploited. The allocation of technology and personnel was done by physician groups making requests which were negotiated with the national government. The structuring of those requests kept the system biased toward high technology (budgeting requests were dominated by physicians in regional hospitals) and specialized medicine (specialists made the requests). General medicine, and primary care in general, appeared at the bottom of the list. When the list was "pared down," it was the primary care budget that was cut (Härnqvist, 1978; 1983; Lindholm, 1978; Tibblin, 1979).

Even with these aspects taken into account, it is still a fact that the cost of medical care was rising at a rate that could not be sustained over the long run. The demand for medical care continued to increase, driven by the rapidly growing population and the rapid aging of that population. There is also evidence that the cost of sickness was rising, even without the aging process. Utilization was increasing at every age and the burden of sickness seemed to be increasing as well, as measured by work loss because of sickness.[15] Even if some costs could have been shifted to the social security budget and some of the more expensive extravagances could have been reined in, producing a decline in the percentage of the national wealth spent on medical care, the longer-range problem remained. The costs of medical care were increasingly difficult to meet. It was to be expected that some increased attention would be given to cost containment.

There is no one obvious path that had to be taken to control costs, however. One possibility would have been to increase control of allocation by better planning. One could, for example, use the existing allocative mechanisms to shift the emphasis from hospital care to ambulatory care, from curative medicine to preventive medicine, or from high-cost delivery settings to low-cost delivery settings. Especially given the low unit costs of the Swedish system, there were enormous savings to be made within the existing system.

The direction, however, was different. As we will discuss, it was to dismantle the very structures that made cost control possible. First, it was a move toward a more privatized, competitive, and market-oriented system. The stated assumption here was that planning was the problem and freer competition among providers would result in a more efficient use of resources.[16] Second, it was a move to decentralize to units that would be more accountable for their balance between income and expenditure.[17] Here the assumption seemed to be that the delivery units were operating inefficiently. While there were features of the system that were not providing optimally cost-effective services, and there was reason to want to make the system more efficient in that regard, it seemed not to be the case that the Swedish system was less efficient than those already organized along market principles. Quite the contrary. If compared with the United States, the units delivering medical services were more cost effective in Sweden.

Alienation

In Chapter 2, we described the alienation of patients in the professional–patient encounter as having four dimensions: clinical, organization, economic, and interactional. Clinical alienation is a function of expert knowledge and is inevitable to some degree if one is to have a medical profession. It is not a form of alienation normally thought of as problematic. Indeed, when people are symptomatic they typically do not know what the underlying problem is or what to do about it. It is for that reason they seek out a "competent treatment agent," one they believe can help. Most of the authority to define the nature of the problem and to set a course of treatment is delegated to the professional, both by the patient and by those with whom the patient interacts (Twaddle, 1979). As the gap widens between the knowledge of the patient and the knowledge of the physician, the autonomy of the professional increases as does the alienation of the patient in that encounter.

Economic alienation is largely a function of ability to pay. This has become more problematic in this century, as payment has been more formalized and restricted to a cash economy. Older forms, such as barter or the direct exchange of services, are no longer in use. This issue is more salient in countries where medical care has developed in the context of a service provided by free professionals. In Sweden, the public provision of services has a long history, particularly for persons with few economic resources. As that system expanded in this century to encompass the whole resident population, it made the economic terms of delivery a minor issue for almost everyone.

The other dimensions are not as inevitable. It is there that the alternatives described in Chapter 2 (professions, markets, democracy) for organizing medical services become salient. The organizational and interactional dimensions of alienation are the ones of most concern.

Turning first to the organizational dimension, it will be recalled it has to do with the shift of medical practice from settings controlled by patients (e.g., the patient's home) to those controlled by physicians (e.g., hospitals) (Twaddle, 1982). At issue was the locus of decision making about the ways in which services were to be provided. It will also be recalled that when a professional model of organization applied, decisions were made by experts in the knowledge applied by the organization with a goal of providing the most effective services. When a market model applied the decisions were made by business interests with a goal of profit, providing the most cost-efficient services. When a democratic model applied, the decisions were taken by politicians with a goal of providing the most equitable services. These dimensions seemed to underlie the debate in Sweden in the early 1990s. We begin with the situation as it was as of about 1980.

Organizationally, there was much concern expressed over whether the medical care system was as responsive to public needs as it could be. This discussion did not refer to issues of technical quality. It was taken for granted that when anyone was in the care system they got the best application of knowledge available anywhere in the world. Instead it was on issues of quality of care that concern was expressed.[18] That is to say, it was the organization of services that were at issue.

One issue was queues, or waiting lists, for treatment. Especially in the large cities patients experienced long waits for some elective procedures. Among them were coronary artery bypass surgery, angioplasty, cholecystectomy, inguinal hernia repair, arthroplasty, cataracts, and the like. While from a medical perspective these conditions may not have been life threatening, from a patient perspective they required urgent treatment. To have to wait six weeks to three months for treatment posed a problem (Socialstyrelsen, 1993b).

Treatment in hospital settings was said to be "cold" and "bureaucratic." Patients complained about being treated impersonally, "like a piece of meat." Indeed, when asked, most people seemed to express anger about their own treatment or the treatment of someone they knew well.[19] At the same time, people expressed generally positive feelings about the medical care system, which they regarded as competent and efficient (Zetterberg, 1979).

EFFECTS OF CHANGES ON FINANCING AND ALIENATION, 1983–1990

Taken together, the reforms of the 1980s, as described in Chapter 1, expanded the private sector and laid the groundwork for further expansion in the future (cf. Rosenthal, 1989). The Health and Sickness Care Law of 1982 turned over to the counties the responsibility for organizing private practice, which had been tightly contained earlier. The result was a rapid expansion of private practice which was reigned in by the Dagmar Reform of 1984. In shifting primary care for the aged to municipalities, the Ädel Reform of 1992 again expanded opportunities for private physicians to enter into contracts to provide that care. The Point of Service Reform of 1993 further opened the door to private practice by allowing private physicians to become family physicians on the same terms as public physicians and lifting restrictions on where primary care practices could be located.

A second effect of the combined reforms was to reduce central control over the distribution of technology and personnel. Coming particularly from the Health and Sickness Care Law of 1992, decisions on the location of expensive technology and on the numbers and types of physicians to be trained and their distribution, once made by the national government, were transferred to the counties. The result was a "downward press" of technology. Machinery once limited to regional hospitals was found not only in county hospitals but also in local free-standing clinics.[20] Duplication of specialized personnel and technology could no longer be controlled.

A third effect was a decentralization of administration and financing. The Health and Sickness Care Law of 1992 transferred all administrative authority and almost all financing authority to the counties. The national government retained the right to set standards and exercise oversight with respect to those standards. They surrendered all operational control of the system. The Dagmar Reform tightened national control of the expenditure of national health care funds in private medical care by shifting to a block grant system in place of fee for service. That provided more predictability and reduced expenditures from the national budget without direct control over the delivery system. Indeed, national control over allocation, once distribution was made to the counties, was almost totally surrendered. The Ädel Reform further decentralized some primary care activities to the municipalities. The Point of Service Reform provided for the "free establishment" of private physicians, eliminating even county and municipal control over their distribution.

As of 1994, there seemed to be a continuing commitment to the principle of universal access to medical services and maintaining a strong public system. This was clearly a priority for the public and political support for the principle seemed to be solid in every party to the left of the Conservatives. At the same time, the balance was clearly shifting toward a more privatized system.

While none of these decisions directly reduced the medical surveillance of children and pregnant women, it seemed likely that the same physicians would not be involved. There was a clear trend toward general practitioners replacing maternal and child health physicians in much ambulatory care activity.

It seemed the technical quality of Swedish medicine would remain high, but there was no longer a protection against the duplication of technology or specialized physicians. As primary care expanded, there might be a force holding down costs, but it seemed likely that the duplication of services would act to inflate the cost of medical care, perhaps dramatically. A hypothesis that the unit costs of Swedish medicine would increase in comparison with other countries seemed a safe bet. When that happened, the national government would be without means to control those costs.[21]

The ratio of general to specialized services was substantially improved during the 1980s, but not because of the reforms under consideration here. Reforms in medical education in the early to mid 1970s had capped most specialty training and expanded enrollment in medical schools. The number of primary care physicians grew rapidly throughout the 1980s as a result. The development of Care Centers in the late 1970s had provided a better work environment for primary care physicians and eliminated most of the earlier access problems.

Two countervailing processes with regard to costs were in force by 1990. On the one hand, there was a shift toward primary care and restriction of private medicine. Indeed, after the Dagmar Reform, Sweden was one of the only countries in the world where the percentage of GNP spent on medical care actually declined. On the other hand, cost controls were abandoned and private practice again expanded. One would expect this to cause the total cost of the system to rise.

As of 1995, there was no evidence that the quality of care declined, with one notable exception: the care of the aged. Even there, most of those able to live in their own homes seemed to be doing well. There was evidence, however, that when the municipalities took over nursing homes, the quality of care deteriorated. Indeed, a flow of horror stories about abuse and neglect in nursing homes appeared in the national morning press. Studies documented very poor care in the nursing homes of Uppland. The first report on the effects of the Ädel Reform targeted the quality of care in nursing homes as an area of great concern (Socialstyrelsen, 1993a).

In interviews in the spring of 1993, we picked up a number of anecdotal reports of elderly people with easily treatable life-threatening conditions being turned away from *Söder Sjukhuset* in Stockholm on the grounds that they were "too old to be treated." Whether that was simply a policy decision by the hospital, a glitch in the county–municipality relationship, or the dark side of the Ädel Reform could not be resolved. Nor could we tell whether this was a local problem or an emerging national one. It is certainly a matter worth further investigation.[22]

Paradoxically, given that one of the primary goals of all the reforms was to increase the efficiency of the medical care system, it may be the case that the system will become less efficient. If unit costs go up and a substantial shift cannot be accomplished away from high-technology hospital care, Swedes may end up paying considerably more for less service. Again, it is too early to make an assessment. It is a situation worth watching. What can be said is that between 1994 and 1995 the cost of primary care exploded as a result of the free establishment of physicians.

As of 1994, the major activity was for larger political units to shift costs to smaller units. The Health and Sickness Care law and the Dagmar Reform limited national expenditures on medical care and shifted responsibility to the counties. The Ädel Reform shifted one of the areas of rapidly expanding cost from the counties to the municipalities. In neither instance was there a transfer of funds corresponding to the magnitude of the shift in responsibility.

One obvious conclusion is that the reforms of the 1980s were much more concerned with the crisis of financing than with the crisis of alienation. The changes introduced into medical care were administrative and fiscal. They were intended to generate financial savings by making the system more efficient. The major mechanisms were decentralization, introducing market elements into the public system, and providing more opportunity for the private sector to take a larger role. While it might be argued that an expansion of primary care and the introduction of a care guarantee might address issues of alienation, the reforms were not presented in that light. Instead, both were presented as means for addressing financial problems. Increasing the relative use of primary care would, it was argued, reduce the relative use of more expensive hospital facilities. Introducing a "guarantee" that elective procedures would be carried out within three months was presented as a means of providing financial incentives for specialty clinics to operate more efficiently. Indeed, the reforms seem to have ignored any suggestion of a crisis of alienation. Before concluding that such a crisis does not exist, however, we should look at the political debates on medical care.

THE POLITICAL DEBATES, 1993

Substantively, the hot political topic in early 1993 was the *Husläkare* reform. This was an "old warhorse" of the *Folkpartiet liberalerna* (the Liberal Party), which had introduced a proposal for a primary care physician in 1978. It was before the *Riksdag* again in 1993, in an altered form, as discussed in Chapter 1. An examination of the debate can be informative, but only in a larger context.

It will be recalled from Chapter 3 that interviews were done with representatives of a variety of interest organizations (physicians, nurses, blue collar and white collar umbrella union organizations, and the blue collar and white collar municipal employees unions), governmental organizations (the Ministry of Health and the Federation of County Councils), politicians representing all the parties on health policy, and some scholars taking an active role in the health policy debates. Each respondent was asked, "Is there a medical care crisis?" "What is the nature of the problem in medical care?" and "What are your (organization's) goals for the medical care system?" The latter question was designed to elicit issues without necessarily defining them as constituting a crisis. Together, the questions should allow us to discriminate the priorities of different interests for changing the medical care system (Table 4.4).

Is There a Crisis?

While there had been some effort to portray changes that put pressure on medical services as if they constituted a crisis (e.g., Landstingsförbundet, 1993c), almost nobody would accept the label "crisis" when asked directly. Hans Bergström (1992), the editor of the influential daily newspaper *Dagens Nyheter* in Stockholm, attempted to outline the "pressures behind the Swedish health reforms."[23] One such pressure was the "overheating" of the Swedish economy in the 1980s followed by stagnation in the early 1990s. He asserted that the capacity to raise taxes had reached its limit, particularly as municipalities were prohibited from raising taxes. In addition, the cost of medical care was increasing as was the cost of medical technology. Wages of medical care workers were low and the medical care system was said to be insensitive to demand factors.

In this context, Bergström pointed to several specific problems with the medical care system. There were long waiting lists for elective surgical procedures. Physicians had "low productivity." There was a "lack of humane care" for the aged. There was an increasing public demand for

Table 4.4
Problems Noted with the Swedish Medical Care System in Interviews with Key Decision Makers and Opinion Leaders, Sweden, 1993

Availability	Accessibility	Acceptability	Affordability	Effectiveness	Flexibility	Other
None noted.	Waiting lists for elective procedures—increasing demand for medical care; "bed blockers" in acute hospitals.	Decrease in quality of care for aged.	State debt.	Bureaucracy.	No choice of physicians or hospitals for patients.	Care teams.
		Privatization.	Overextension of welfare state.	Managerial system—administrative control of hospitals.	No freedom of establishment for physicians.	County Council Monopoly —No separation between representatives of people and administration of system.
		Fragmentation.	Rising costs—increase in aged population; technological growth.	Unthoughtful use of incentives.	Hospitals too large.	Increased employment of women—reduction in uncompensated care.
		Continuity of care.	Inefficient use of resources—hospital over capacity and over staffing; over specialization; budgetary system; decreased physician productivity.		Political control of system.	Unemployment of physicians.
			Fragmentation—loss of budgetary control.			
			Lack of standards for medical audits—vast differences in use of resources by area.			

choice and personalized care. He held that politicians could not manage both the financing and delivery systems, administrators wanted to be free of politicians, and professionals wanted greater autonomy. All of this coalesced in a new consensus that to be "modern" one had to endorse market-oriented changes. The Federation of County Councils had gotten out in front of the reform to salvage their influence. The public was said to be dissatisfied with the system and had unrealistic expectations of what medicine could accomplish. At the same time, almost all the people interviewed shied away from calling anything about the medical care system a "crisis." When asked, they stated that there was no crisis in medical care.

Governmental Organizations

Representatives of Landstingsförbundet (1991a; cf. Berleen, Håkensson, et al. 1992; Mollstedt, 1992) saw problems for the health care system resulting from the tight economy, a rapid rise of demand associated with the large and growing aged population, the cost of new technologies, and the putative inefficiencies of a planned economy. These were portrayed as factors that led to increased waiting times, increased public dissatisfaction with the system, impersonality of care, and powerlessness of patients. In their view, industry had become more critical of costs, productivity was low, and health services were not integrated with social insurance benefits. Insurance costs had grown more rapidly than the costs of care. The documents held that the financial system did not encourage good management, leading to a conclusion that the County Councils got too little money for care and people got too little care for their money. Berleen noted that general practitioners had been poor gatekeepers, allowing overutilization of specialty services and unexplained variations in utilization from one region to another. Mollstedt focused on the competition from the European Community as a pressure for change.

While portraying a system that had "no choice but to change," the representatives of *Landstingsförbundet* interviewed shied away from characterizing the situation as a crisis. The following statements, transcribed from interviews, illustrate.[24]

> The first part is to define what is a crisis. If you call it a crisis that you have rationalized medical care in Sweden to such an extent that you have unemployment . . . among doctors, then there is a crisis. But that is not what I, or the employers, *Landstingsförbundet* as an employer, would call a crisis. I deny there is a crisis. But if you feel that you get less money, then that is right, because we have diminished the costs for medical care, even in fixed prices. Inflation last year was about 2–3 % on the average and we have balanced that. But I wouldn't call that a crisis. (Bengt Mollstedt, President of the Board, *Landstingsförbundet*)

> There is no crisis in health care. The crisis is concerned with financing health care. That's the crisis. We are not allowed to finance health care the way we have done it over the years. This is the first time it has happened in decades that the increases in county councils became a decrease from 1991 to 1992 by 1.2%. (Olof Eliasson, Director, Department of Health Services, *Landstingsförbundet*)

The Ministry of Health seemed to share in the analysis presented by those promoting changes. They also declined to call the situation a crisis.

> So, there have been many changes, but the ideological question, the question of whether there has been a fundamental shift, . . . I don't think so. . . If you mean a fundamental shift of going back to the 1880s or going back to some kind of free market or even to change the present Swedish system of general welfare policy within a general welfare policy system, most discussion at present is not in favor of leaving the general welfare system and going to a more restrictive system.
>
> But there is a discussion whether we should change one essential part of the general welfare system, that part that has to do with giving compensation, some kind of proportion of your former income, and change that system to one where you have a flat rate.[25] That, of course, is still a general system, because it's a general policy. . . . But I have not talked about health care yet. Is there a crisis in health care? . . . No, I wouldn't say so. We have one of the best systems in the world. . . . We have a very high degree of equity. We have a very good level of prevention, especially in maternal and child care. . . . We have good access for people irrespective of their income. We also have a good measure of equity in results. (Bo Könberg, Minister of Health)

Interest Organizations

The physicians union (*Läkarförbundet*) was the only nongovernmental organization with a seemingly major role in politically defining the problem of medical care. They noted long waiting times for elective surgery, less than optimal continuity for patients, lack of patient choice, and inefficiencies posed by geographic boundaries for seeking care. They also had concern for the working conditions of physicians. Milton (1991) noted that the tasks of primary care physicians were poorly defined, with little variety in their work, heavy workloads, rigid organizational forms, and organizational units that were too large. The growth of primary care physicians had been slow and job satisfaction was low. Hasselius (1991) noted the same factors and attributed the problems to politically planned medical care. However, Anders Milton, Secretary General of the Physicians' Union, held in an interview that there was no crisis in medical care:

> When we started . . . the public debate, or proposals that led to a public debate, the reason was not that we felt . . . the health care sector was falling apart. I mean that was not the case, because it wasn't at that time and it still isn't.
>
> So within the profession there was very much discontent. You have probably seen the inquiry that *Landstingsförbundet* sent out to heads of clinics about four, five, six years ago. . . . What they asked was "what are your greatest problems?" and out of the two thousand, 80% said our relation to the politicians is our greatest problem, meaning that the owners, *Landstinget*, . . . their bosses didn't speak the same language. . . .
>
> We started to try to see whether or not one could not change the system in a way that would be more efficient. I am not using the word "efficient" in a very strict sense, but a system that would be more rational in the way it works. . . . The minister, Gertrud Sigurdsen, was heavily criticized because of the [inefficiencies] and she had no means to address them. When she turned to *Landstingsförbundet* they only said "give us more resources—more of the same—and everything will turn out fine." And so after a while she got tired of that answer. This criticism also got back to *Landstingsförbundet*, and that's why they started the Dagmar reform. Within the Social Democratic Party, they were very critical of the situation and they realized they had to do something. What they did was Dagmar. I think it was a fair attempt to vitalize the debate. . . .
>
> You can hear people tell you these anecdotal things—like . . . that there was a city in Southern Sweden where you had to set your alarm clock for six in the morning in order to call *Televerket* in order to get in line . . . for the local health care center . . . in order to get a time for three weeks later. Then you have an access problem. Then if the politicians have decided you can only go to this *vårdcentral* then people are not satisfied. . . .
>
> It cannot be possible that you have 10%—it used to be 10%—of all we produce in Sweden and you cannot do one thing to make it efficient. I mean that's improbable. It's [the percentage of GDP spent on medical care] going down, not because there are people being fired. It's going down because we are redefining it. You see, we start taking away things that in other countries are not on the health care budget, or that are done through other channels. Then we get down to something like 8% (7.5%) so we are adjusting to the European average. . . .
>
> So I think the general background was not a background where we saw everything falling apart, but where we felt there was room for improvement. That's why we started our recent work in this field. (Anders Milton, Secretary General, *Läkarförbundet*)

Respondents from organizations representing workers in health care almost all recognized problems in medical care, but none would call it a crisis. The *Tjänstemännens Centralorganisation* was the "peak" organization representing white-collar labor unions. While they had not taken a role in the debates on medical care, they were clearly interested. Anders Forsman, an economic historian, offered the following opinion:

> Well, from an American point of view, there isn't. I mean it isn't the kind of mess you have.
>
> The basic problem is demographic. . . . We have 18% of the population 65 years old and over. . . . It's so many old people, so much new technology, so we have heavy queues for heavy medical care. That's a kind of crisis, if you like. It's a strong word.
>
> We have a kind of cost containment in the Swedish health care system because of the rule of the *Landstings* budgets. We were in Germany a year ago and they have problems with cost increases, but they have no cost containment. A lot of health politicians come here and study the *Landstingsmodellen*, because it's possible to contain costs within this kind of system. You don't have that in Germany. . . . I'm an expert on this issue, but I wouldn't say it's a crisis. (Anders Forsman, Chief, Socioeconomic Analysis Unit, TCO)

Sture Nordh, President of *Kommunaltjänstemänsförbundet (SKTF)*, the union representing white-collar public employees, responded to a question about a medical care crisis with a detailed analysis of the shifting political climate in Sweden. While he saw some major problems they were not with the medical care system.

Nor did respondents from organizations representing blue collar workers see a medical care crisis. *Landsorganisation i Sverige* is the "peak" organization of blue-collar labor unions. Per-Olof Edin was an LO economist with a major role in the national debates on economic policy. He offered the following viewpoint:

> I can't see it. Of course we have, and always have had, problems. Of course we have a system that can be improved in many ways. That's true, but as I see it, if you look at the overall situation in Sweden, we have a splendid system.
>
> We . . . distribute medical care according to need instead of according to wallet. . . . I think we have a medical standard that is as good as any in the Western world. If we see how the normal Swede is treated in the medical care system, the level of technology and knowledge and so on. . . . We do it at a cost that is much lower than in the United States. . . . The basic organization of our medical care system is very good. . . . I would say "keep the fundamental system and do some marginal changes." (Per-Olof Edin, Economist, Political Economy Unit, LO)

From a more local perspective, Tommy Petterson was a youth worker in Linköping and an active member of SKAF, the Swedish Union of

Municipal Employees. He saw many more concrete problems associated with the Ädel Reform. Even so, he shied away from the term "crisis":

> Not yet. I am only in the [municipality]. We did a change in 1991. We call it the Ädel reform. Then we had the beginning of a crisis, I think, because then you lost . . . medical competence, skill. . . . Physicians and nurses are very few, now. We are not in that old organization, *Landstinget*. They have the medicine skills. [Municipalities] have schools and such things. We haven't the medical skills. They did it very quickly and we had very little money. We lost much skill on the organizational level. But it's not a crisis. That's too strong a word. (Tommy Petterson, SKAF, Linköping)

The only interest organization to take the position that there might be a crisis in medical care was the Nurses Union. For them, the crisis was in the new approach to public services, not the medical care system, although they acknowledged that the system had not been as responsive at it could have been:[26]

> Maybe not a crisis, but the ideological grounds for the system are threatened. People want a greater say, greater choice. Public health care has neglected public demand for a greater say and choice. There is economic pressure on the health care system to do more for less cost. And there is the growing aged population putting pressure on the system. Also, expectations of people are growing out of hand. People expect health care to solve all of their problems. . . . The better educated people with higher standards don't think equality is enough. They want to have a greater choice. Equality is a value that has become unfashionable. People take it for granted, but when it is threatened they don't want to lose it. (Inger Ohlsson, President, *Vårdförbundet SHSTF*)

It is important to note that no representative of an interest organization interviewed for this study took the position that there was a crisis in the medical care system that caused or explained the change in political direction we are exploring. Several pointed to crises outside the medical care system as factors: either the performance of the economy or a shift in political ideology. We will return to these in the next chapters.

Politicians

None of the politicians we interviewed, who included representatives of every political party in Parliament, spoke of a medical care crisis. To gain insight into the parliamentary perspective, we interviewed a cross section of the members of the Health and Welfare Committee of Parliament.[27] We present their statements from right to left.[28]

The nature is there is no shortage of doctors or hospitals or money or other persons. There is just a lack of common sense. (Leif Bergdahl, New Democrat)

Well, there is and there isn't [a crisis in medical care]. The Swedish health care is basically very good, but the economy makes it impossible to meet all demands, and the demands have gone up faster than the resources, in terms of money. . . . We have greater resources than we thought we had because we have not used them very cleverly before. Many things you can do today are very expensive. Earlier you put in some money and you got a big good result. Today you can put in very much money and the differences in quality and so on are very small. (Leif Carlsson, Conservative)

Do we have a crisis? I would say not yet. What we have is that shock therapy is going on at present in Sweden. We were building up welfare, not only the health care system. I think we must see health care in the perspective of the total welfare system that was very ambitiously built up in Sweden over . . . about 60 years. These were 60 wonderful years, very wonderful years. . . . Our taxes went up almost 60% . . . those who are economists have convinced me that the taxes cannot be increased. If we increase them there will be no more money in the basket. . . . And now begins a painful process, which is, I would say, not a crisis, but shock therapy, and different aspects of welfare have to be reduced. . . . Sweden is a corporative country. . . . We have very strong organizations that guard our different interests. . . . But nobody defends health care because there is no organization, for natural reasons, for sick people. (Jerzy Einhorn, Christian Democrat)

I don't think it is a crisis, but of course people need medical care and I think we have had the wrong organizations for that. . . . If you have good contact with a family doctor you can save a lot of money, I think. . . . I also see that we educate many young students as medical doctors and they stay in the hospitals. In Sweden, only four percent of our educated doctors are in primary care. In Canada, New Zealand and other countries . . . they have 40% of the trained physicians in primary care. (Ulla Orring, Liberal Party)

We lack money. That's the greatest problem right now. In the Center Party we want a new insurance system . . . a guaranteed level for everybody. We want a higher level. We think everybody has to build upon that with a voluntary insurance. (Rosa Östh, Center Party)

Yes, we had a debate over medical care in Sweden for the past two years where people said the Swedish model was in crisis. There were five health economists, one from the USA and one from England . . . who said that the Swedish medical care system could not be said to be in crisis, but it had problems. . . . My position as a Social Democrat is that Sweden is generally in good shape and we hold that we will not drive in privatization and the neoliberal things the Conservatives want. I believe the next elec-

> tion will be referendum on the welfare state. (Bo Holmberg, Social Democrat)
>
> Sweden has a very good health care system and we need to be very careful to keep what we have that is good. But it needs to be made more efficient and the costs need to be kept down. . . . The process of privatization is more urgent for the Conservatives than is the issue of making the system better for the Swedish people. (Eva Zetterberg, Left Party)

The politicians did not claim there was a crisis in the medical care system even when they were sponsoring a change in that system, although some said a crisis was looming if changes were not made.

Those who came closest to responding positively to the question of whether a crisis existed were the New Democratic and the Conservative politicians. Leif Bergdahl (New Democrat) claimed there was a sharp drop in productivity among physicians as a result of a lack of incentives for seeing large numbers of patients. Leif Carlsson (Conservative) and Jerzy Einhorn (Christian Democrat) claimed the economy could not support the growth of medical care costs.

The other bourgeois politicians disclaimed the idea that a crisis was present or imminent, but referred to problems they thought needed solutions: the underdevelopment of primary care (Ulla Orring, Liberal), and the income-replacement principle for social insurance (Rosa Östh, Center). The first could be seen as a medical care system issue, the second could not.

The socialist politicians were emphatic in claiming that the medical care system was not in crisis. Indeed, it was in good shape and had to be defended from those who threatened it for their own ideological ends. Bo Holmberg (Social Democrat) and Eva Zetterberg (Left) took this position. For them, whatever crisis existed was in the threat to the Swedish model posed by neoliberal ideologues.

Others

There were three others interviewed because of their unique roles in the debate on medical care. Two of these, Gösta Tibblin (Professor of General Medicine, Uppsala University) and Johan Calltorp (Docent in Social Medicine, Caroline Hospital), took the position that there was no crisis in medical care organization. Johannes Vang of the World Health Organization (WHO) said there was.

Tibblin was a cardiologist who, in the 1970s, was so concerned with the need to develop general medicine that he took an almost unprecedented step and resigned his professorship in cardiology to found the first professorship in general medicine in the country. His response was as follows:

> It depends on how you are using the word "crisis." Maybe in Sweden, in this very happy and calm country, you can call it a crisis. . . . I think it is more of a crisis in the US than it is here,—but the important thing is that we start realizing there are limits to the welfare state. We have expanded too much and we have too big a costume for us so we must reduce it. People are now used to high salaries, to a summer house, to traveling around, and so on. Therefore they are complaining. You see, it's the reduction in the standard of living, but 93% of the population are working and have a good salary, social security, and so on. It depends on how you define "crisis." If you look around you, you see a very high standard of living, but there is an increased number of unemployed, especially the young people.

While clearly pointing to problems, they are problems of the general economy, not those of the medical care system.

Johan Calltorp was a researcher in social medicine who made important contributions to understanding the changes taking place in the Swedish medical care system, especially with reference to setting priorities and making political decisions (see, especially, Calltorp, 1989b). He deflected the specific question on whether there was a crisis to provide a broader perspective:

> This powerful process going on needs be put into perspective and reflected on. . . . Suddenly we have a new situation with very rapid changes. My own view is that when we suddenly face, for different reasons, such strong pressures and tensions in the system that are difficult to handle, . . . then there is a sort of reflex mechanism that we are used to doing organizational changes. We have a problem, we do an organizational reform. I think many people regard the kind of policy changes that are now performed as some technical measure of the same kind as shifting the authority from state government to county councils. For example, using competition ideas and economic incentives in health care is, in my view, much more powerful than politicians think. The general view among politicians so far is there is not much [to] fear about economic incentives in health care. Most politicians think it is something that can speed up productivity, which I think is naïve. They say ugly things that we hear about in America won't appear here in Sweden. Swedish physicians are clean and have a good sense of ethics. My view is that Swedish physicians are like American physicians and economic incentives are so powerful that they can overwhelm medical ethics, or at least shake them.

Clearly, Calltorp did not see the most important problem in any crisis of medical care delivery, but in how politicians and others in key decision-making roles are responding to problems in medical care delivery. More explicitly than anyone else interviewed, he posed a conflict between market and professional interests in the medical care reforms.

The contrast between all those discussed so far and the perspective provided by Johannes Vang was striking. Vang was a physician who worked for WHO in Denmark, but who took a leading role in the Swedish debate by coauthoring the *Landstingförbundet*'s influential *Crossroads* report (*Landstingsförbundet*, 1991). He presented a classical conservative case:[29]

> I think one of the bigger problems in Sweden is the definition of equity has sort of slid towards "equal" instead of toward "fairness." . . . I can only see that the tendency in Sweden has not been fairness. It has been equality, people getting equality in a manner of measurable equality. For instance, you got the same amount of money if you get a child, almost independently of how wealthy you were or how poor you were, because that was equality. That's not fair, because we would assume that for a poor person there is a problem. It would be fair that he would get more than somebody who is stinking rich.
>
> The traditional problem in Sweden is that one didn't want charity. Charity goes to a time when you had to hold out your hand to get some money. So when the social system was invented just after the second World War, charity had such a bad connotation. Therefore everything should be given to everybody without thinking about whether they need it or not. It was a right. If it's a right, you cannot give it to one group of people and not to another group of people. If you make a service into a right, it has to be a right for everybody. Therefore a way developed out of fairness towards something which is equal. . . . I think that sliding away from charity . . . and making health services almost a God-given right was one big point.
>
> The other big point was, of course, . . . the new system was based on a political slogan of *folkhem*.[30] The idea was that the family was concerned about each other, looked out for each other, [and was] not concerned about rights. You were concerned about the future as such or your responsibility as such. So it was a society, a vision of a society in which we would all go around thinking about our responsibilities toward the group. . . . The problem was that the glue . . . in that context would be loyalty towards your fellow men and society. You could do that in a small society where people knew each other, . . . but as the society became more and more developed . . . what we saw was that as health care developed and became more and more effective we needed larger and larger units, more hospitals, more and more centralization.

In another context, he said, "They like to tell you Swedish health care is decentralized. It isn't and it wasn't. It is starting to become so now. . . . Formally, of course, different *landstings* had the right to do whatever they wanted, but they never did. The politicians would go together."

Not to put too fine a point on it, Vang described a set of developments in which the medical care system became a bureaucratic giant removed from the everyday needs of people and nonresponsive to their concerns. He portrayed a system that had grown from good intentions to one that no longer served the people. People were now "fed up" with the rigidities and wanted true decentralization and a means of influencing their care. Without using the word, he portrayed a system in crisis. While embedded in broader social changes, it was also a specifically medical care crisis. While many Swedes would agree with many of the trends Vang portrayed, few would have put them in the same context or agreed with his interpretation of them. His perspective was in that sense unique.

Problems in Medical Care

To say there was little to no sense of a crisis in the medical care system is not to claim there were no problems in medical care delivery. Indeed, every one of our respondents noted problems. There were, of course, differences in the kinds of problems defined depending on the role of the respondent vis-à-vis the medical care system. At the same time, there were areas of near consensus. At this point, we are not assessing or evaluating claims that there were or were not "real" problems with the medical care system. We are presenting the views of our respondents.

Government Organizations

Both the Ministry of Health and the Federation of County Councils had, as noted, seen similar problems with the medical care system:

> We have now, for the third consecutive year, a decrease in production. . . . If it continues for several years, of course, Sweden can't keep the welfare system of the present. . . .
>
> One of [the problems] was . . . a big lack of choice for patients, choice within ambulatory care and choice of hospitals. . . . Another . . . was the problem of long queues for treatment. . . . Another has been a problem with mostly elderly people in acute hospitals who have been medically treated and need something else, some nursing home, . . . *färdigbehandlade*. . . . We had, I think two years ago . . . about 4000 people where the doctor, the chief of the clinic, had said that we cannot do anything more with you with the resources we have here. You need something else, going home, or some people having you at home, or a nursing home, or something. That was 4000. What do we have, 42 or 43,000 beds? Almost 10%.
>
> What has happened this year, for the first time in Swedish modern history, people have been discharged from their work in the health sector. . . . I can't remember any time before when the county councils haven't been able to keep people occupied within the sector. . . . To these people who have never seen such problems it is a shock. It was a shock for all people. And, of course, if it will be in 1994 that we will have maybe 4 to

> 5% less resources than we had last year.
>
> Our proportion of the national income is now about 8.8%. It's dropping: 9.5–9.6% was our top. . . . Here I have the figures for the United States and Sweden . . . So let's say we have the same [percent of GNP spent on medical care in the US and Sweden] in 1980. The Swedish figure has decreased some, definitely less than nine, and your figure is definitely higher than 13. So, the non-socialist parties and the opposition criticized the costs of the system, especially, of course, the Moderate [Conservative] Party. In Sweden that criticism has diminished. In my opinion there is no big debate today in Sweden that the health care system costs too much. It was [there] two or three years ago, but not today, really. (Bo Könberg, Minister of Health)
>
> There were very good services, but for the patient it was too much a bureaucracy, which even applied to health care. (Ingrid Petersson, Assistant Minister of Health)
>
> It's the costs for health care. . . . we now live under completely different economic situations than before. That is the crisis. The crisis in Swedish health care is concerned with financing, not with anything else. Before in Sweden we have paid for health care 100%, 110% if you want, by taxation. That way isn't open. We had to look for new sources for financing. . . . There are three ways to go: raise more money in the traditional way, redefine what public money should finance in health care, [or] make the sector work more efficiently. . . . You have to work all three things at the same time. (Olof Eliasson, *Landstingsförbundet*)

Interest Organizations

The general secretary of the physicians' union laid out a viewpoint that there was widespread discontent with the medical care system on the part of physicians and the general public:

> So the reason that there has been discontent within the medical profession is more due to the fact that one has felt that the organization of health care has not been efficient, meaning . . . the budgetary system, which in effect is very similar to the ex-Soviet system where you have administratively decided the budget. . . .
>
> The second thing is the monopoly the county councils have had has not been effective because they have decided if or when they would like to have competition. And of course the first thing is that the managerial system has . . . not been very efficiently set up, because you have given responsibility to certain individuals, doctors in this case, but you have not given them the possibilities to bear their responsibility. You have to match responsibilities and authority. . . . A couple of years back, *Expressen*, one of the large evening newspapers . . . studied the surgical

theaters at Huddinge hospital for 24 hours. Three of them were actually used during that 24 hour period and three were used only eight hours per day. . . . You had surgeons who could not operate because there were no operating rooms running. The patients were waiting in lines. The reason was there was a lack of assistance in the operating theaters. . . . You had a boss, a head surgeon. He had responsibility. It was his area, but he was not given the authority to go in and say "let's recruit these 35 who are needed; let's raise salaries by 1500 SEK or 1000 SEK per month in order to recruit them." He was not allowed to do that because that was decided by the board, which is way up, meaning that if they made that decision they would have to raise the salaries not only for the 35 or 55 or 100 involved in the surgical theater in Huddinge, but for the 4000 employed in that section in the Stockholm County Council, and then you can't afford it.

This created a situation where there was a lot of discontent among the patients. You had waiting lines; you had access problems; you had continuity problems; you had problems in the service area. People were not satisfied with the level of service they got, . . . the medical attention they got.

While not discussing directly the issue of rising costs, the physicians' union was aware of the problem. . . . We had to look into the question of cost control, because that is a crucial issue. (Anders Milton, *Läkarförbundet*)

The nurses, as we have noted, saw the problems more in the reforms themselves and in the ideological support for strong public services. Nurses provided an analysis of the medical care system and a program in a document published in 1990 in collaboration with the Municipal Workers' Union. They focused on the aging of the population, the growth of medical knowledge and technology, the growth of medical care need outstripping the capacity of the economy, and the demand for medical personnel exceeding the even potentially available supply. All this has led to long cues, premature discharges from hospitals, patients being turned away from care, increased severity of conditions treated in clinics, personnel burnout, and understaffing of care. In essence, medical care was very effective, and its very effectiveness was creating problems.

Among union leaders, the growing costs were also among the concerns of people in the peak organizations, LO and TCO. They were much less salient in the major organizations of public employees, who were more focused on the effects of changes on their membership, and they were more tied to political decisions that had created economic pressures on medical care.

If we go to the health sector now, we can see that at the beginning of the '80s . . . the landstings, the County Councils, were trying to save money. They had rather great reserves in their budgets at the beginning of the

'80s and had so for a long time in the '70s also. But from the beginning of the '80s to the end of the '80s all the reserves were emptied. From the '90s on the county councils had to borrow money to operate. At the same time the state was keeping down the possibilities to raise taxes, because we already had high taxes in Sweden. . . . When people are not paying taxes any more, when unemployment is going up, . . . it's very difficult for health care programs, social security programs, to finance themselves when at the same time you have to pay a lot of people unemployment benefits and your resources are [depleted]. So during the 1980s there has been a need for saving money in the health care sector. . . . If everything had been going well, that might have happened . . . but when reform was attempted all these things happened at the same time. There was a shortage of labor in the municipalities and also in hospitals. The reform[31] was set in motion when it was not possible to get the personnel you needed in the municipalities. Nor could you raise money to finance the new small hospitals, not even the service apartments we had been building since the 1960s and 1970s. There was no money for it any more. People who should take care of the people at home, you couldn't finance them any more even if you could get them. . . . What we had was this. These are the people who are over 65 and these are the people who are over 80. This is a measure of the social service for these people. These are the people who have some kind of care in their homes. You can see that this figure is really going down, but the population over 80 and over 65 is going up. . . . Patients who are moved out of hospitals are not very simple patients. They are much heavier than the population that used to be there. So you shouldn't take notice only of the age factor, you should take notice of the reform factor. That's heavier. I think you could say we have doubled the burden, the need for care in the homes. It's not only elderly people who need a lot of care, it's also the psychiatric patients who need a lot of special treatment and care. In fact, what is happening is that the county councils have tried to get rid of some of their problems in some of these reforms, but the municipalities couldn't do what they should have been doing in order to make the shift go smoothly. So now we see that there is a declining care level—rapidly declining care level—in the municipalities. (Jan Edling, LO)

We have 18% of the population 65 years old and over, so we are a couple of decades ahead of the development coming up in Germany, France, Japan and Switzerland. . . . That is one of the basic reasons, I think, that medical care costs have increased. Now this 18% will persist a few decades from this point, but for 75 years old and over are getting a lot more. It's so many old people, so much new technology, so we have queues for heavy medical care. We have a kind of cost containment in the Swedish health system because of the rule of the *Landstings* budgets. . . .

A lot of people, including myself, who are consumers of some health care, . . . think there are changes to be made. If you are sick, you are pretty helpless. If you get to *Akademiska Sjukhuset* you can be frightened. I mean it's so huge and it's difficult to find the right place. The service—maybe they could be a little more service minded. (Anders Forsman, TCO)

A 1990 report prepared by SKAF president Arvidson focused on the greater health risks faced by workers (cf. LO, 1991) and the danger of lowering the standard of living to afford health care. Problems included a lack of long-term beds, a shortage of personnel in both the public and private sectors, and heavier and more stressful work in medical care. It was said that proposals for change would increase differences in health and medical care and result in a more hierarchical organization. A market economy would be inappropriate for a medical care system. Primary care needed strengthening.

Underlying causes included the increasing difficulty of financing work by higher taxes, a stagnant public insurance budget, overdependence on hospitals, deinstitutionalization of mental patients coupled with a reduction in long-term beds, aging of the population with need increasing faster than communities can raise resources, and shortened work hours for physicians. Counties had a greater incentive to reduce patient days than to make long-term reductions in sickness episodes or loss of production.

When I was in my ward working as a nurse assistant, we also had these questions. We had to save money, we can't let money fly out in this way. But doctors who led the clinic, they said: "We know that we have to save money, but we know that we will get new money next year." I think it was about 1986–87 that they started to say we had to save money, because our economy is not good. And suddenly they change the government . . . very quickly . . . and they say we have to close down . . . and put people out of work. I think there is a small economic crisis. I think so. (Per Rudin, SKAF)

Sture Nordh, president of the white-collar Union of Professional Employees, representing most health workers with skilled levels of training, said the problem was primarily political:

There was at the end of the '80s a climate where it was an "established fact" that public spending was too high, the public services too big, the health care system inefficient. . . . Yes we do face some difficulties, and the difficulties deal with the age of the population . . . and the attitude from a lot of politicians, at least the national government politicians. . . . They don't really see, if you talk as a whole about the financing of health care systems, they don't see the difference between Sweden and other countries when it comes to age and when it comes to trying to figure out how much your system truly costs compared with the Swedish one.

Basically, it's a matter of resources. It's a matter of structural change. That is necessary. We have to get rid of some of our hospitals. We have

> too many hospitals throughout the country. . . . We had some development within the services that was some kind of stagnation. The difficulties of measuring productivity and efficiency within the services, the lack of competition, the lack of knowing. I mean you can state to any of our members "You are inefficient. The service you work in is inefficient." You can state that from an ideological point of view and we can never show, give evidence, that this is wrong. (Sture Nordh, SKTF)

Politicians

The New Democrats and the Conservatives were actively pushing market reforms. The other governing parties were supporting those reforms, often with some reservations.

> They diminished the number of patients treated per day from 30 to 40 to just below 10 and at the same time they doubled their salary. . . . You got the money even if you didn't work. It's like Russia. Why do you have to work? . . . Before [1970] you were paid per capita: the number of patients and the mode of therapies you used, what you did. At that time the patient paid seven crowns. Now the patients pay 150–200. Then they paid seven crowns and then the doctor got two to three times more from the *försäkringskassa*. [Changes in economic incentives are what has] caused enormous costs. The Swedish . . . are working as private specialists and there are also private general practitioners talking about the *vårdlag*. That's socialistic. That's a team, a health care team. You don't visit the doctor, you visit the team. . . . There's a professor who's writing about Nicaragua and things like that. He's a pure Communist. He has written books about this *vårdlag*, "*vårdlag begreppet*." That means that the doctor isn't important. (Leif Bergdahl, New Democrat)

> We can say that the demands of the people have gone up like this and the resources have gone so. Then, because the people generally have better and better education, they also demand more and more and . . . there is no limit to it. . . . Everyone is afraid of pain, sickness, and death, and the technical advances have made many believe there is no limit to what the health care can do. So we have to do something. Even a good health care, we must save it. We have not the resources to do it. (Leif Carlsson, Conservative)

> The problems are that we have a growing number of elderly people. . . . We, together with Japan, have the highest mean age in the world. Elderly people need more health care. . . . In Sweden 93% of the women between 30 and 50 are employed. In countries where half the women are employed, they can take care of sick people and help people at home without pay. But in the hospitals the society has to pay for it. So there are a number of factors that put tremendous economic pressure on the present health care system. . . . Our health care system was totally gov-

erned by budget and until recently the country could decide about taxation. . . . Now the state restricts the possibility for county governments to raise taxes. But we had no market for medical care. We just had the budget. . . . In a market economy you have the patient, the hospital or whoever provides health care, and the patient pays by the insurance or directly. Now in Sweden this was cut off and we had here the politicians. . . . The influence of the patients was very much reduced. (Jerzy Einhorn, Christian Democrat)

People have been asking for medical care and I think we have had the wrong organization for that. I come from the North of Sweden, Västerbotten, where we have Umeå University for the education of doctors. I thought during this time that if we only got more and more money sometime we could strike a balance between demand and the facilities we can offer. But now I see we have the wrong organization. Therefore I am very happy . . . we are going to have this *husläkare* law for doctors where we say we try to get the doctors out in primary care. Because if people are used to going to the specialist first, no country can afford this. If you have good contact with a family doctor, you can save a lot of money. (Ulla Orring, Liberal)

It is certainly the case that we lack money. It is very expensive. There are lots of personnel and it is well built out there. We are now trying to reduce that and that has created conflict between the personnel and the politicians, because they want to keep their jobs. The public is upset because they think they will have poorer care. And it is clear that we cannot provide the exact same care for less money. . . . There is a shortage of money and we have lived far beyond our means. We have built somewhat too large facilities and we must pay for them. They cost a lot of money. That is part of the problem. But it is clear that we will reduce expenditures by 400 million within three years.[32] That is a lot of money—we will collapse in our county. That is tough. (Gunlog Bratt, Liberal)

We lack money. That is the greatest problem right now. In the Center Party, we want a new insurance system. We want a guaranteed level for everybody. . . . That level would be higher than today, both in the health insurance, the parental insurance, and the unemployment insurance. We want a higher level. We think everybody has to build upon that with a voluntary insurance. (Rosa Östh, Center)

The opposition parties, while recognizing problems and taking an active role in seeking solutions, opposed market solutions:

[The] problem in Swedish medical care, is that we have too many hospital beds, and we are promoting a policy in which we reduce the number of hospital beds. And we support the provision of (1) primary care and (2) continued specialty training, higher specialization.

> If one sees how much money is spent in different parts of the country one can see the differences are huge, sometimes so large, in psychiatry, for example, to indicate a problem. We perhaps do not have a single solution, but there is municipal self-governance that causes unequal allocations.
>
> The other problem is that I meet many politicians who say that the Swedish medical care system is quite open, that physicians go to conferences in the USA and Canada and England, and bring in new technology, and that speaks to openness in the system. Social Democrats do not want to see medical care or welfare as a large and heavy system, but want an openness so that quality and knowledge come in. [If we find evidence that is lacking] we want to make immediate changes and open it up. Is it a system failure that there are things we need? (Bo Holmberg, Social Democrat)
>
> Sweden has a very good health care system and we need to be very careful to keep what we have that is good. But it needs to be made more efficient and the costs have to be kept down. (Eva Zetterberg, Left)

Others

Professor Gösta Tibblin, who founded the first department of General Medicine in the nation at Uppsala University, generally supported the argument that the medical care system needed to be scaled back, but had reservations about the point-of-service (*husläkare*) reforms:

> We have expanded too much and we have too big a costume for us, so we must reduce it. People are now used to high salaries, to a summer house, to traveling around, and so on. So therefore they are complaining. You see, it's a reduction in the standard of living, but 93% of the population is working and has a good salary, social security, and so on.... I think that people in the health sector need to reduce their numbers in a way so you can get some employment. They are certainly crying and saying that it is wrong and so on. What people are not talking about is that we have a state debt up to a thousand billion Swedish crowns. We have borrowed a lot of money. The interest is very soon up to 200 billion, so we have solved the problem. The welfare state costs a lot of money from taxes and we couldn't raise the taxes; we decreased the taxes and decreased the income and then you must borrow to compensate. Therefore we have such an increase in the debt. I see a reduction. We are not so rich, so we must reduce ourselves....
>
> Then in the 1970s it changed. Then we started talking about primary care. In 1975 we started building primary care and the number increased. Now, there is a slight decrease of outpatient visits at the hospital, but still nearly half of all outpatient visits are done in the hospital. This is

> the typical Swedish characteristic you will not find in any [other] country. . . . Therefore it is a new thing, primary care. They hadn't thought about it. It's so new, let's say the last 10 years or so. It has worked very well, primary care, but there is a shortage of doctors. I have been working since 1976 and I think we now have excellent doctors and very well equipped health centers. But we still have a shortage. . . .
>
> [Physicians] are seeing fewer patients, but they are working a lot. It means they are sitting in on meetings, they are phoning, . . . and so on. At least in primary care they are working a lot, but it is a work not linked to patients. . . . They have a lot of teaching, a lot of training, and so on. . . . They are not having any individual patients during this time, but they are working as doctors or they are working in the medical field.
>
> In the hospitals you have employed a lot of people, a tremendous lot of people in the day. In the night there are very few. So it's overstaffed in the hospital and, I think, they have less patient-linked time in the hospital than in primary care. . . . If you could pay these people part of their salary related to production—if you say that 90% of the salaries is just—but if 10% of your salary is related to what you are doing, all this problem would disappear. . . .
>
> If you would like me to talk about real problems, it's our way of guiding or leading—steering all the time. This is the politicians. We should get rid of all politicians below the level of Parliament. We have a lot of crazy politicians, useless politicians. All of the activities of the health centers are built upon political decisions. . . . They are badly trained and they are following directions from above. I would like to get rid of them and use the combination of administrators and a few experts.

Johan Calltorp, a prominent researcher in social medicine, had done several studies aimed at improving the assessment of medical work:

> Here in the Stockholm County Council . . . two weeks ago it was announced that there is a program of privatization here in the county council. It's not final yet but the County Council plans to get an international management company, a French company linked to a for-profit American company, American Medical International, to manage St. Görans Hospital.[33] . . . To explain the pressure . . . the overall health care budget was very effectively contained during the '80s. Actually, we dropped from 9.7% of GNP in 1982 to . . . somewhere between 7.2 and 8.5%. . . . We have a totally new situation in health care. The big issue, if Sweden continues in this way, we will soon have a privatized health care sector. That's a big political issue, of course, which is not yet recognized either. . . . The big issue is if we are moving to a two or a three tier health care system. If you look at the newspaper and the public debate you don't find that debate at all.

> Another big issue in the health care sector is the county council model. . . . The government committee on health financing, an expert committee headed by Bengt Jönsson, has published a report giving three scenarios, which are not under discussion. They say that in the future we will have one source of financing, either government financing or county council financing. . . .
>
> I think it is true that the right wing coalition . . . is very eager to demonstrate something. . . . There is a political will, but there is also inevitably economic pressure, resource pressure. You have the elderly and you have growing needs and you have growing technology and then you have pressures within the system that are difficult to handle with these models. . . . You have a lot of bad things and if you look from a macro model at the Swedish health care, its real success is cost containment, maybe too much. It's equity is better than most systems, but it's also inflexible, this system.
>
> When I came to this hospital, for example, . . . I didn't believe my eyes how old fashioned the routines were for handling personnel and so on. So there really is a need for a shake-up in the system in many ways. . . .
>
> The more we move into a fragmented system we tend to lose . . . the rationality of controlling technology and so on. . . . The main problem regarding the hospital structure is that we have many hospitals. We have too many hospital beds. There are enormous tensions in many county councils to change the structure. . . . We have a potential for out-patient delivery of services that is very large, but it's difficult to close down hospitals. . . .
>
> What I see in this hospital is a tremendous rigidity. . . . I think it's interesting in health care where we generally have weaker hospitals than in your country. It's size that is negative for innovation. Sweden is much more affected by the general political swing in the world than we have recognized. . . . Some people say that the socialized parts of the system is something we have to get rid of—it's associated with the values of the Eastern countries. And that's, of course, a tremendous mistake.

Johannes Vang, the WHO physician who coauthored the *Landstingsförbundet's Crossroads* report, voiced the most ideologically consistent classical conservative position:

> We lost many, many so-called normal hospitals, small hospitals of maybe 150 beds with . . . a department of medicine, sometimes not even that. Beds were used up. Surgical patients and medical patients could lie in the same room. . . . Basically [it was] a very small organization. People knew each other and there was a strong social control. Now these hospitals have disappeared because they were "not effective." From an administrative point of view they were not effective, but from the point of view of medicine they were quite effective. But at that time the administrators started to take over from the physicians and . . . this changed the judgment of what was important.

Up to the war, if you had a hospital you had a physician as the head of the hospital. He was in a staff position, not something that would be an administrative [one]. . . . He had somebody who would take care of buying the necessary things you needed. . . . [That] turned around when they started to build hospitals and they became more and more complicated. They moved the administrator up as boss and moved the medical head down as sort of a medical director . . . and that changed the focus. . . . It changed ethically in the sense that while the physician would always still have maintained the view of the patient being the center of attention, [for] the administrator . . . that was a distributive issue. He was concerned with distribution, or at least rationing, of something. That changed focus underlined even more the faults of the administrative system because the patient became less and less important as centralization became also more and more expressed, as hospitals became bigger and bigger, and you got large distances to the big hospital.

Then, of course, loyalty wasn't really anybody's strong glue any more because you didn't know the people . . . and the glue that had been loyalty became the bureaucracy, the rule system. . . . When we got to the point that people realized it, it was because the service became worse and worse. Those who worked in the hospital, although they were very nice people, . . . were not concerned about patients the way they were earlier. They were not concerned about them as customers. They were part of the bureaucracy that served people like any other bureaucracy.

Waiting lists developed. . . [People] got used to the wait for getting to the doctor, and the doctor rushed by, . . . very busy. He wasn't really busy, but giving the impression of busyness to give importance to his work. . . . This is also very often the power of bureaucracy, withholding information, withholding time, and that sort of thing. . . .

Moreover, in Sweden there was an unholy alliance between politicians, who are supposed to be those who represent the people, citizens, but as they were also basically the hospital owners, they had dual loyalties. . . . The senior politicians were very much concerned about running the health care system and they were very insensitive to criticism from those they represented.

At the same time as the patient/customer lost importance, it always appeared as a total monopoly. In our situation here, we had a total monopoly. It was the *landstinget*, the county councils. They financed it. They produced it. They controlled some of it. The product was very bad. And they could even improve the demand, if they wanted to, simply by increasing taxes.

Themes

Several themes can be discerned among these responses. While each respondent had their own special emphasis, and some themes, such as seeing care teams as a manifestation of communism, were idiosyncratic, most were shared by a number of respondents. Few were the province of a single interest group and many were broadly shared. Here we will note the themes and identify by whom they were held.

For this analysis, we will group the responses by a listing of criteria for an effective medical care system found in the public health literature going back to the 1950s. It will be seen that the problems with the Swedish medical care system, while encompassing most of those dimensions, were seen by the respondents as focused on the issue of affordability.

Drawing on some of our earlier writing (Twaddle, 1980) the criteria are (1) availability, the existence of relevant services; (2) accessibility, the ability of people to get available services and the absence of barriers to care; (3) acceptability, services provided in a manner compatible with people's values and desires; (4) affordability, services at a cost that does not threaten other social goals (i.e., will not bankrupt the society); (5) effectiveness, they meet the needs of patients and are relevant to the medical problems presented; and (6) flexibility, they are adaptable to local circumstances and/or individual needs. We also have an "other" category for responses that do not fit these criteria. For the most part, these "other" responses seemed to be connected with the listed criteria, but at the same time had an ideological centrality that set them apart. We will try to make that statement clearer when we get to that point. Table 4.4 has columns that list the criteria, under which are the themes noted in the responses.

It is noteworthy that no respondent mentioned availability as an issue. Sweden had a system in which anything technically possible to medicine anywhere in the world was present. There was no problem with the technical development of the system.

One issue was raised involving accessibility, the waiting lists for elective procedures (Milton, Vang). Indeed, this had been a problem, but one already resolved at the time of the interviews by the *vårdgaranti*, the "guarantee of care," in which anyone not treated for a list of specified conditions within three months could go anywhere else in the country and have their treatment paid by their home county, and the portion of the Ädel Reform that forced municipalities to pay for hospital beds "blocked" by people whose medical treatment was completed (Könberg).

The biggest issue raised about acceptability involved the result of the Ädel Reform, the sharp decline in the quality of care for the institutionalized aged (Edling). The reform had transferred responsibility for the care of the aged from the counties to the municipalities, which had no experience with organizing medical services, and banned municipalities from raising taxes to cover the additional expenses. The result was a "deskilling" of medical services to the aged and a decline in the quality of nursing home care from a standard among the highest in the developed world to one that would be unacceptable in most Western countries (Petterson) (cf. Thorslund and Parker, 1992).

Other issues raised in the context of acceptability were the fragmentation of services, where people had different physicians for different problems, creating an issue in continuity of care (Orring, Calltorp),[34] and privatization, which some thought would lead to a "two-tiered system" or a "2/3 society" with the United States as a negative model (Calltorp, Ohlsson).

By far, the criterion that was most important to the respondents was that of affordability. The general concern was whether Sweden could meet the growing expenses of providing comprehensive medical care when the economy was no longer growing. Some noted the problem without attempting an explanation (Östh, Zetterberg).[35] The concern as expressed by other people had several dimensions.

First was the issue of the large state debt (the source of which we will discuss in Chapter 5). For a number of reasons, the national government had borrowed heavily and was forced to use a larger portion of its resources in debt service. That money was no longer available to provide human services, making the financing of medical care more difficult and more in conflict with other expenditure needs (Tibblin). It may be important to note at this point that nobody attributed the state debt to the medical care system.

Second, as in the rest of the world, medical costs were increasing rapidly (Eliasson, Edling, Bratt, Carlsson, and Könberg, who thought the problem was largely solved). This was primarily a function of the rapid growth of the aged population, particularly the population over the age of seventy-five. It produced a sharp upward pressure on medical care need and on the cost of providing services to the society (Ohlsson, Edling, Forsman, Nordh, Einhorn, Calltorp). Upward cost pressures also came from technological developments which expanded the use of costly equipment in diagnosis and treatment (Forsman, Carlsson, Calltorp). While widely discussed, neither was seen directly as a political issue.

Third, some, mostly on the political right, claimed that the welfare state had become overextended. These people expressed the view that Sweden "was living beyond its means" and needed to scale back its ambitions in the human service arena (Tibblin, Bratt).

What was more controversial was the alleged inefficiency of the medical care system. Especially as primary care developed, bed blockers were removed, and the care guarantee took effect, it became apparent that there was an overcapacity in the hospital system and an overspecialization in medicine (Tibblin).[36] There was a widespread consensus that hospitals would have to be closed to reduce capacity with an acknowledgment that this would be a politically unpopular move (Nordh, Holmberg, Tibblin, Calltorp).[37] Some attributed these problems to the budgetary system of funding, which, they said, did not allow for local adjustments in allocations, removed incentives for cost reduction, and generated wasteful use of resources (Milton, Rudin, Bergdahl, Einhorn).

Another theme under affordability was the alleged decline in physician productivity. That physicians were seeing fewer patients per day than they had a decade or two earlier was not disputed (Könberg, Bergdahl, Tibblin). Most of those who noted this as a problem did not attempt an explanation. According to Gösta Tibblin, there were many more physicians in primary care and the new team organization, which provided greater effectiveness and higher quality services, required more time in meetings to coordinate services.

Two additional themes were the loss of budgetary control as a result of the reforms of the 1980s, resulting in a new problem of duplication of services and overuse of expensive technology, and the lack of practice standards, resulting in vast discrepancies from one setting to another in the handling of virtually identical medical problems (Nordh, Holmberg, Tibblin). That lack of standards also made medical audits extremely difficult. The result was a lost of control over costs (Calltorp).

With regard to effectiveness, some respondents thought the system was hampered by a growing bureaucracy in which administrators had taken control of the hospitals (Vang). There were problems of people being given responsibility without adequate authority (Milton). There was also the problem of a headlong rush into making system changes without adequate reflection, study, and research (Calltorp), raising a potential of making major and damaging errors of judgment.

On the issue of flexibility, it was alleged that patients had no freedom to choose physicians (Könberg, Milton, Calltorp) and physicians did not have freedom to establish private practices where they wished (Könberg, Milton).[38] Freedom of choice was also raised in the context of choice of the level of treatment, rather than choice of personnel (Ohlsson). Further, hospitals were too large and rigidly organized, and politicians controlled the system (Tibblin, Calltorp, Vang). The latter argument was linked to support of the greater use of the market as a means of organizing and financing medical care.

Other themes included the following:

1. Care teams (*vårdlag*) were a leftist form of organization (Bergdahl).
2. County councils had a monopoly on medical care in which they simultaneously served as the representatives of the people and administrators of the system. They were hence compromised in their ability to serve as the people's advocate against the system. This argument was often raised in connection with objections to budgets as managerial tools, inefficient use of resources, and a lack of flexibility in the system (Milton, Calltorp, Vang).
3. Women had entered the labor force in such large numbers that there was little opportunity for the kinds of uncompensated care the system had previously depended upon. As a result, there were new needs for expenditures (Einhorn).

Political Agendas

While there were several problems with the medical care system noted by different respondents, and virtually nobody saw them as serious enough to be characterized as a crisis in medical care, it was nonetheless the case that some sought reforms of the medical care system that could be seen as making fundamental changes in the organization of that system. That is to say, some of the reform proposals were put forward as if there were a crisis. For the most part, however, the proposals were more modest and more in keeping with the problems noted.

Governmental Organizations

The main proposal from the Ministry of Health was the point-of-service reform, which they referred to in English as a "Family Doctor" reform.

> The family doctor system is not really an ideological question. It's not a question . . . about value judgments. Of course . . . some of the people in my party would like to have it as an ideological question. That is, the real social liberalism is the family doctor system, and I suppose I have made some speeches myself that it is so. But . . . in most of my speeches I have used a more pragmatic approach, that it is good value for money. . . .
>
> Maybe with one exception, the right-wing populist party. Maybe you could say that there are ideological arguments against family doctors. They want a system that is completely free. They see America's, your system, as . . . worth striving for. . . .
>
> Of course the Social Democratic Party is against the right for doctors to establish themselves, . . . to have the right to money from the social insurance. . . .
>
> But there is a discussion of whether we should change one essential part of the general welfare system, that part that has to do with giving you compensation, some kind of proportion of your former income, and change that . . . to a system where you have some kind of flat rate. That, of course, is still some kind of general system, because it's a general policy. I myself am in favor of the first system and not the change at this point. . . .
>
> The main field which I think has too little resources, or we don't use the resources in the best ways, is in the psychiatric field. Otherwise much has to do with getting more value for money within the county council system, or a system with more competition. We are introducing competition with the *husläkarproposal*. That's the debate we have with the Social Democrats. We are trying to get more competition between the public clinics, also in some cases between public hospitals and private hospitals, etc. . . . But I think the field, the sector, that needs much restructuring, changes, is the psychiatric sector. Many, many people are getting

> too little help with their problems. We have closed down many beds in psychiatric hospitals. I think we had more psychiatric beds in the sixties than any other country in the world. We were at the top of the list. In almost all countries they have closed down beds. We have done it too. In some places it has worked well. People have good care in their homes, etc. In many cases they are very lonely and not being rehabilitated. . . .
>
> The most important split is the one introduced in the national health system in the United Kingdom, what they call purchaser–provider. That is, there is a national or county health system which tries to split themselves into buyer and seller. Some of the people in the right wing of the political debate tell you that this is not the real competition, the real buying and selling, just a stimulation. It seems that even so small a change has led to big increases in production. . . . Of course I cannot see that this process continues all the way around. You can come to a system in which the money is used not on the medical needs of the nation but all the doctors and nurses getting more wages. . . . We are not intending to change the system similar to the system of the United States. We are trying to use, within this general proposal, market mechanisms to get as much value out of the money as possible. But of course there are risks, and I suppose that we are going to make big mistakes, mistakes that I hope will not be too big and that we can correct as fast as possible. (Bo Könberg, Minister of Health)

The Federation of County Councils, in their 1992 *Crossroads* document, had set a goal of generating public discussion on medical care organization and financing. They offered three scenarios: a population based model, in which financing would be regional and based on some form of capitation in which regions would monitor their own systems; a national model, where a national insurance fund would replace the current county taxes, central and regional agencies would monitor the system, and services would be provided by any level of government or private organizations; and a coordinated model, where municipalities would finance and provide care for children, and a national health insurance fund would cover adults and contract with providers.

While that document stated no preferences, subsequent documents began to spell out a position. Berleen, Håkansson, et al. (1992), writing for SPRI, advocated greater use of market mechanisms, reduction of bureaucracy, greater emphasis on primary care and explicit rationing of tertiary care, and more freedom of choice for patients (meaning that patients would not be tied to particular providers or geographic areas). Bengt Mollstedt (1992), President of the Board of the Federation of County Councils and a Conservative politician, wrote that goals should include a separation of production and financing (different units, rather than counties doing both as in the present system), population-based resource allocation (e.g., capitation) to provide work incentives to physicians, and public competition.

The representatives from *Landstingsförbundet* interviewed also talked about the point-of-service reform. They, however, had reservations about it:

> If we talk about the *husläkar* system, there have been two big issues. The first is free enterprise, because the Social Democrats feel that this is changing a pattern that is in existence. The second thing is that some people feel it could be very expensive. And then some people feel that you don't have enough doctors in general medicine. . . . The listing has been discussed, could it be active or passive. . . . The Conservatives are advocating an active listing. That is, it is the patient who should take the first step. The Liberals have advocated that you must have possibilities for passive listing, because if you don't have that, you won't cover all the drunks and some social aid cases, some unintelligent people who haven't made the effort to list themselves and so on. . . . Another point which is discussed is the possibility to see a specialist. I am always advocating that patients are not stupid. If you have a problem with your ear, you know that you should see an ear specialist. But I think the problem can solve itself. Either you should see your house physician all the time, and then get a referral to a specialist, or you should have what I call an escape route so that you could see a specialist on your own, so that you don't have to pass through the house physician.
>
> The other big thing that is discussed is the way to use the old health center system, *vårdcentral*, . . . The Social Democrats . . . feel that the house physician system will break up the working health centers. They have pointed especially to the district nurses, because the house is based upon, not a single practice necessarily, but the doctor working as an individual. He is responsible for his supporting staff. He will get paid so he can have assistants. In the proposition now they have covered parts of this but the people are anxious about the maternal health and the child health system that we have had for many years. I don't think that there is any problem in the bigger cities, because there you have pediatricians and obstetricians running the system. But it could be a problem in the countryside where you don't have these specialists involved in the health aspect.
>
> Then, of course, you can always find doctors who don't like this system for different reasons. One group feels that buying and selling is unethical. They oppose the system because of the ethics of it. Another group is opposing the system more because of the technology of it. DRG-like systems are tough systems to handle and actually we don't, to my knowledge, have any real DRG system anywhere in Sweden. . . . And then some nurses are opposing it, but that is to some extent the role of traditional district nurse that is at stake. Then some of them are afraid they will lose their jobs. The unions have agreed to work with rationalizations of different kinds, but they are afraid today. We have reduced the staff of Swedish hospitals by about 30,000 people out of almost 400,000 people employed. . . . So the unions are opposing the changes. . . .

> [My goal is that] the family physician system will be working, meaning that in five years all Swedes will have a connection to a personal physician. We don't have that today, although some have it out in the countryside. . . . Its importance in the system is that the doctors will take a more personal interest in individual patients. . . . Many small hospitals will disappear. We can't afford to have . . . the same quality all around the clock everywhere, and that means that some small hospitals will disappear as acute hospitals. Others will change to more specialized hospitals for acute care. The financing system will be changed in a way that works closer to the patient than it does today. The insurance, or you could call it the individual tax system, will introduce some sort of competition in the system. . . . Hospital care and compensation for loss of earning must be coordinated.
>
> One of the problems . . . is the economy of it. Any system with some sort of third party payer is a vulnerable system. If the patient and the physician have a common goal to squeeze more money out of the system, it's a dangerous thing.
>
> Another one is the duplication of services. We have bragged about the Swedish system that it wasn't particularly expensive because we have very little duplication. The more competition you have the bigger is the risk for a rapid expansion of duplicate technology. . . . You always run the risk if you have a free market that people will demand a higher level of care than they really need. (Bengt Mollstedt, President, *Landstingsförbundet*)

Those responsible for the operation of the Federation of County Councils were equally concerned with the Commission of Inquiry on funding the system. They were clearly poised to defend the county council system against the other alternatives offered by the Commission:

> To make the health care sector work more efficiently. That is what we are working on day in and day out, and we are seeing good results. We can really prove figures that productivity has been raised in health care during the last two years, very much so. . . . What we are doing now is putting more money into primary health care. That could be a good business. We could reduce secondary and tertiary care to at least the same level, but we haven't seen that yet. That's an historical problem in Sweden that we have worked with for decades as well, to force the primary health care on costs of the secondary and tertiary care level. . . .
>
> There is a discussion about the pros and cons of moving [primary care] to municipalities. . . . They started a trial in seven municipalities in Sweden (where) the county council and the municipalities have agreed for a period of three or four years to let the municipalities handle the primary care. . . . We are more doubtful about this, but we want to give those seven municipalities a fair chance to prove it, if there is any good to it, and also to look upon the maybe negative consequences. The problem is, of course, that if you have one source of finance you have some

> control over the total costs. If you have two sources of finance, one for primary care and one for the other health care, you can put yourself in a situation where you lose control of the total costs. . . . We also believe that the shift toward primary health care must be corresponded by cuts in the other, hospital, health care. . . .
>
> We are occupied to . . . convince the Swedish government and the Swedish parliament that the future of health care in this country is the reformed county council model and not the comprehensive insurance model or the primary care steered model. . . .
>
> What's going to improve and what has improved is productivity. What you have to be very keen to look upon is efficiency in the broader sense of efficiency. I mean if this is doing things right, efficiency is doing the right things. I mean that's a problem with the model we are shifting over to. . . . On the other hand, we know very little about efficiency in health care, what is the right thing to do. . . .
>
> We are trying to combine the planned political model with market incentives. We have not found the right proportion of those, but I think we are moving toward a better situation where we try to use both of these things. The professional goal, to be at least as good as any colleague, is working in both of these models. This is a very good thing which we haven't really used as much as we could. . . .
>
> I do believe that you have to ration the same way you have done in Sweden and other countries for years. That is a combination of different things. Ultimately, it's always the doctor who has the patient in front of him who is doing some sort of rationing. I do believe, also, that . . . we have to find new sources of finance. I believe that maybe we shall see an increase in Sweden in patient fees. . . . That reduces demand. The question is does it reduce demands that also correspond to needs or does it just reduce demands that do not correspond to needs. . . . Maybe it's not, as you suggest, a total less demand on health care, but you can at least manipulate where this demand is taken up. (Olof Eliasson, Federation of County Councils)

The direction of the national organization of county councils, then, was to pursue a course that would strengthen the private sector and introduce more competition into the public sector. Second, it was to preserve a county-based system of medical care delivery.

Interest Organizations

The physicians had a longer list of goals. Milton (1991) provided a list that might be categorized as follows.

The first stated goal was to provide good patient care by providing a free choice of physician, strengthening the supply of basic health and medical services, and maintaining access to specialty services. The first two were consistent with Federation of County Council goals. The last may be in conflict, although the issue had still not been explicitly joined. It would seem to position physicians to oppose attempts to ration access to specialties, especially for the aged.

The second goal was to create a system that provided a better work environment for physicians. This would include a financing system that is "producer neutral." That is, it would fund private physicians on the same terms as public physicians. It was contended that such a system would improve recruitment of physicians to primary care, encourage rural practice, provide work incentives for physicians without promoting unnecessary care, and promote preventive medicine. It would serve a related stated goal of creating an organization "characterized by high work satisfaction, independence, and good income for physicians."

The third goal was to separate financing and delivery of care, consistent with the Federation of County Council goal. The objective was to have a mix of financing, including capitation, patient fees, and DRGs for special services.

Included in the discussion was an assumption that district nurses would be coordinated by and work under the direction of physicians and an assertion that "social medicine" is outside the scope of primary medical care.

Hasselius (1991) incorporated all of the goals from Milton's report and specified some of the goals to include framing health insurance so that money follows the patient, giving physicians freedom to set up practices anywhere they choose, reimbursing physicians according to "productivity," and establishing medical criteria for treatments as a means of cost control. General Secretary Anders Milton underscored all of these points in an interview:

> What we did was put forward a proposal on primary health care and we put forward a proposal on an insurance based system with universal coverage. . . . First we discussed how the system should be organized. Once we have done that, then we can get back to doctors, nurses, nurses helpers, etc., how they should be remunerated. . . . The second thing we decided was that we had to look into the question of cost control, because that's a crucial issue. . . .
>
> Those were the two starting points, and then we had to decide what was most important. Is it to propose a system that would be good for patients and/or should the system also take care of the interests of the local politicians that today run health care? We decided that the patients were the primary concern and the welfare of politicians was something that was not on the agenda. When I say it this way it sounds, at least to me, quite natural. But . . . if you say it in the way politicians say it, "democratic control"—but what it is all about, really, is whether or not they should have the positions still there. . . . You see a lot of layers of bureaucracy and you create a lot of confusion within the command structure of health care that is not efficient. . . .

> We proposed a system that . . . gives the patients a much stronger position than they used to have, meaning the patients make the choice. They choose the doctor they want to see. They carry the money with them, meaning that their choice has a budgetary implication. Also, on the provision side, there should be free competition . . . within quality boundaries. I mean once you pass the society's need when it comes to quality, then it should be a free market.
>
> We also said we should try to have a system where you would not tend to have doctors see patients very often in order to make money. You should not have a system with incentives to see 50 patients a day just because you needed the money. Rather, you should have a system to promote preventive work, meaning that capitation should be, say, 70% of the total income of the doctor. On the other hand, there should be some part that is related to how often you see the patients in order not to have a disincentive. I mean 70/30. If that's a right mix, nobody knows, but that's the way we reasoned.
>
> We proposed an economic barrier . . . between primary care and other open specialist care in order for patients to go through their GP if they need to see another specialist. . . . You have to decide within the profession what a GP should do. That's a professional judgment. But once you have a consensus on what GPs should do, then patients should . . . go with all their problems that fall within these boundaries to their GP. It would mean you have few people going to other open specialists. You would have fewer patients waiting at the emergency rooms of the hospitals.
>
> Then we said we did not want a total referral system like in Great Britain. We said the patient should have the right to see another doctor, for a second opinion or whatever reason. But then we set an economic barrier so they would pay, instead of 100 crowns they would pay, let's say 200 crowns when they bypass the GP. Then you decide a capitation fee. We said 1000 crowns. If you would have that capitation fee this whole system would cost 8.5 billion crowns, which is much less than it costs today. . . .
>
> We proposed a system that would be insurance based, where you would take the present . . . money that goes into *Riksförsakringsverket*, the national insurance scheme. Then you would decided (Parliament would decide—Parliament or an agency decided upon by Parliament, *Socialstyrelsen*, for example) on capitation, and there would be local variations according to geography or according to age, for example. Parliament would then decide that all producers of primary health care, whether it's a *landsting* or a private practitioner or a foundation or whatever, regardless of the legal boundaries or legal structure of the producer, he or she would get the same amount of money. They would be dependent on the number of patients that listed themselves with this or that doctor. . . . That was our basic proposal . . . to make all the financing "producer neutral."

Nurses had set a policy goal (SHSTF, 1990) on first promoting good health. Work environments needed to be improved to reduce injury by increasing the flexibility of jobs, increasing worker participation in decision making, and providing for the personal development of workers. Within the medical care area, workers needed to be brought into the planning process early enough to participate in goal setting.

A second goal was to strengthen the decision-making capacity of politicians, giving them more control over the direction of the system, particularly vis à vis the physicians. Only politicians could deal effectively with the linkage between the knowledge base of medicine and the demand for care. They were the only ones who could make the difficult choices among quality, quantity, and cost effectiveness. One objective, then, was to shape a system of political control that enables counties, municipalities, and hospitals to use the most effective methods, as well as a labor market that recruits the needed workers to achieve the goals of medical care.

A third policy goal was to increase the degree of experimentation with medical care organization. Several counties were trying out different means of financing and organizing services. This should be linked to increased research on cost effectiveness.

A later report (Boden, 1992) looked at changes being proposed by the physicians and the Federation of County Councils to identify issues of concern to nurses and other health workers. The main problem was uncertainty about the meaning of "privatization" and the new forms of production. That report noted an absence of research on the implications of the changes, anxiety about the speed of change, and uncertainty about the consequences of change for workers and employees. The policy goals identified included fighting for the interests of union members (whatever the form of organization) developing a system of economic control that keeps the product central, and seeing that decentralization of responsibility is accompanied by authority, placing emphasis on ethics, and conducting research on cost and quality control in different kinds of production forms. It was seen as imperative that nurses be included in planning and prioritizing.

A third report (SHSTF, n.d.) was designed to respond to the point-of-service (*husläkare*) proposal from the Ministry of Health. The problem was that "the proposal for a family physician has the benefit of meeting popular demand for a physician who is freely chosen and who will stay with the patient, but the cost may be the sacrifice of preventive health care provided by nurses and physical therapists. Primary care must not be organized under [the direction of] the family physician."

Policy goals in that report included changing "care centers" of physician group practices to "health centers" staffed by nurses, physical therapists, laboratory technicians, and so on. Financing of health centers should be separate from the financing of family physicians. Nurses should have more autonomy, including the right to prescribe. Maternal and child health nurses should have independent responsibility for patients, and a role for laboratory assistants should be developed within primary care.

> We need to have more producers involved in the production of medical care (meaning more non-physician workers). It is a question of being creative. . . . Not only doctors can produce medical services.

> We must work inside the organization, now. We will make people sit down in small groups and let them discuss their positions. Then we will ask them to form goals, then discuss strategies to achieve the goals. We need to get our members to see ways out of the problem rather than to despair. Female health workers are conditioned to do what they are told. They are not alert to having power. Physicians are a strong group all over the world. Nurses lack high self esteem and they lack class consciousness. . . . Our members have not discussed the organization, delivery, or financing of health care. One of the Swedish problems is letting the physicians organize medical care to the needs of their specialties. . . . So many people's problems are quasi-medical and even non-medical, things like home help, counseling, prevention. (Inger Ohlsson, Vårdförbundet SHSTF [Paraphrased from notes])

LO had not prepared a document specifically on the medical care system. They made reference, however, to a more general statement of principles and goals written in 1986. There, they laid out several models of social policy (residual care of the poor, social insurance, and a general security system). They presented the argument that certain activities were legitimate public monopolies, among them medical care. They noted a danger with monopolies in that they could become less efficient unless there was oversight to make them handle resources well. The goals of security and equity could not be met with a private profit-driven system or a private collective system of production and distribution.

There were exceptions on very specific issues, however. LO (Kolk et al.,1991) prepared a report challenging the contention from the Federation of County Councils and the government that Sweden had high rates of absence from work associated with sickness. Two other documents responded to the Ministry of Health proposal to introduce uncompensated sickness days into the social insurance system. This was a plan, subsequently enacted, to terminate salary replacement for the first one or two days of each sickness episode. One (Edling, n.d.) presented data on costs of sickness by length of episode, concluding that a so called "Karens day" would have little meaningful effect on sickness insurance costs. The other (Edling, 1992a) looked at alternatives to the Karens day and recommended a lower level of payment instead of days with no payment. A fourth document (Edling, 1992b) attacked the Ministry of Health proposal to reduce compensation for work-related injuries. While acknowledging the rapidly growing costs of work injuries, Edling suggested that rather than reduce compensation, the policy should be to improve the work environment for workers.

In interviews, LO officials seemed not to have thought through a specific policy for medical care. In spite of the ferment in the land, they did not seem to make it very high priority; education seemed to them a much more salient concern. Nevertheless, the interviews showed some broad concerns with health issues.

> It was a reflection of discussion by many economists saying that we should have a system where we have a publicly organized insurance [with] a system of vouchers. But our analysis was that it's an awful system because . . . you get a fundamentally wrong incentive system. . . . It gives the hospital an incentive to treat the healthy people very well and the sick people very badly. You can't avoid that. Every system where you give overall guidance to profit . . . will give that incentive to treat the healthy people very well and the sick people very badly.
>
> Therefore I think it is very important that the basic or fundamental culture of the doctors' world be preserved. They are there to cure people. It's the basic culture not to earn money, not to make a profit of it. And I would say we have that in Sweden. . . . We have to keep the basic culture of that system. I don't think you can do it by making profit centers out of hospitals, but you can introduce competition without doing that, internal competition.
>
> But it needs some kind of evaluating system. . . . It will certainly take at least 10 or 15 years to do that. . . . If you want to [have a] system . . . to measure production, the result must be almost 100-percent accepted by the professional staff. . . . If it is not accepted, they will use 20 percent of their time proving it's a bad way of measuring the results. They have to be totally involved with the process of measuring. I think it will take time, but in the long run it will be a good system. . . .
>
> In the end, politicians should be able to say what to do, not how to do it. We usually try to avoid leading the professional in saying how to do it. . . . We haven't been so much involved with the technical or professional medical problem. Of course, if you go to our union organizing medical care staff, they have more dealing with those questions of how to organize people or staff within the hospital and medical care system. I don't think they are too deeply involved in the method of doing it.
>
> I don't think the Swedish people want privatization. On the margin, if you got five percent, seven percent, 10 percent, it could perhaps be, but in the end, I am rather sure 70 to 80 percent of the Swedish people really do want a public system. . . . On medical care, we have basically such a good system it won't be a very big change before people see, and the politicians will say let's keep the core of the Swedish system. (Per-Olof Edin, LO)
>
> We are spending too little money on the elderly people. . . . We also have other initiatives from the *Landstings* to save money. [The Ädel reform]

is only one of them, but the others are connected with them because they are trying to develop new models to become more efficient. Most of these models are adopting their philosophy from the market. The DRG system, for example, is one of the things they want to cling to, because they want to find some system of measuring and maybe pricing things they have been doing in the health system. Of course, everyone says we shouldn't just take over the DRG system. We must develop some quality measures also.

What we are trying to do now is find a system where we could combine the passive system of paying people with active measures where we can try to prevent diseases, shorten the duration of diseases. We think that the social security system in the future should finance some of the *företagshälsovård*. . . . It was an agreement between the parties on the labor market. This system is also destroyed at the moment since the state contributions to the system have been withdrawn. . . . Now the system is going through a whole new change and the companies will be responsible for paying them. Of course, the power will be shifting from the parties in the labor market to the companies and the health care in those systems will be shifting from prevention care to maybe some kind of primary care.

So what I see in the long run is that the base for all health care should be where the people are. It should be the *vårdcentral*, really. It should be the occupational health care system, maybe. . . . When there is a need for hospital care or specialized services, that money should buy those services from the special health care sector. . . . But in order to make that work, you should try to avoid a system where you have prices on everything. You must get this system functioning in preventive care, also. It is difficult to make incentives in the system that do what is right for the society as a whole, not only for this sector here. . . .

That's the reason for our idea to make a connection between active and passive measures in the social security system. If you only take passive measures, you could pay anything, almost, but you couldn't restrict the money that goes out from the system if you don't have active measures. . . .

You get a very difficult situation where you have a democratically run producer organization fighting against a democratically run consumer organization. . . . That is what is happening here. You have to find out where the main democratic decision should be. I think it should be where the needs are, where the people are, and not among the producers. We shouldn't mix them both. . . .

We still want a general system for everybody. We think there are a lot of advantages having high taxes for people. I mean high taxes is a kind of insurance system. Anybody who gets a disease or who gets old can cope with those problems without going under. And to make other people in solidarity pay for that, I think, in the long run will be cheaper and you will reach more people. We have high taxes in Sweden, . . . but when we have paid our taxes we don't have to—we didn't, at least, before—pay

> very much extra for hospital care, private insurance. We had all this paid already. . . .
>
> So, I don't see that privatization is really a solution, but I don't think what we have today is so very good, either. I think there is a real need for structural change within the public sector. The structural change that should be going on is a change that would make different parts of the society go together, not working separately in financial sectors that are only making their own results. (Jan Edling, LO)

SKAF, the blue-collar municipal workers union, was much more engaged in the issue of medical care reform than was their peak organization, LO. Indeed, they were in the debate from the beginning. By 1990, they had set goals that included keeping medical care in the public sector to preserve equality of access, opposing market mechanisms in medicine, strengthening primary care, generating policies to reduce class differences in health, reorganizing to make better use of human resources, setting priorities to increase healthy years of life, and eliminating special privileges such as queue jumping (Arvidsson, 1990).

In a later report (Arvidsson, 1992), the municipal workers offered their response to the point-of-service proposal. The problem with that proposal was said to be that while it addressed the needs of physicians for autonomy and independence, the needs of other workers in primary care were ignored. There was a risk that incentives would be reduced for workers other than physicians. According to SKAF, policy should be aimed at (1) completing the proposal by delineating consequences for workers in primary care other than physicians, with special emphasis on the content of work, possibilities for influence, and job security; (2) addressing issues of preventive and rehabilitative medicine important to LO members and which could reduce overall costs; (3) delineating implications for the distribution of primary care and the quality of care; (4) calculating the economic consequences of the proposal and how it would affect the care offered at that time; and (5) including all affected groups in any reorganization of medical care.

> You can't go back. You can't row the boat back because there is nothing left there to go to. You have to build something new, better than what we have. And that, I think, has to be a mix of the right wing's saying of individual liberty and mix of our way to take care of each other in groups. It must be a better mix of it. . . .
>
> Yesterday I was in a home for older sick people and there you have one woman who has senile dementia, 106 years old. But you also have a woman who is 50 years old and she has cancer and there are not so many nurses' aides. These people can't go out. I want a society that can take them out in the sun. They do not have time to talk to them. . . . That's because we are saving too much too fast in this welfare system.

> That's not good, I don't like that society. We see, we know these problems.... We are not opposing changing, but it is going so fast you don't have the thinking with it from the employees. (Tommy Petterson, SKAF)

> They talk nowadays about . . . higher competence. They have to take away nurse assistants. They have to change to nurses in our primary care and in hospitals. And we say, "Why?" And they say it's an economics question, we have to save money. If we take one nurse instead of two nurse assistants, we get more educated people, and she can do a lot more things. And we say this is wrong. We talk about the employed; they have to grow in their work, they have a feeling that they can do more, that they have more responsibility, and we say try to educate them, not into nurses, but try to educate them as nurse assistants. . . . But we say, "No, it's not an economic matter, and it's not a matter of higher competence. It's just that you say we take nurses instead of nurse assistants." And we say if you let the *vård* take real decisions, I think we can all save money, if that's the most important question now, save money. . . . We have said if it needs to be a very high competence, where just nurses can do it, it can be OK, but we have to have a discussion first, so that we have got an agreement.

> We have the opinion that primary care must take a big part of the total. It has to do that, because the patient shall not be treated at a too high level. I worked in primary care before I came to work with the union, and I know that we can take care of rather difficult things. And also, I think that the suggestion from the government now, about the *husläkare försäkring* is a good way, but it just talks about the doctor. There are also other people, nurses and nurse assistants, in that system who also have to be in on that decision. . . . I think they are in the wrong way, the government, when they just talk about doctors. . . .

> They say the market asks for it, the market has the answer. Then I must say, "Who is the market?" Is it you and me or is it someone else, or is it just an idea? I must say, I really haven't an answer. . . . It's also interesting to see they talk about freedom, but they don't talk about freedom for all. They talk about freedom for just a small class or a small sum of people. . . . And I say, if they talk about freedom for everyone, then I know that our members are ready to get aboard. They are interested in taking part in that freedom. (Per Rudin, SKAF)

TCO had joined in the analysis of work absences from sickness prepared for LO by Edling (n.d.). Otherwise, they had a low profile in the debate in 1993.

> It's an old institution, *Landsting*. Maybe it was good from the beginning, because it put health care policy in a better position. The county council has had just health care as their task, but maybe it's outdated. It's both too small and too large. Every *Landsting* wants a heart transplant institution. That's way too many. We should have that kind of

resource allocation on the national level. And in some respects it's too big because it tends towards huge hospitals. Primary health care is underdimensioned, I think.

We have a congress . . . and there we take stands on the welfare policy and say fairly clearly, concerning health care, that this should be a public affair. There are some private parts in it, traditionally. We take a stand for this kind of system we have had traditionally. Market influence should be kept at the level it is now. It's a matter for politics and democratic control. . . . Some kind of possibility for people to choose—that's good, I think—which you can, even today. You can choose from different *vårdcentraler* and so on, hospitals. . . .

The crisis has led to huge deficits in the public budgets. . . . A lot of proposals for cutting in public spending have been put forward. Within the next four or five years a lot of the traditional Swedish model will be questioned, I think. . . . I think it's a political matter. Under this economic debate are huge differences, political views. Lindbeck[39] will cut public spending down to 45% or something and we won't. We can afford a decent health care system. We can afford decent schools and social insurance. We are still one of the richest countries. . . .

I think you have to raise taxes. You have to rationalize certain kinds of social insurance system, perhaps higher fees. The leader of the *Folkpartiet*, Bengt Westerberg, also says we are going to have to raise taxes. We can't solve it in another way to secure our welfare system. (Anders Forsman, TCO)

SKTF saw the issue as primarily political, both in the sense that the reduction of social welfare was a Conservative plan for which they had mobilized considerable power, and in the sense that decision making had been changed to a process that excluded workers:

We analyzed the situation in 1980. We were seeing the difficulties that the public sector, public services, were apt to face because of what was happening in other countries, because of the tiredness of taxation, etc. What we . . . have been trying to do has been to find forms for making the services more efficient. We as a union, together with some other unions, have had a number of activities and campaigns to promote efficiency within our services, to make them more listening to the citizens needing the services, suggesting to local governments and to the county councils changes in organization, etc. . . I think within the entire trade union movement there is an awareness that the solutions to the problems within the service system is not only more money. It is also looking into methods, looking at what professional groups we are working with. . . .

One of the possibilities for the health care system in Sweden now is that by new medical techniques, methods, etc. I think they're going to continue to increase their productivity, while within the municipalities—they have taken over the responsibility for the elderly people—it is going

> to be very difficult to create the same kind of increase in productivity that we will have in direct medical treatment. So the municipalities are going to face much more severe financial difficulties for the next few years. What we are doing now is we are trying to analyze and to show what is happening because of policies, politics against the local governments. When it all ends up in just higher unemployment to very much the same cost for the entire government budgets as a whole, there isn't much sense in such a policy. What we are aiming at . . . is you have to rely upon that the improvement in the health care sector, in the social services, in the educational system must be based on the experience of people working there, analyzing what are the true problems more than the big structural changes of privatization, of *köp-sälj*, where no one really knows anything about how it's going to end up.
>
> The huge experiment that is taking place in *Stockholms Läns Landsting* right now, no one knows how it is going to end. . . . We could just end up in a huge mess. It could end up with us in this area having to pay more tax for a health care system that is less efficient than it used to be.
>
> Our message is "You have to rely on people working there and our will to make these services better and to give us that possibility. We have to accept if you do cutbacks in the services, but let us do it for a longer period of time. Please, try to define. This is the cost that we intend to spend in the next coming years within the health sector services, within local government as a whole. Have an agreement between government and the Social Democratic opposition and let us work toward that goal. At least give us some time, because we can save services. We don't have to face the same number of unemployed as we are facing right now." (Sture Nordh, SKTF)

Politicians

The members of the Parliamentary Committee on Health and Welfare were the ones who handled all bills on medical care. They were the ones with the official responsibility for carrying out their parties' policies in this area.

The right-wing populist New Democrats were sponsoring the most extreme free market position. Indeed some very modest nonideological reforms of the past appeared to them as left wing:

> *Ja*, the *landsting*. We don't like that they are running this. We want to separate buying and selling. We want to have a general insurance system where you have an insurance and if you have this insurance you are welcome to the hospital and the hospitals are competing, "You come to my hospital." Not like they do now: "This is not your area hospital, go there." Then you are welcome and all these waiting lists you have, it's like in Russia, the shops, there are long waiting lines. People are standing outside waiting because there is no free market.

> [Now] they are not paying the doctors more or like that. What they are doing is selling from one place to another place. One department is selling to the next and it's an enormous bureaucracy.
>
> [The people at *Landstingsförbundet*] are pretty much like us. They have the same opinion, even if they have not understood the dynamics, how much it means to pay people to do more. That's something even the Moderates don't really [understand]. If you tell them, they agree, but not officially. It's just that a New Democrat has told them it's very important. . . . I think the *Folkpartiet* would [agree], but they are a little socialistic, especially their leader, Bengt Westerberg. He was an FLN member. . . . That's the Communist organization. You know, they were on the streets against the United States, doing things outside your embassy, throwing eggs and things like that. And you must remember that the Vice Prime Minister belonged to this organization, like Birgitta Dahl in the Social Democratic Party. (Leif Bergdahl, New Democrat)

The Conservatives were very much in tune with the reform proposals coming from *Läkarförbundet* and *Landstingsförbundet*:

> We try to be more effective, to make it possible to know what good treatment is. There's nothing politically controversial about that. Everyone, of course, likes to be treated in a way that has some good effect. And look at the structure we have in Sweden with many hospitals, rather weak primary care, and a few doctors in the first line. That is changing, but it has gone too slowly, and that means that people in Sweden are used to going to a hospital, a rather expensive way to treat the sick. So we have to . . . possibly take away a few, 15–20, hospitals. That is almost politically impossible. No one wants to lose the hospital in his town. Everyone will agree that on a national level it is OK, but don't touch us. . . .
>
> I personally believe that it is necessary for people to have a hospital close to them for simple things and for elderly people. It's not humane to let an elderly person travel many miles. He can't be visited by his relatives. Many who are older have no drivers' license. They often have very simple diseases that can't be cured in his house, but which need very simple x-ray resources. That should be close to the people. . . .
>
> When you have to move, with today's communication, no problem to go five or ten miles. The borderline is whether to go or not. Could you cure it close to your home or have you to go. Then it doesn't matter to go a few more miles. There you could have much more cooperation between *länsjukhus*. Everyone today tries to cover the whole spectrum and that's not possible with a small population. . . . These *läns centrallasarette* have a great deal of highly specialized care. That means in a small, sparsely populated country like Sweden it drains people from the university level. There is a risk that we do not have quite as good care as we could have for more rare diseases and we can't have new modern methods because the university clinics don't get the people they need. . . .

> Until today, the workers health care could do a good job or a bad job. . . . There is no reward system for good work and a hospital or clinic that has done good—has shortened queues and so on—has lost money. The only way to prove that it was important was to show political leaders they had a long queue, needed more people and more beds and so on. If you were very clever, worked everything fine, cut down the costs, you were punished. That meant that no clinics worked as well as they could. . . .
>
> [Privatization] is one aspect of what we talk about, competition too. We have in Sweden in principle a monopoly. The society has had all health care and that made it expensive and reduced opportunities for the patient to have a choice. We say that we shall keep a great deal of the care in the hands of . . . the government. We have to have other care given, private, cooperatives, other non-profit funds, to make it possible to compete with quality, with costs, and in service and to make it a reality for the patient to choose "what is best for me." . . .
>
> I think the trend in Sweden is that the *landsting* will vanish. We have three levels that take out taxes: the municipality, the *landsting*, and the state. This level, the *landsting*, is sick. . . . If the municipality were responsible for primary care, *husläkare* and so on, and either the municipality or congregation took care of the hospitals and so on, or the state, and we got rid of this middle level it will be . . . even more close to the patient. Democracy is much more identified with the municipality, where he lives, than with the more diffuse level. (Leif Carlsson, Conservative)

The representative of the Christian Democrats was a physician who entered politics to defend medical interests. He set his party's agenda on medical care. It is interesting that while he shared some of the analysis of *Läkarförbundet*, he was not in accord with the physicians' union on all issues.

> We have very strong organizations that guard our various interests. They are very, very strong and very influential and very well organized. And they are subsidized, usually, also by the society. . . . And they are acting and they are defending everything that we try to cut. But nobody defends the health care, for natural reasons, for sick people. Who would like to belong to an organization for sick people? There are organizations of women with breast cancer and other organizations, but they are weak. . . . We can cut as much as we want from health care. Nobody cares. Nobody. So we try to defend health care. . . . When there are polls in the opinion everybody says health care is more important or the next most important, but when it comes to decisions, there are no pressure groups. . . .
>
> In addition, the state is stronger than the counties . . . because the legislation is with the state and the division of resources is with the state. When the state comes stronger than the counties, so the state withdraws money from the counties because the state does not have formal responsibility for health care. . . . If a hospital is closed here in Stockholm, nobody blames the government. Everybody blames the county, the lo-

> cal government, and there are meetings, but nobody blames the government. . . .
>
> We need more influence for the patient and more incentives to make the work effective. . . .
>
> We have one more problem I forgot to mention, and this is quality assurance and quality control. For some reason, when we had this system that was monolithic control, everything, there was . . . a natural quality control. (Jerzy Einhorn, Christian Democrat)

The Center Party seemed to have little in the way of specific health policy. They were, however, the main defenders of the counties as providers of medical care:

> We don't want the County Councils to be abolished. We want to have them in the future. . . . They are very important, we think, because the municipalities are too small to have the responsibility for health services. If you transfer responsibility to them, we ought to have an *övergripande* organization, . . . an organization that will take over from the municipalities when they are too small.
>
> The most important thing is to find a system for setting priorities. . . . We propose a mix between public and private. . . . We want solidarity in payment in the future so everyone can have his . . . level of health care. (Rosa Östh, Center Party)

The Liberals were focused on passing the *husläkare* law establishing a family physician system:

> If you have a good contact with a family doctor you can save a lot of money. . . . In Sweden only four percent of our educated doctors are in *primärvården*. . . . *Husläkare*, I am happy for that, but I am also a realist. I see now that we have some problems with it. I see so many doctors sitting in a hospital. Many of them do a very good job, but many are staying in the hospitals and I think it is important they go out where the people stay and help them in their common situation. . . .
>
> *Ny Demokrati* has made some proposals we have taken dealing with the tax for the doctors. If you are a doctor and a surgeon and you had to do more for the patients than only looking and listening, and then you had to do something in practice, it takes more time and then the doctor can get more money for that.
>
> Competition is very good. For so many years you had no choice. If I go to the doctor and he doesn't listen to you or give you help or take the money. . . . And I pay with my fee. So now you can, as a patient, have a real choice and perhaps that will be something for the doctors to think about, because they have been small gods sitting still and people have

called and been very unhappy with the doctors. But, of course, there is a risk you can go too far. If you are a very honest doctor and you don't give the patient everything he wants, you might lose your patients. (Ulla Orring, Liberal Party)

The Social Democrats were trying to rationalize the system by reducing hospital beds and developing primary care. They were committed to maintaining strong public services, democratic control, and fiscal viability.

> We have too many hospital beds and we are driving a policy to reduce them and to provide primary care and continued specialty training, higher specialties. But it is a great problem to close hospitals. . . .
>
> Then in medical care policy we want to begin more work in evaluation, and with the help of the medical profession look at a number of methods used in Swedish medical care, to see that they hold to scientifically proven means. . . . There is an organization that has started in Sweden, a little unit called SBU [Swedish Council on Technology Assessment in Health Care].
>
> Then as Social Democrats we will certainly also work to continue to define quality in medical care. We believe that people more and more will demand or want to know what is good medical care, what does it really look like? There is a growing interest among Swedish physicians to measure what they do. . . .
>
> Then as Social Democrats we want to provide a little more for the elderly, because we have so many old people. We believe we need more housing in service homes or group homes. But we oppose the idea that economic considerations should control our decisions. . . . In the Social Democratic Party we respond to the Lindbeck Commission's contention that only economics should steer decisions. We think that it would force democracy backward. . . .
>
> There is a fear in the population that democratic institutions will not have enough money: that sickness care will not have it, that child care will not have it, so they will not be sufficient. One also wants medical care and care for the aged. If one feels that they have begun to collapse, there is real anxiety in the Swedish population. And I think you can mark that. And I personally will agitate within the Social Democratic Party for a clear democratic perspective and for the Swedish model. . . . I have the party's mandate to look at the governance system in municipalities and counties, where one sees economic control more and more. That leads to economists dominating politicians, physicians don't have the same influence. Politicians become more passive. I note that when I travel out and question politicians, that they can do fewer things. And the political parties become more passive, because economic forces control the money, where one has prices on everything, buy–sell, buy–sell. (Bo Holmberg, Social Democrat)

The Left Party wanted to improve the information on which decisions were being made and to retain the gains of the last generation. They were generally opposed to the reforms supported by the New Democrats and the Conservatives:

> Now the limit is 10,200 Swedish crowns. You cannot spend more than that [out of pocket] for health care. People with big needs who pay this much do not have to pay any more. We want to keep this.
>
> We would like a scientific survey to get a scientific picture of what elderly people really need. I oppose the statement that people should be left to choose their health care. That is a slogan of the Conservatives. It is a false way of discussing the problems with the health care system. Choice means that you have a lot of information and knowledge, lots of sources of information, and that you know how to compare firms. Who can do this at age 75? Most elderly people do not care about the choice issue. There are basic needs of the elderly that the society should provide for, regardless of choice. Choice is not an issue. (Eva Zetterberg, Left Party)

Others

Other people interviewed were less participants in the political process than they were interested observers. None of them presented an agenda in a form similar to governmental agencies, interest groups, or politicians. At the same time, they presented analyses that often had political implications.

Johannes Vang presented no political agenda. However, from the analysis he offered, as presented, it would be safe to say that he supported efforts to privatize and/or create "market mechanisms" in medicine.

Gösta Tibblin, with a chair in general medicine, favored reforms based on the analysis of practice patterns. Research by SBU had shown vast differences in treatments prescribed by different physicians for identical medical problems. Educating physicians to use the most cost-effective treatment would rationalize the system and make more effective use of existing moneys, which he thought were sufficient. He supported efforts to abolish county councils:

> As I see it, it is not a question of money. Money is not a problem. It is more the distribution of money. The health care system costs us 140 billion dollars, just about 140 billion, and the cost of the sick leave and the pension. . . . It is about 90 billion. So the society, or we, pay all together about 230 billion for what diseases do to people. But there is no relationship, there is no link, between these two boxes of money. What I think we should do is put this money together and then work in order to decrease the early *fortidspension* and decrease the sick leave, and this is possible. . . . There is a trend, so the good boys and girls are spending less money than the bad, if you look at the quality of their decisions. It's

a fantastic variation, a ten-fold variation in cost in front of the same patient. If we could get doctors to optimize their diagnosis and treatment we could save a lot of money. . . . There is what we call a lot of air in the system. . . . Certainly it will cost jobs, but on the other hand we will save money so they can get other jobs. I'm pretty sure that this is a solution, but it costs the doctors. The doctors will be unhappy. . . . We need to double the number of GP doctors. Then it will be just fine. . . .

What I am afraid about, a little, is that *husläkare* means you must be a businessman and we are not, up to now, recruiting businessmen.

Johan Calltorp was concerned that the reform effort was moving too quickly with too little reflection and analysis. While seeing value in undertaking a reform effort, even along lines of introducing market mechanisms into the public sector, he wanted a more research-guided process for making decisions and selecting options. The danger was that the achievements of the past generation might be destroyed in the process:

The main problem I see in Sweden right now is to relate the situation, the kinds of problems we have, or think we have, to other countries and to health care. That's a fundamental problem for Sweden to see that we have a very good health care system. I personally fear that we will throw out the baby with the bath water, so to say. . . .

In the department here we regard the implications for quality, what is happening with patients, the outcome of health care issues is a very healthy interesting effect of the internal market concept. If we don't get a reform that throws everything overboard, we could develop something quite interesting by creating an internal market concept within the public sector. It's an interesting concept, but, of course one feels now that there is—the ghost has gone out of the bottle. That's quite a lot my feeling. . . .

The main issue is how to maintain an equitable system. That's number one from my perspective. . . . I mean we have a tremendous value base in the health care system. . . . We have a very strong value in health care which is at risk.

We are confronting an inevitable change of financing health care. Tax money will not fund growing demands on health care. We have had a restriction. We will not have enough tax money to finance the health care needs. When we have different flows of money into health care, how will we avoid a fragmented two-tier system where we can retain equity. That worries me most. . . . I don't think we have an answer. So far, I think it's important to voice the issues.

SOME CONCLUSIONS

We are now in a position to offer some answers to the questions we posed at the beginning of this chapter (see Table 4.5 and Table 4.6):

Table 4.5
Comparison of Interest Groups on Selected Dimensions of the Medical Care "Crisis" in Sweden

Dimension	Physicians	Nurses	LO
Is there a medical care crisis?	No	Yes	No
Is there an economic crisis?			
Short term	Yes	Yes	Yes
Long term	Yes	No	No
What is the nature of the problem in medical care?	Rigidity of system, freedom of choice, cost of care.	Ideological, Professional monopolism.	Cost of care, rigidity of hospital sector.
What are the causes of the crisis?	Perverse incentives, public monopoly.	Economic depression, loss of principles of solidarity.	Economic depression, overly rigid public hospitals.
What are your policy goals?	Freedom of choice for patients, provider neutrality in funding.	Expand role of nurses, freedom for patients to choose level of care, protect the weak.	Fight unemployment, stabilize economy, keep strong public system.
What do you see as major opportunities?	More flexible, cheaper system.	Making costs visible, more flexibility.	Making costs visible, more flexibility.
What do you see as major dangers?	People left outside the system.	2/3 society with weak excluded from services.	2/3 society, reduction in quality of care.

Table 4.5 (*continued*)

SKAF	TCO	SKTF	Lanstings-forbundet	Ministry of Health
No	No	No	No	No
Yes	Yes	Yes	Yes/No	No
Yes/No	No	No	Yes	Yes
Deskilling of services, protection of elite workers at expense of members.	Increased demand for services, cost of care.	Political, attempt to dismantle welfare state.	Inefficiency, cost of care, rigidity, non-responsiveness to patients, financing care.	Cost of care, non-responsiveness to patients, inefficiency.
Economic depression, unemployment.	Demographic, European Community, over-specialization.	Top-down decision making, loss of solidarity.	Public monopoly, lack of economic incentives, legislative cap on funding.	Budget deficit, unemployment, bank crisis.
Support use of low-cost workers, keep public system strong.	Control privatization, control expensive technology, deep strong public system.	Reduce hospital sector, involve workers in increasing efficiency.	Make patient decisions economically consequential, increase efficiency.	Family physicians, national health insurance, improve psychiatric services.
Possibility for workers to influence changes.	Prospect of raising taxes to cover budget deficit.	Prospect of making boundaries between occupations more adaptable.	Increase flexibility, freedom of choice, more cost effectiveness, increase productivity.	Increase efficiency and effectiveness, more financing closer to the people.
Unemployment for members, more costly system, probability worker's input will be ignored.	2/3 society.	Unemployment, attacks on democracy.	Patient and physician interest in squeezing more money out of the system, duplication of services.	Funding going to enrich providers instead of services.

Table 4.6
Comparison of Politicians and Researchers on Selected Dimensions of the Medical Care "Crisis" in Sweden (A. Politicians)

Dimension	New Democrats	Conservatives	Christian Democrats
Is there a medical care crisis?	No	No	No
Is there an economic crisis?			
short term	Yes	Yes	Yes
long term	Yes	Yes	Yes
What is the nature of the problem in medical care?	Decline in productivity, loss of medical dominance, care teams.	Inefficiency, cost of care, rigidity, nonresponsiveness to patients.	Cost of care, funding.
What are the causes of the "crisis"?	Lack of economic incentives.	Unrealistic public expectations, increased demand, poor use of resources.	Growth of welfare state beyond tax capacity, lack of political voice for patients, growth of aged.
What are your policy goals?	Abolish counties, create buy-sell system, general insurance.	Reduce number of hospitals, reduce specialist care, increase primary care, introduce competition & privatization, abolish counties.	Keep adequate funding for medicine, make system more efficient.
What do you see as major opportunities?	Create more competition in medicine.	More efficient medical care system.	Not answered.
What do you see as major dangers?	Not answered.	Those not profitable may be dropped.	Not answered.

First, is there a crisis in the organization and/or operation of the Swedish medical care system? The short answer is "no." Neither the data nor the opinions of those engaged in the health care reform debates supported the notion that the medical care system itself was fundamentally flawed. While there were problems, some of them serious, that could become the basis for claiming a crisis if not addressed, none of them had yet reached

Table 4.6 (*continued*)

Center Party	Liberals	Social Democrats	Left Party
No	No	No	No
Yes	Yes	Yes	Yes
Yes	Yes	Yes/No	No
Cost of care, threat to district medicine.	Non-responsiveness to patients, cost of care.	Increased demand, reduced funding, attack on welfare state.	Attack on solidarity and equality of care, cost of care.
Lack of money (state and individual).	Wrong organization for medicine, poor health habits of people (diet, exercise, etc.).	Neo-liberal dominance, increased aged population, confusion in SAP.	Not asked.
New basic insurance system, keep counties, limit privatization, keep district responsibilities.	Reorganize around family physicians, health education.	Preserve strong welfare state and medical care model, protect democratic process.	Preventive medicine, make system more efficient, keep cap on out-of-pocket cost.
More responsive to patient needs.	Continuity of care.	Not asked.	Decentralization, more direct democracy.
Loss of quality of care.	See only positive effects, perhaps distribution problems.	Destruction of unions, loss of working class voice, increased class divisions.	Privatization, 2/3 society.

a state where the term "crisis" would be appropriate. Several agencies, among them the Federation of County Councils, the Physicians' Union and, to a much lesser degree, the Ministry of Health, had presented arguments that the current mode of operation had reached the limits of its usefulness and could not adequately address those problems. In so doing, they tried to create a climate in which a need for change was ad-

Table 4.6 (*continued*)
(B. Independent Researchers)

Dimension	Johannes Vang
Is there a medical care crisis?	Yes
Is there an economic crisis?	
short term	Yes
long term	Yes
What is the nature of the problem in medical care?	Bureaucratized care, nonmedical management, inefficiency, lack of choice.
What are the causes of the "crisis"?	Confusion of fairness and equity, loss of individual initiative, professional management.
What are your policy goals?	None
What do you see as major opportunities?	Greater efficiency and fairness.
What do you see as major dangers?	Return of paternalism.

dressed with a sense of urgency. Every spokesperson for each of those organizations, however, backed off from the characterization of any problems faced by the medical care system as a crisis.

Second, what problems did the Swedish medical care system face and how well was it organized to solve them? There are many parts to this answer. The system faced some important challenges. There was a large and rapidly growing population of elderly people whose needs for medical and related support services were stretching the resources allocated to medical care. The system was built quickly without adequate reflection on cost implications. One result was a medical care system too much focused on high technology, tertiary care hospitals, and highly specialized medicine. Another was an overcapitalized system that delivered most units of care in more expensive settings than were technically necessary. Indeed, it was observed more than eighteen years earlier that the system had the potential to be self-bankrupting.

There were also some inefficiencies in the system that needed attention. Most important, there were long waiting lists for some elective surgical procedures. This was only in part a system of rationing according to need. Much delay came from complexities in scheduling and getting

Table 4.6 (*continued*)

Gösta Tibblin	Johan Calltorp
Yes	No
Yes	Yes
No	Yes
Cost of care, over-specialization, unemployment, debt.	Rapidity of change, lack of thought and research as basis for decision making.
Limits of welfare state, consumption outstripping revenues.	Naiveté in applying economic theory to medicine.
Improve distribution of money, link sick leave and pension funds, set practice standards, medical audits.	Have policy decisions based on solid research.
Linking salaries to productivity.	More efficient and effective system.
Not asked.	Fragmentation, managers interfering in clinical decision-making.

the right resources to the right place at the right time. The result was that expensive resources, among them operating theaters, lay idle, not because appropriate personnel were unavailable but because appropriate supplies were not at hand or because the beds were being blocked by patients whose treatment had been completed but who had no appropriate place to go. By instituting a care guarantee and requiring municipalities to pay for "blocked" beds, these waiting lists had already been reduced by the time our study began.

Some of the reforms of the previous decade or so had made the problems more difficult. By relinquishing control over the allocation of technology and personnel, the state gave up the most essential tools for cost control. Unless that control could be regained, there were few means available to the national government to cap the rapidly growing cost of medical care. Capping payments to the counties, forbidding municipalities from increasing taxes while increasing their medical care responsibilities, and the like would do nothing to alleviate the problem. Privatization would further decrease the ability of the society to cap costs. Market mechanisms, unless closely tied to solid knowledge about how decisions are made by real people facing real-life medical care decisions (patients and providers alike), have a potential for creating perverse incentives that would make the system more inefficient and of markedly lower quality. Indeed, such measures could increase the stress under which the system worked.

The short answer, then, is that the system faced some serious problems, not least of which were poorly thought out attempts to make it more efficient.

Third, what were the competing political agendas for changing or defending the Swedish medical care system? Representatives of the Physicians' Union, the Federation of County Councils, and the Ministry of Health, and some journalists tried to present a case that there was a new consensus in Sweden that the Swedish model had failed. It had created an elaborate bureaucracy that stifled initiative and generated costs beyond the taxation capacity of the state. To be modern, one had to endorse markets, competition, and privatization as the solution.

Whatever the merits of the case, it was certainly a distortion to speak of a consensus. The push for market solutions in medical care came from the three sources identified with considerable support from a neoliberal think tank, *Studieförbundet för Näringslivet och Sämhälle* (SNS), located in Stockholm. SNS had close ties to the Swedish Manufacturers Association which had been promoting a shift toward a market economy for decades. Once you looked beyond that group of interests, the evidence for a new consensus evaporated.

White-collar and blue-collar unions, including unions of health professionals other than physicians, uniformly expressed skepticism about the value of market reforms. Blue-collar unions were more unambiguously opposed to them. All gave the impression of being "hunkered down" to protect the interests of their members in a period of great uncertainty.

New Democratic and Conservative politicians were in favor of strong market reforms. Other parties in the government (Christian Democrats, Center, and Liberal party politicians) were in favor with substantial reservations. Left parties (Social Democrats and Left Party politicians) were opposed.

Some outside observers, such as Johannes Vang of the WHO, were providing ideological support for market reforms, and had indeed become part of the Federation of County Councils planning process. Others saw many of the problems the proponents took as the reasons behind the reform effort and had reservations about the pace of reform and the degree to which consequences had been thought through.

Our short answer, then, is that there were competing agendas and little evidence of a consensus. The proponents of market reform seemed to have taken the initiative, but they had yet to convince a majority that they had an answer.

Fourth, was there any reason to fundamentally change the nature of the organization of Swedish medical care in order to solve problems internal to the medical care system? Again, our short answer is "no." There is no reason to believe, with the evidence at hand, that a system of medical care delivered as a public service by county councils under a national mandate could not solve the problems it faced if the state could regain control over the allocation of personnel and technology. Indeed, the evidence suggests that the more the medical care system is handed over to a market, the less cost control is possible. Without stringent safeguards that would introduce a new set of constraints on the development of the system, equity, universality, and acceptability might be sacrificed.

If the problems faced by medical care were to be solved, a strong public system consistent with the Swedish model would seem to have a strong advantage over a more privatized, competitive, market approach. In this we join with a panel of international economists whose recommendations have been largely ignored in the current debate (Cuyer, 1991).

Our overall conclusion is that the pressure for change in the Swedish medical care system did not come primarily from within that system. Indeed, our respondents have repeatedly pointed to problems in the general economy and/or in political ideology. It is to those areas that we now turn.

NOTES

1. I have as authorities Jan Sundén, a medical historian who searched on my behalf for such a historical overview and found none, and Björn Smedby, Claes-Göran Westrin, and Johan Calltorp, all of whom have used historical materials in their work and who knew of no such overview.

2. A reform of medical education in the mid-1970s vastly expanded the size of medical school classes and capped opportunities for specialty training. In the late 1970s, the primary care system reorganized to reduce the number of primary care districts and to provide primary care in "Care Centers" (*Vårdcentraler*), where several general practitioners, pediatricians, dentists, maternal health physicians, pediatric nurses, nurse–midwives, and community nurses could be under one roof, sharing staff and facilities. These reforms improved access to primary care and dealt effectively with most of the problems reported by district physicians in the late 1970s (see Twaddle, 1986; Tibblin in Twaddle, 1994b).

3. We have in mind here the kind of work Rosemary Stevens did on the development of medicine in the U.K. (1966) and the United States (1971), and Paul Starr (1982) did for the United States.

4. The United States may be a unique case in the lack of licensing laws for medical practice following the Thompsonian movement. The expansion of medical knowledge in the United States was retarded by several competing sects providing curative services (Kett, 1968; Twaddle and Hessler, 1987) and the very poor quality of mainstream medical schools, most of which failed to teach the scientific knowledge that was available (Flexner, 1910).

5. The so-called "Proletarian writers" created stories of late-nineteenth- and early-twentieth-century agrarian and working-class peoples (e.g., Lo-Johansson, Johansson) which depicted a level of poverty at which healing was almost en-

tirely an indigenous folk tradition practiced by women. The growth of demand may have been retarded somewhat by the late entry of Sweden into the industrial revolution and the late emergence of a broad-based middle class. The only competing healing tradition other than the folk was naprapathy, about which we know little. It is said to be a manipulative therapy and may bear comparison with osteopathy and chiropractic in the United States. Recently, a College of Napropathy was established in Stockholm, indicating that it may be in the process of professionalizing.

6. Two thirds of all the medical schools in the United States closed between 1910 and 1936 because they could not meet the standards proposed in the Flexner Report and enacted by state legislatures across the country. The American Medical Association managed to cap the number of places in medical schools until the 1960s, holding down the number of physicians in training while the population grew and aged. Physician incomes grew from twice the average wage to between eight and forty times the average family income between 1920 and 1980.

7. We caution that demand is not the same as need. Need is defined by the health problems people have in the form of disease, illness, and sickness (Twaddle and Nordenfelt, 1994). Demand is generated by decisions taken in response to need. The decision to seek medical care is typically taken by the patient, as influenced by her or his family, friends, and acquaintances. Once in the medical care system, effective decision making is largely confined to health care providers, most often physicians.

8. In the United States, 41 percent of all physician were in primary care specialties at that time.

9. One third of the positions in Göteborg in 1978. Physicians preferred to work in smaller localities, particularly when they got the same pay for less work in such places.

10. Averaging, in 1978, 18 thousand persons in Göteborg with a range from 2 thousand to 24 thousand.

11. This was only one of the factors associated with the perspective of district physicians that their work was dull and uninteresting (Twaddle, 1986).

12. Sweden's medical care system was among the most expensive in the world as of 1980, rivaled only by the United States, which continued to increase to over 14 percent of GNP in 1993. The decline in relative cost of the Swedish system in 1982 is associated with the Dagmar Reform, augmented by the Ädel Reform in 1992, which transferred care of the aged from the medical care budget to that for the care of the aged. While part of the decline is artifactual, some of it is real.

13. In the 1960s, the Kaiser Permanente Health Plan in Portland, Oregon, showed it was able to deliver medical services to a voluntarily enrolled population at a cost some 40 percent below the national average. This generated a myth that they practiced more aggressive preventive medicine than did other services, giving the prepaid group practice the label health maintenance organization (HMO). The Kaiser Permanente plan achieved its savings, not through preventive medicine (nor, as charged by the American Medical Association [AMA], by denying patients needed treatment), but by delivering each unit of service in the cheapest possible setting. Nothing was done in the hospital, for example, if it could be done as well in a nursing or outpatient facility (Saward, 1970). At that time, 40 percent of the medical beds in the Massachusetts General Hospital were

occupied by patients who technically did not need them, but whose insurance would not pay for out-of-hospital procedures.

14. These are the data that seemed to be accepted in the Ministry of Health (Könberg and Pettersson, 1993; cf. Twaddle, 1994b) and by most researchers in social medicine. It should be noted, however, that there are other figures showing a continuously rising percentage of GNP devoted to medical services. Most of those data came from the Business College (*Handelshögskolan*—often translated as the Stockholm School of Economics) in Stockholm. Gerdtham and Jönsson (1992), for example, provided a table (p. 8) from their own calculations showing the increase between 1980 and 1990 in current prices at 144 percent (from 62.0 billion crowns in 1982 to 123.2 billion crowns in 1990), and in constant prices at 28 percent (from 52.7 billion crowns in 1982 to 64.7 billion crowns in 1990). It is not clear how their calculations differ from those in official statistics or OECD compilations.

15. These data are difficult to interpret without additional research. It is clear that payments from sickness insurance were increasing at all ages. Whether this is because of increased disease (which is unlikely with the kind of workplace environment protection in Sweden), illness (in part a function of alienation, which is likely with the rollback of workers' decision-making rights at the workplace), or sickness (reflecting a change in the social definition of what is an acceptable level of health) cannot be resolved with the data at hand.

16. This is a position promoted most prominently by Alan Enthoven (1980; 1986; Enthoven and Kronick, 1989), whose "pro-competitive strategies," organized through the Jackson Hole Group, provided the frame within which the Clinton health care reforms were being developed in the USA. That Enthoven had visited Sweden several times to promote this strategy is not irrelevant, but the specific impact of his marketing of ideas has not been assessed. *Caveat emptor.*

17. The Swedish term was *resultat enhet*, literally a "results unit." In usage it seems the equivalnt of the Amercian "profit center."

18. Technical quality refers to the effectiveness with which the state of existing knowledge and technology is brought to bear on health problems. Quality of care refers to the extent to which the needs and desires of individual patients are accommodated by the care system. See Twaddle and Hessler (1987).

19. These complaints can be found in any country among any people in contact with hospitals, particularly the large teaching hospitals. They are in the "double binds" that characterize all patient–physician relationships (Bloor and Horobin, 1975; cf. Twaddle, 1980).

20. Privatization is a factor here, as several high-technology private clinics were formed, partly to provide quicker access to elective surgery, partly to market Swedish medicine to non-Swedes, and partly so physicians otherwise blocked from highly specialized practice could have an opportunity to specialize. The profit motive need not be mentioned.

21. In fact, there was a sharp increase in medical care costs between 1994 and 1995. It was not clear, however, that runaway technology was the culprit.

22. My work did not include interviews with the general public, so this was not a matter to be systematically followed up in the project. I did hear the story from health care officials outside of the Stockholm area and my wife, Sarah Wolcott, heard such stories in her interviews, which focused on the teaching of reading in the lower primary grades of the Linköping public schools.

23. In this, he was laying out a position favoring changes supported by *Dagens Nyheter, Landstingsförbundet, Läkarförbundet*, and the Minstry of Health.

24. Complete transcriptions of the interviews can be found in Twaddle (1994b).

25. This refers to a debate on social insurance, where income replacement while sick, pensions, and so forth are paid as a percentage of working income, the so-called income loss principle. The Center Party was sponsoring proposals that a flat level of payment be given to everyone, the so-called basic security principle.

26. While all other quotations are from transcriptions of tape-recorded interviews, this is transcribed from field notes.

27. We are grateful to Chairman Bo Holmberg for arranging the interviews.

28. The New Democrats are difficult to place. They seemed libertarian on most issues and biased toward small business on tax issues. Their stance was a kind of populism and seemed to us to be ideologically contradictory. In part this may have been because they were a new political party that was still seeking its stance on most issues. In placing them at the far right, we may be giving too much weight to their anti-immigrant positions.

29. Unfortunately, the tape of this interview was difficult to transcribe, making it impossible to provide all the arguments complete in his own words.

30. This was Hjällmar Branting's image of Sweden as "the people's home" (*folkhemmet*), where everyone looked out for the welfare of everyone else and the state became the means for so doing (Isaksson, 1985).

31. Referring to the Ädel Reform.

32. In the County of Östergötland.

33. This deal fell through during the study period.

34. In some studies in the United States, continuity of care seems to be a greater concern for providers than for patients. We know of no such studies in Sweden.

35. This should not be taken to imply that they did not have explanations, only that they did not offer them in response to open-ended questions.

36. Foreign observers had noted this almost two decades earlier.

37. It seemed to us that the overcapacity was in the high-technology tertiary care facilities, with possibly a need for expanding local, low-technology hospitals. Instead, the political thrust of the right–center government has been to target small hospitals for closing, leaving the more expensive ones untouched. Two large, high technology hospitals have been targeted. One was a hospital in Stockholm that the county tried (without success) to sell to private interests. The result was that its twenty-four-hour emergency department was closed. The other was the hospital in the home-town of the Social Democratic Chair of the Parliamentary Committee on Health and Welfare.

38. In fact, patients could choose which care center they wished and many had indeed chosen to get medical care closer to work than to their homes. Physicians were not limited in whether they could enter private practice, only in whether they could link their practices to national health insurance.

39. Professor of Economics at Stockholm University (see Chapter 5).

CHAPTER 5

The Crisis in the Economy

While almost without exception those advocating reform of medical care said there was no crisis in the medical care system, many held that there was a crisis in the general economy that made it impossible to support the welfare state as it had developed in Sweden. They held that Sweden had created "a costume that was too big"[1] and the public sector had to be reduced in size. Medical care was the largest component of the public welfare system. It had to be reduced, not because it was ineffective or inequitable (although many claimed it was inefficient), but because the economy could no longer support it. A cursory review of Chapter 4 will confirm that this position was widespread among our interview respondents as well as in the *debatt* literature on public policy (see Tables 4.5 and 4.6). The severity of the economic crisis reported varied.

Among those holding that the crisis was a major one that required large-scale restructuring of the medical care system were representatives of the Federation of County Councils, the Physicians' Union, the New Democratic Party, the Conservative Party, and Johannes Vang. Representatives of the Ministry of Health, the Liberal Party, the Center Party, the leadership of the Social Democratic Party, and Gösta Tibblin all held that there was a long-term economic problem that required some adjustment in the medical care system, but not a major reform. Representatives of LO, SKAF, TCO, SKTF, the Social Democrats in the parliament, and the Left Party all held that there was no long-term economic crisis, only a short-term problem coupled with a depression that encompassed all Western economies. As these divisions tended to replicate traditional political positions, we will refer to them respectively as the right, center, and left views on economic crisis.

In this chapter, we take a closer look at the economic situation in Sweden as of 1993. It is not our intent to present our own technical analysis of the economy to render an independent judgment on the existence and/or degree of crisis, but to identify the data and arguments of those representing different positions and to assess the debate.[2] We begin by looking at the components of the short-term crisis on which all those in the debate seemed to agree: the sharp rise in oil prices in 1973–1974, the "overheating" of the Swedish economy during the early 1980s, the worldwide economic downturn in the economy during the late 1980s, the insolvency of Swedish banks associated with a crisis in the real estate market, a large budget deficit, and the emergence of massive unemployment. We take note that even while there was general agreement that the crisis of the early 1990s contained these elements, there was a difference of expert opinion on the underlying causes. The right position was that they reflected a long-term structural problem that required radical reform. The center–left position was that the crisis was short term, resulting from a changed external environment, poor decisions in the private sector, and bad decisions taken by the government. We will look as well at some of these policy decisions; most importantly, a tax reform in 1990 and a decision to join the European Union.

The left also contended that there was a deliberate campaign on the part of right-wing economists to marginalize Marxist and Keynesian theory and make a neoliberal stance the sole approach in Swedish economics. In what amounted to an ideologically motivated political campaign, the competition of ideas was severely truncated, if not eliminated. To the extent that such is the case, the apparent consistency of advice given to the political decision makers may provide grounds for suspecting its adequacy, in that the ideas may not have been well tested in debate or challenged in the political arena.

Against this background, we can assess whether the state of the economy was either necessary or sufficient to explain the new pressures for medical care reform through promotion of markets, competition, and privatization.

THE ECONOMIC CRISIS: ELEMENTS

"Oil Shock"

In 1973–1974, the newly formed OPEC consortium restricted output and sharply raised the price of crude oil. Being highly dependent on oil to fuel its economy and entirely without oil reserves of its own, Sweden was particularly sensitive to that development (see Figure 5.1 and Figure 5.2). Indeed, most observers held that the country entered into a recession that lasted until 1982 and concluded that the OPEC initiative introduced

Figure 5.1
Trends in per Capita GNP in Sweden, OECD, and Seven Rich Countries (1960 = 100, 1985 prices and exchange rates)

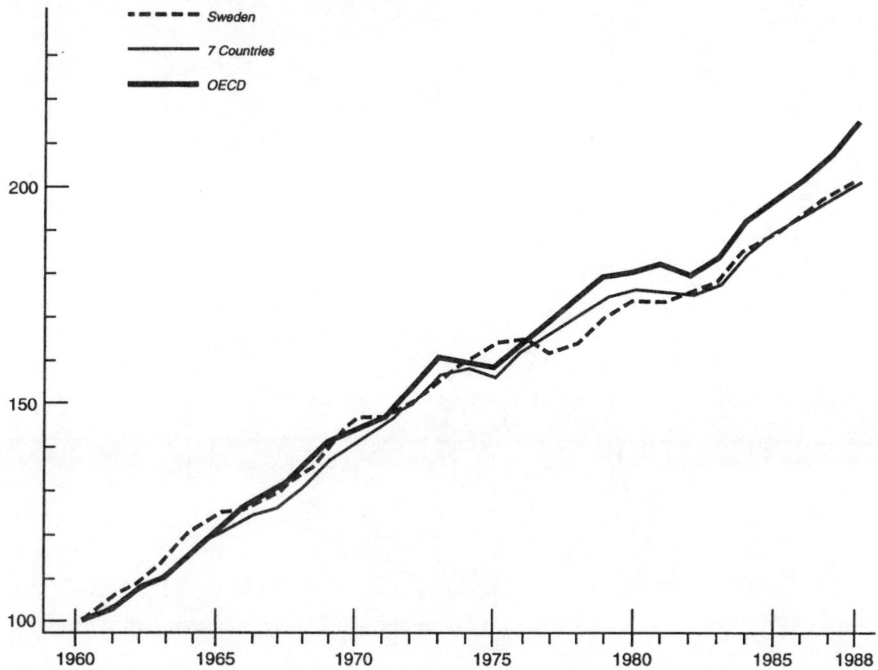

Source: Walter Korpi, 1992. *Halkar Sverige Efter: Sveriges Ekonomiska Tillväxt 1820–1990 i Jämförande Belysning* (Stockholm: Carlssons).

a "permanent" burden on the Swedish economy (Långtidsutredningen, 1990; Korpi, 1992; Olsson, 1993; Ekonomikommissionen, 1993; Hamilton and Rolander, 1993).

The increase in oil prices raised the cost of production directly dependent on petroleum fuels and shifted the burden to more expensive and environmentally damaging fossil and nuclear sources of electricity. Basic costs of production were not only higher, but less under the control of Swedish industry. According to some observers, this resulted in a shift of attitude on the part of Swedish manufacturers toward a more antilabor stance, as that was an area where substantial cost savings could be realized.

Overheating and Inflation

Beginning in 1982, the economy recovered. Production increased in absolute terms through 1993, but the rate of annual increase slowed dramatically after 1984 (see Table 5.1 and Figure 5.2). Unemployment fell

Figure 5.2
Changes in Productivity (GNP per employed person) in OECD and in Sweden (annual percentage change)

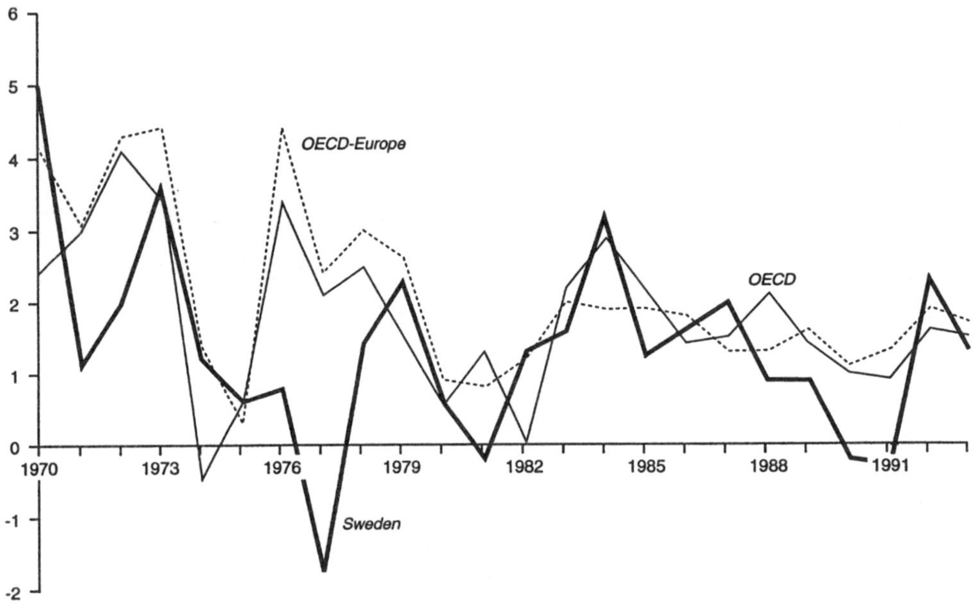

Source: SOU 1993: 16, *Nya Villkor för Ekonomi och Politik—Ekonomikommisionens Förslag* (Stockholm: Inrekesdepartmentet), 12.

until 1989, after which it rose to record levels (Figure 5.3). Real wages rose in constant *kronor* and disposable income rose even faster until 1990 (Figure 5.4) (Långtidsutredningen, 1990; Ekonomikommissionen, 1993). Indeed, growth was so rapid that there were inflationary pressures and the government took measures to slow it.

It was in this context that the Social Democratic Party shifted its political goals from expansion of the welfare state to "consolidation" of the system. It was also during this period that the Conservatives became the leaders of the nonsocialist bloc. The 1985 elections were framed as a contest between consolidation and dismantling of the welfare state (Olsson, 1993).

Recession/Depression

If there was one item on which there was unanimity in 1993, it was that Sweden was in the midst of an economic depression which was not limited to the Swedish economy but encompassed all of Europe and North America. As compared with other OECD countries, Sweden's economic performance was not particularly poor. Indeed, from 1973 to 1989, Sweden showed economic growth that was somewhat below that of Norway, Japan, Canada,

Table 5.1
Timeline of Recent Economic Events Affecting Sweden

Date	Event	Meaning
1973-1974	Oil Shock: OPEC restricted output and raised prices of crude oil.	Sharp increase in cost of production in country without own oil resources.
1980-1982	Recession.	Raised unemployment to nearly 3 percent.
1985-1990	Banking reform.	Created real estate and banking crisis.
1989	Shift of emphasis in Finance Ministry from full employment to inflation.	Sharp increase in unemployment to highest levels in twentieth century
1991	Tax reform.	Created massive acute budget deficit.
1993	Decision to enter European Community.	Intensified pressure to reduce welfare state.

Figure 5.3
Unemployment in Sweden, 1963–1992 (percentage)

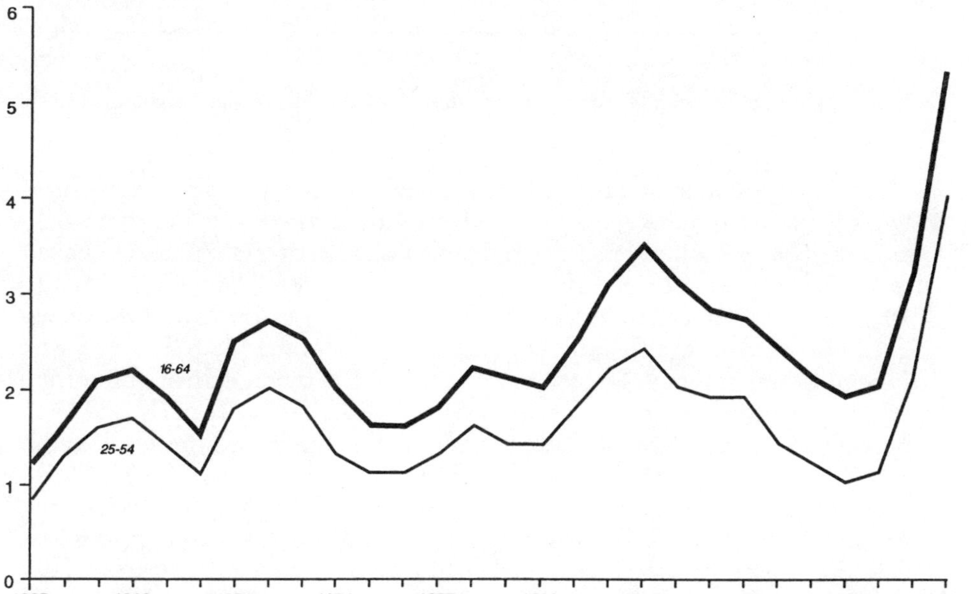

Source: SOU 1993: 16, *Nya Villkor för Ekonomi och Politik—Ekonomikommisionens Förslag* (Stockholm: Inrekesdepartmentet), 1.

Finland, and the United States, but higher than Germany, Austria, Italy, Denmark, France, Australia, Belgium, England, Switzerland, Ireland, the Netherlands, and New Zealand (Figure 5.5) (Korpi, 1992, 107).

Figure 5.4
Real Hourly Wages after Taxes and Real Household Disposable Income, 1974–1990

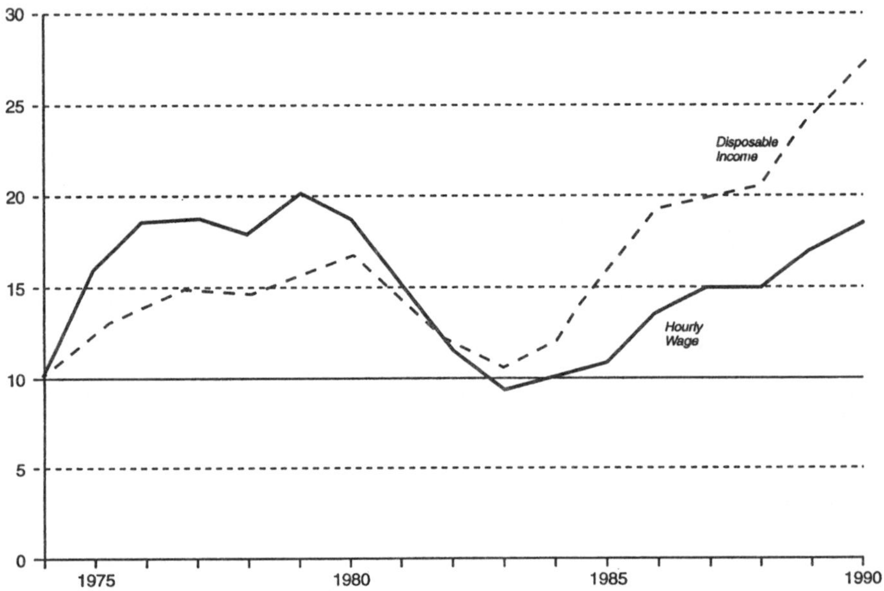

Source: LTU90, SOU 1990: 14, *Långtidsutredningen 1990* (Stockholm: Finansdepartmentet).

Throughout most of this century, Sweden's economy was robust, maintaining higher than average levels of growth and, on any international comparison, very low levels of unemployment. After 1970, as we have seen, there were some signs of weakness. Productivity fell between 1970 and 1977, recovered unevenly until 1979, fell again between 1979 and 1982, rose until 1984, and fell again throughout the remainder of the 1980s (Figure 5.6). Unemployment remained well below the OECD average throughout the whole period, rising to about 3 percent in 1983, falling to well under 2 percent 1989, and then beginning to rise again (Ekonomikommissionen, 1993; Calmfors, 1993b; Langby, 1983; Korpi, 1992; Olsson, 1993). The growth in number of hours worked fell between 1984 and 1987, rose until 1989 and then fell sharply, actually declining in 1992 (Figure 5.7). The gross national product, which had grown until 1990, began to fall thereafter (Figure 5.8).

There was also little disagreement that the economy worsened dramatically in the early 1990s. Here, however, one found profound disagreement on the reasons. The right, coalesced around a group of neoliberal theorists led by Assar Lindbeck, held that there was a long-term crisis in the economy that demanded radical revision. Following Langby (1983) they saw Sweden following a pattern that could be found

Figure 5.5
Average Anual Growth of GNP Per Capita in Eighteen OECD Nations (in crowns, 1985 prices and exchange rates)

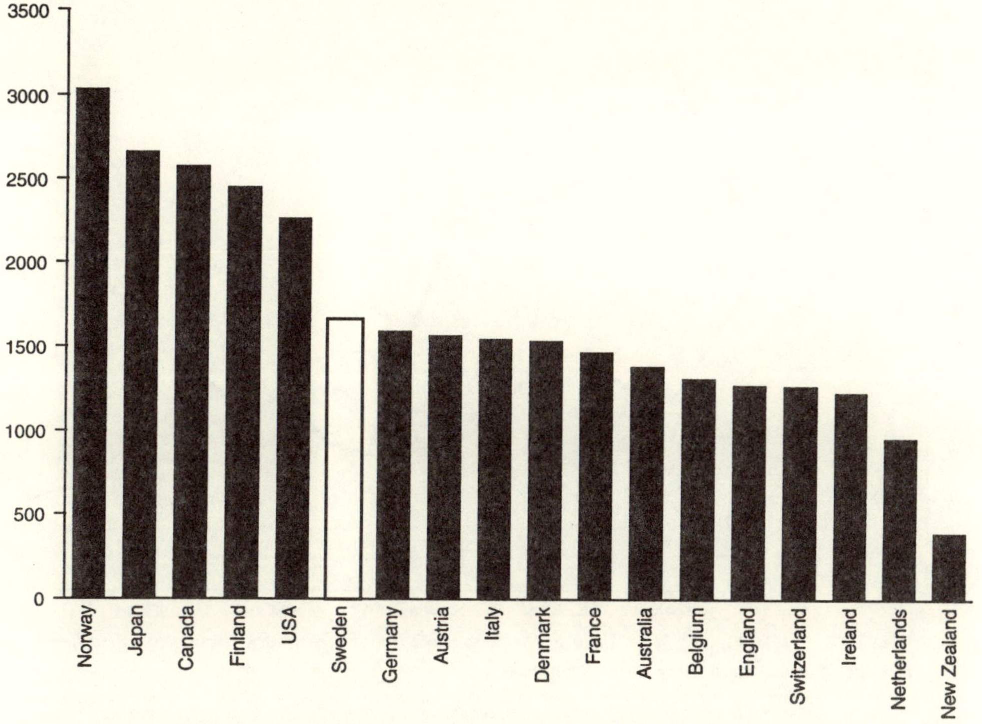

Source: Walter Korpi, 1992. *Halkar Sverige Efter: Sveriges Ekonomiska Tillväxt 1820–1990 i Jämförande Belysning* (Stockholm: Carlssons).

in ancient Athens and Uruguay in the late 1950s and early 1960s. That is, the public sector had been allowed to grow to a level where it produced stagnation in the economy. The solution, according to this line of thinking, was to sharply reduce public services and expenditures, to reestablish a market economy for goods and services, and to restrict democratic control of the society, particularly in economic matters (Ekonomikommissionen, 1993). Villy Bergström summarized the right-wing position:

> The fundamental problem in the Swedish economy was partly "over consumption," partly a number of "system shortages" in the Swedish economy, among them the tendency of companies and households to learn the "reaction patterns of government," which reduced the possibility of stabilizing employment and prices by means of economic policy.... Economists agree in recommending "... fixed norms in stability policies and a minimum of discretionary use of stabilization policies." Economists are also in agreement nowadays that the government can not—as earlier thought—buy for itself high employment at the price of high

Figure 5.6
Relative Cost of Labor (RULC) and Market-Share Changes, 1970–1991
(1970 = 100)

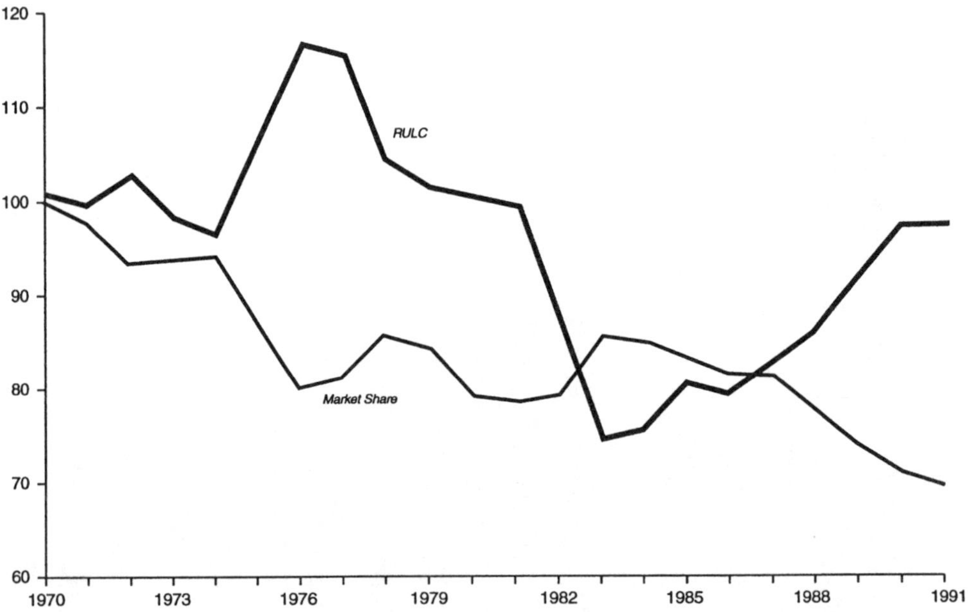

Source: SOU 1993: 16, *Nya Villkor för Ekonomi och Politik—Ekonomikommisionens Förslag* (Stockholm: Inrekesdepartmentet), 2.

inflation, but in the long run it is impossible to be under the "natural level of unemployment." (Lönnroth, 1993, 11)

The center position repudiated as extremist the arguments put forth by Langby and Lindbeck. They did not generally think the Swedish model needed to be completely abolished. They thought that making reforms in the public sector would be sufficient to ensure economic stability and growth. Some programs would have to be scaled back, most would have to be made more efficient. At the same time, the principle of providing basic security to all Swedes was sacrosanct.

The left position was that the problem with the economy was short term. Sweden had been caught up in the recession that had swept over all of the Western world in the 1980s, and, perhaps, had aggravated the problem by some political decisions. From this perspective, the economy was not "broken" and did not need fundamental reform. New developments, at the same time, required some new political decisions that would make adjustments in the management of economic affairs. Anything that was amiss could be fixed within the existing system: "Another of welfare

Figure 5.7
Municipal-Sector Consumption and Employment (working hours)

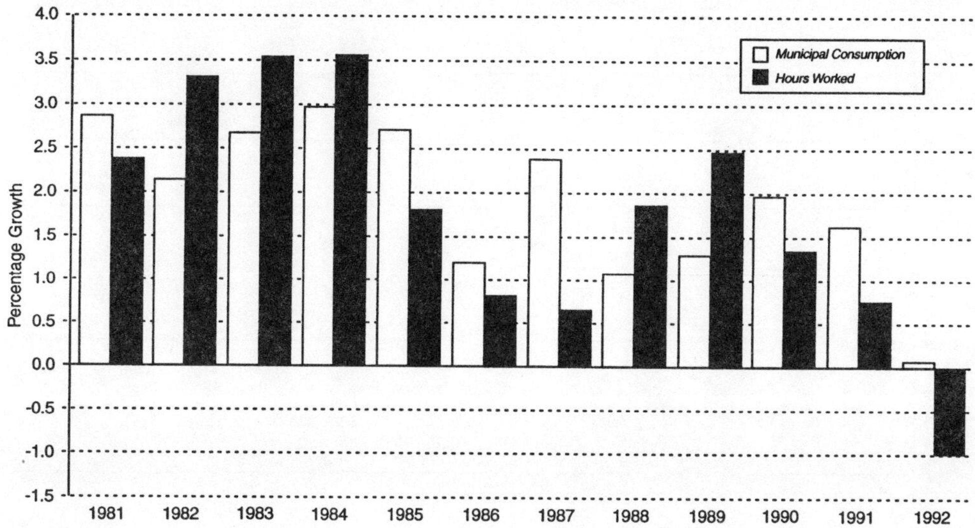

Source: LO, *Om viljan Finns . . .: Los Program mot arbetslöhet* (Stockholm: LO, 1993), 23.

policy's tasks is to function as a motor in the social production process. Regardless of which stage of economic development a nation finds itself in, its production needs the support that the society's welfare policy can give" (Socialdemokratiska Riksdagsgruppen, 1993: 1). That did not imply a lack of appreciation of problems in productivity and growth. Indeed, the case was quite the contrary:

> One of the most important conditions for retaining and developing welfare policies is that production increases in tandem with the growing need for welfare. During the 1980s the need for welfare payments grew rapidly both from the growing number of aged people and from the fact that female employment continued to grow at the same time more children were born in Sweden than had happened for some time. While this was going on, productivity grew at an ever slower pace and then gradually declined. (Socialdemokratiska Riksdagsgruppen, 1993: 6)

While there was agreement as to what was happening, there was a sharp division on the response. The right sought to decrease public spending and to provide more "freedom of choice" for the private sector to "become the economic engine." The left sought to decrease unemployment, increasing the tax base to raise the funds for the public system to be the engine (see, e.g., Jonung, 1989; LO, 1993).

Figure 5.8
GNP Sweden, 1985–1992 (seasonally adjusted, first quarter 1985 = 100)

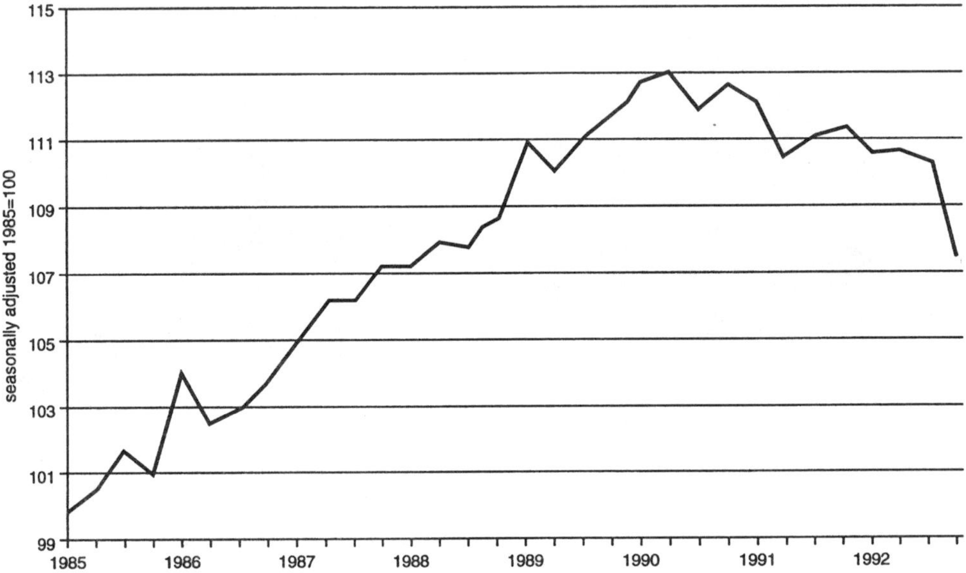

Source: LO, *Om viljan Finns . . .: Los Program mot arbetslöhet* (Stockholm: LO, 1993), 53.

Some observers thought that Sweden had made some poor choices that compounded the effects of global recession. As expressed by Jan Edling (1993), economist with LO,

> The economy was going quite well in the beginning and there were a lot of profits made and orders were coming in from all over the world.[3] We could export our products. The problem was . . . that labor was made very cheap compared to capital and some employers the day before devaluation thought they had to substitute capital for labor. The day after . . . he says "labor is much cheaper, now. I don't have to invest in machinery and things like that." . . . We made the first mistake in 1982 because we didn't make the investments in industry grow fast enough during the '80s. . . . When you don't invest money you become more labor intensive. . . . The low price of labor compared with other countries went up and productivity was not growing at the same time. . . . What happened was that all of the structural changes that should have come during the '80s came at one time, about 1991. The recession in Sweden, compared with Europe and the United States, was much heavier. . . . We got all the problems that we made in the '80s at the same time as the recession came.

Clearly, a recession of this magnitude made it difficult to sustain a high level of public expenditures for very long. It created a situation in which a rationale for cutbacks would have plausibility to the general public.

The issue would seem to have been whether public-sector savings could free money to fuel a private-sector expansion sufficient to pull the country back to prosperity or whether a direct attack on unemployment might generate the tax revenues needed to maintain the level of public services. In this, however, we are ahead of our story.

The Real Estate and Banking Crisis

In the mid-1980s, legal restrictions on mortgage loans, especially those outside of Sweden, were relaxed, creating a chain reaction that resulted in almost every bank in Sweden going into receivership. There is agreement on the following:

- Banks greatly increased their mortgage loans during a period of moderate inflation. This was a period in which real estate values were high and rising, making real estate seem a profitable as well as a safe investment.
- Banks failed to hold enough in reserve to cover their loans adequately.
- The real estate market became badly inflated and went bust, with a sharp decline in real estate values.
- Most banks found they held mortgages that exceeded the value of the property they had mortgaged.

The factors leading to the housing and banking crisis are in some dispute. On the one hand, Gabriel Urwitz and Staffan Viotti (1993), writing for the *Ekonomikommissionen* summarized the crisis as follows:

> The financial crisis is fundamentally shaped by a real estate crisis, which in turn is the result of a dramatic reevaluation of real estate capital. Without going into a deeper analysis of the causes behind the financial and real estate crisis, we offer the following summary:
>
> - An inflationary economic parade with a somewhat toughly regulated and powerfully subsidized construction and real estate sector led to work in real estate being regarded as virtually risk free. This led to high loans and low interest rates on mortgage loans.
> - A money and securities market with a small number of large players, who demanded too little risk compensation for their loans to the construction and real estate sector.
> - A tax system that encouraged high financial risk-taking and large debt when the financial system was deregulated and the foreign lending market became free. (p. 395)

These factors were compounded by the government's actions to curb inflation.

> Deregulation in combination with the altered tax system, a very quick and deep depression and an unexpected quick reduction of inflation led to a unique sharp

and powerful decline of real estate values with extensive consequences for the whole financial system.

Something that is special about the Swedish financial system is that Swedish savings were (and still largely are) so concentrated in a small number of large institutions and that collective savings patterns play so meaningful a role. (pp. 395–396)

Carl Hamilton and Dag Rolander (1993) portrayed the banks as taking a more active role in creating the crisis:

[In] 1985, when the ceiling on bank loans was removed, loans for real estate exploded. Everyone who had earned any money during the stock market rise or in the economic expansion got advice from their bankers to borrow additional funds and put the money into real estate. Banks prioritized real estate loans ahead of all traditional business activity; it was easier to calculate on a real estate deal. Over three years, bank loans increased by 350 billion crowns above the normal level. In small cities real estate speculators could point precisely to which official in the town's insurance office would buy their house and at what price. The rules under which insurance companies placed funds had also changed. Now they wanted to place their capital where it would earn more than in apartment obligations. Real estate provided an alternative. Housing prices rose to unheard of levels. And of all the money that inflated the real estate balloon, 80–90 percent came from the credit institutions themselves. . . . banks accounted for interest income—which they themselves financed—as income. . . . During 1985–89 the real estate market was like a pressure cooker. . . . The next step in deregulation was taken—deregulation of the foreign exchange market in 1989—created another shift, this time outside the country. Real estate entrepreneurs, who had earned a lot of money selling their holdings in insurance companies and funds, turned to Belgium and England with their newly obtained billions. . . . Within three years, 1989 to 1991, real estate and stocks overseas were acquired for 140 billion crowns, twice as much as foreign investment in manufacturing. . . .

The cause, fundamentally found among all actors, speculators, bank directors and insurance companies, was a solid conviction: first, that Swedish inflation would not be dramatically lowered; second, that if inflation, against all expectations, should radically decrease, interest would also decrease; and third, that if interest were not to sink the government and the National Bank would be forced to see that they did sink. A real interest rate—the rate minus inflation—of more than five percent was not only an unrealistic alternative. It was unthinkable. . . .

Actors in the real estate market were thinking rationally. But they made a mistake. The believed that the monetary policy was also rational.

Iran attacked Kuwait the second of August, 1990 and oil prices rose to 45 dollars a barrel. The party was over. (pp. 17–19)

The insolvency of the financial instruments meant that public resources had to be diverted to protecting depositors and that money that might otherwise be available for investment was missing. Both made public services more expensive to the society and dampened the potential of the private sector.

Unemployment

If Sweden had one achievement that set it apart from other developed countries in the middle of the twentieth century, it was its impressively low level of unemployment. The country had made an active labor policy its centerpiece, with income security the core of its social policy, and achieved the lowest unemployment rates in the developed world (Koblik, 1975; Milner, 1989; Bergström, 1992).

Since the depression of the 1930s, when Sweden's unemployment rate remained lower than the average of post–World War II rates for the United States, open unemployment in Sweden remained below 3 percent until the 1980s.[4] During the bourgeois government of 1976-1982, unemployment first rose above those limits. By 1982, it stood at just above 3 percent and was a major factor in the return of the Social Democrats to office. Unemployment then declined until 1989, rising again slightly in 1990 and sharply in 1991 (see Figure 5.3). That the Social Democratic Party had reduced its emphasis on full employment in the late 1980s was undoubtedly a factor in their electoral losses in 1992, when a coalition of bourgeois parties was returned to power under the leadership of the Conservatives. By 1993, unemployment was in double digits for the first time in the twentieth century. Unlike the situation in 1982, the mood in Sweden was one of passive acceptance.[5]

What is important is that almost everyone in Sweden was faced with a level of unemployment more than an order of magnitude higher than anything they had ever experienced before in their lives. While on the right there was a sense that high levels of unemployment were necessary to impose discipline on the labor force (see, e.g., Calmfors, 1993a; 1993b; Holmlund, 1993; Ståhl, 1993), on the left this was the major element of the crisis itself (see, e.g., Bergström and Löfgren, 1993, Lööf and Spånt, 1993a).

Budget Deficit

In 1991–1992, Sweden first posted a net budget deficit in the public sector. It was in the neighborhood of 10 to 15 percent of the gross national product and growing rapidly (Ekonomikommissionen, 1993, 42). Indeed, projections by economists on the right, under a variety of scenarios, suggested a growth of debt through the 1990s and, except in the best-case scenario, beyond (Figure 5.9). Economists on the center and left also saw the problem as the state debt grew from 500 billion crowns to 1,000 billion crowns in one year (Hamilton and Rolander, 1993, 119).

Figure 5.9
Public-Sector Debt (percent of GNP)

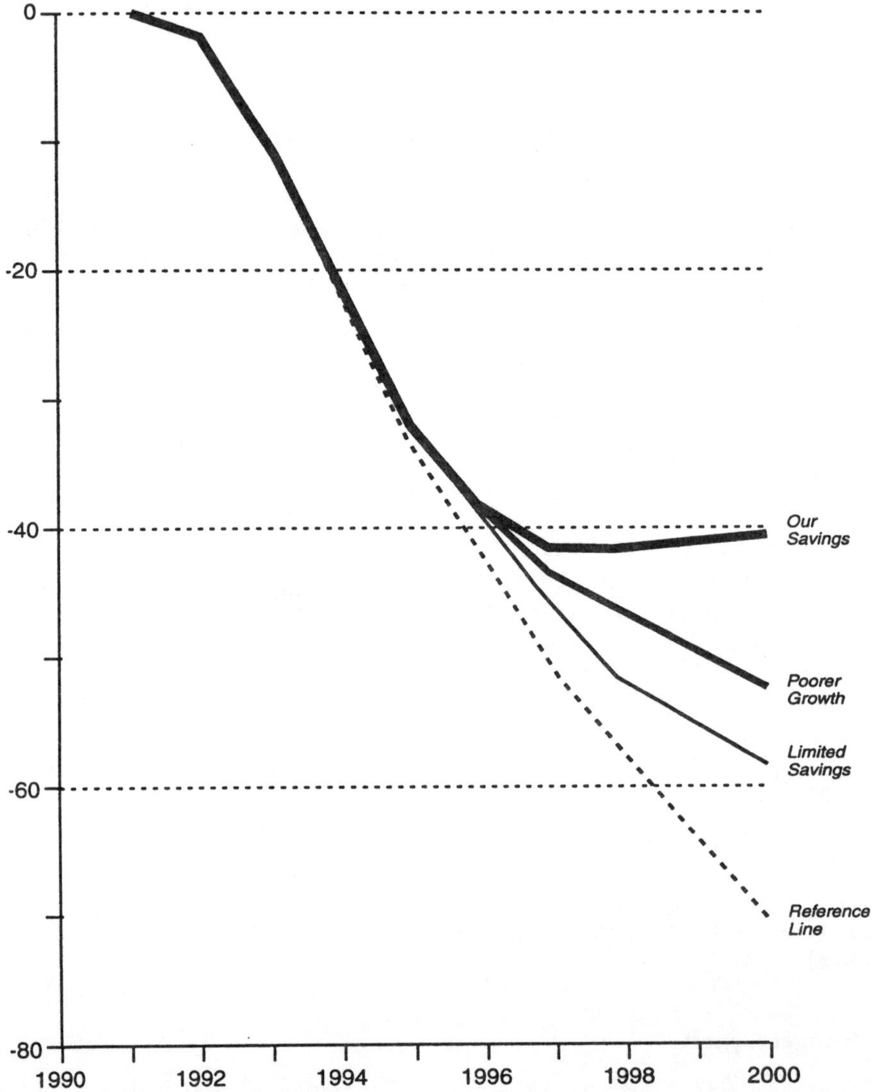

Source: SOU 1993: 16, *Nya Villkor för Ekonomi och Politik—Ekonomikommisionens Förslag* (Stockholm: Inrekesdepartmentet), 57.

As might be expected, there were different explanations of the cause of the debt and different prescriptions for solving the problem. On the right, economists and politicians pointed to the growth of public expenditures. As a percentage of GNP, total expenditure in the public sector had grown from approximately 50 percent in the late 1970s to approximately 65 percent in 1982, declined to the neighborhood of 60 percent in 1989, and thereafter increased (Figure 5.10). In the budget statement for 1992–1993, Finance Minister Anne Wibble (Ministry of Finance, 1992) pointed to the failure of devaluation policies, a lack of flexibility for businesses to adapt to a changing external environment which had delayed structural reforms, and the programs of the Social Democratic Party:

> For many years now economic development in Sweden has borne the mark of a policy that relied on collective, large-scale solutions. This has resulted in a regulated economy with imperfect competition, rising taxes and weak growth. Sweden has lagged behind. . . . More and more resources have gone to public activities, yet many people have not been able to obtain the service and assistance to which they are entitled. . . .
>
> Sweden needs a new policy that generates prosperity. Years of neglect of the growth-enhancing economic forces are to be succeeded by the stimulation of forces that yield prosperity. Instead of the earlier disparagement of enterprise, there is to be a commitment to the spirit of enterprise and creativity. The freedom of the individual and the family is to be widened.

On the left, the view was different. Labor economists noted in interviews in 1993 that the Social Democratic Party had abandoned Keynesian precepts and failed to generate sufficient savings during the expansionary period of the 1980s. They also pointed to a series of what they considered mistakes in both the public and private sectors, including the following:

- Deregulation of the credit market at the beginning of an expansion in 1985 contributed to the overheating of the economy.
- Deregulation of currency led to massive purchase of overpriced real estate in Europe by Swedish interests.
- Abandonment of a full employment policy at the beginning of the recession combined with a focus on fighting inflation.
- The timing of a tax cut generated a massive stimulation for savings at the cost of consumption just when the main economic problem was weak demand.
- Abandonment of policies (endorsed by bourgeois and socialist parties) to provide programs helping small business to meet demands for more technological competence, higher quality, and efficiency.
- Private concerns and investors made poor investment decisions (see section on "Real Estate and Banking Crisis").
- Decentralization of labor–management wage negotiations created wage inflation.
- The international depression made a deficit unavoidable (Lööf and Spånt, 1993a).
- A campaign against inflation after it had already been brought under control.
- The ideological rigidity of the 1991–1994 bourgeois government leading to a failure to seek pragmatic solutions to problems (Hamilton and Rolander, 1993).

Figure 5.10
Public-Sector Expenditures, 1950–1993 (percentage of GNP)

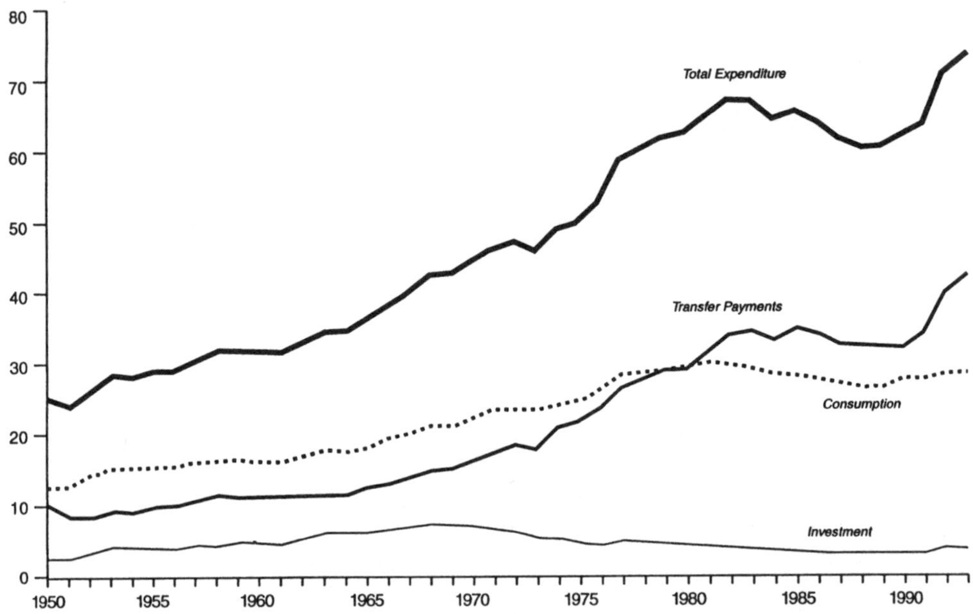

Source: SOU 1993: 16, *Nya Villkor för Ekonomi och Politik—Ekonomikommisionens Förslag* (Stockholm: Inrekesdepartmentet), 88.

On the right, the solution was to reduce the size of the government, particularly by deregulation, eliminate social support programs, and make others more "efficient." On the left, the solution was to make investments and expenditures to stimulate demand. The center was, by virtue of their coalition with the Conservatives in the government, tied to the economic policy of the right.

THE ECONOMIC CRISIS: ECONOMIC OR POLITICAL?

Tax Reform

In 1990, Sweden took the first step in what was described by the Finance Department as "the tax reform of the century" (Åsbrink, 1990). The reforms, which took effect on January 1, 1991, were primarily of the state income tax but also involved changes in value-added and environmental taxes. Coupled with the tax reforms were changes in state subsidies to families with young children and rent assistance for low-income people. Arguments for reform focused on the income taxes. The following assertions were highlighted by the Ministry of Finance:

- Taxes were too high. Sweden had the highest tax rates in the world. They encouraged people to make choices in favor of leisure time as opposed to work, part-time as opposed to full-time work, and education instead of work.
- The investments in commercial life were steered by tax advantages. Big businesses could invest more cheaply than small businesses. The tax structure made it better for individuals to keep stock in a business rather than take money out, encouraging businesses rather than individual investors to invest in other businesses.
- There were inconsistencies in the treatment of interest from outside investments and investments in one's own business as well as earnings from industrial versus other investments.
- Too much energy went into tax avoidance.

It was held that a changed tax system in which there were two levels of taxation, replacing one with several levels and a higher top marginal rate, would be more rational and less driven by inflation. Further, it would give individuals and businesses more power to change their economic situation. It was further held that the tax change would, by stimulating the economy, result in no net reduction in state revenues (Åsbrink, 1990). Sweden's GNP growth compared to OECD is shown in Table 5.2.

With regard to other taxes, the value added tax (MOMS) was broadened to include services and goods previously exempt from taxation. A new tax was levied against the production of carbon dioxide by levies against oil, coal, natural gas, and gasohol replacing earlier ones on coal and oil alone. The net result was a reduction in income taxes and an increase in consumption taxes. The distributional effects are not fully documented but in practice were probably not large, as exemptions for low income were raised and loopholes for the rich somewhat closed. The effects on the state budget were direct and immediate, leading, as similar reforms had in the United States and U.K., to a rapid, unprecedented, and large increase in the budget deficit.[6] Indeed, prior to the tax reform, the Swedish national budget was very close to being in balance. Afterward, the budget deficit was a major threat to the continued provision of public services at the levels Sweden had achieved.

Given this fact, the following statement in the 1992–1993 budget statement seems difficult to understand (Ministry of Finance, 1992):

> The Swedish tax system has been greatly improved by the tax reform, which lowered tax rates and made taxation considerably more uniform. Even so, the total taxation of an additional labor input is still too high in an international context. The taxation of capital also needs to be modified with reference to rates abroad. A successive lowering of tax pressure is therefor required. . . .
>
> Further measures will be taken to make Sweden more competitive for investment and enterprise, increase the stimulation of private saving and generally reduce taxes that are economically harmful. (p. 21)

Table 5.2
Annual Percentage of Growth of GNP, 1970–1993

	1970-93	1970-77	1978-86	1987-93
Sweden	1.5	1.7	2.1	0.2
OECD Countries	2.9	3.5	2.5	2.5
OECD European Countries	2.3	2.5	2.0	2.5

Source: Ekonomikomissionen, 1993, Bilaga 11, p. 353 which cited OECD Projections, 1992–1993 and OECD Economic Outlook, December, 1992.

That is, it is hard to understand unless one considers it in the context of the decision to enter the European Union, another political decision with long-range economic consequences.

The European Union

In 1993, Sweden was involved in a broad national debate over whether to join the European Union. The leaders of all political parties with representation in the *Riksdag*, with the exception of the left party, had agreed in 1990 that Sweden should seek membership. At that level, there was remarkable unity. Within each party, however, the majority of members opposed membership, indicating the decision had been taken by political elites who were not representing their constituencies on this issue.

Proponents of membership argued that closer economic ties with Europe would reduce the chances of war, promote economic growth, protect the environment, preserve Swedish influence in Europe, strengthen workers, promote social welfare, protect women's interests, and facilitate coordination of policies among nations. Opponents argued that membership would threaten world peace, not produce economic benefits, undermine environmental protection, cause a loss of international influence for Sweden, weaken workers, undermine social welfare standards, weaken women, cause loss of sovereignty, undermine democracy, undermine Swedish neutrality, undermine regional politics, undermine animal care standards, remove control over migration policy, reduce consumer protection, undermine public services, and undermine Swedish support of Third World countries.

With the exception of the effects of the European Union on coordination of policies, on which the opposition took no position, and on loss of sovereignty, animal care standards, consumer protection, quality of public services, and support of Third World countries, where the proponents took no position, the two sides were projecting diametrically opposed predictions on the consequences of membership. The issue was being hotly debated and there were few grounds for making informed choices between opposing positions.

The proponents prevailed, and in the fall of 1994, Swedes voted in a referendum to ratify membership in the European Union. Whether the Swedish economy will benefit from incorporation into the European economy, as the proponents predict, or be further marginalized by the power of the German economy, as the opponents contend, will be tested by history (Twaddle, 1997).

Irrespective of the impact of formal membership on the Swedish economy, it is beyond dispute that the increased integration of European economies had already been impacting Sweden for some time. Indeed, the European Union itself is but one manifestation of the internationalization of economies discussed in Chapter 2.[7]

For many years, the Swedish economy had been more and more closely integrated with Europe's. Swedes were investing more abroad and an increasing share of Swedish industry was in the "exposed" sector, competing directly with European countries. Indeed, it was the political pressure from these exposed industries that generated the move to join the European Union. This change generated increased concern about the competitiveness of Swedish companies in the international market and increased concern about the Swedish economy in comparison with other developed countries. The right wing noted that the growth of the Swedish economy was slower than that of other OECD countries and argued that Sweden was falling behind economically (e.g. Bildt, 1992; cf. Ekonomikommissionen, 1993). The rate of growth of the gross national product was slower (see Figure 5.8) and industrial production was increasing slower than in other OECD countries (Figure 5.11). At the same time, the left argued that the growth of the Swedish economy was keeping pace in absolute size adjusted for population and the rate of growth was equivalent to the most highly developed OECD countries (see Figure 5.1).

The state of the Swedish economy in international comparison looked quite different depending on how one looked at it. The right saw an urgent problem. The left saw structural changes that needed accommodation, but no crisis. From the right perspective, the highly developed welfare state, rather than being seen as an achievement in creating a just society, was a problem in that it demanded resources that made Sweden less competitive. Low levels of unemployment and a central system of collective bargaining became a problem to be overcome, rather than an achievement to be preserved, as in the left perspective. The right wanted wages to fall and for investment to be shifted from public social welfare to the private sector. These were the traditional battle lines between the Conservatives and the socialist bloc, with the center parties (predominantly the Liberals) seeking a position in support of both economic

Figure 5.11
Average Growth of GNP per Capita, 1979–1989, in Eighteen OECD Countries (in crowns, 1985 prices and exchange rates)

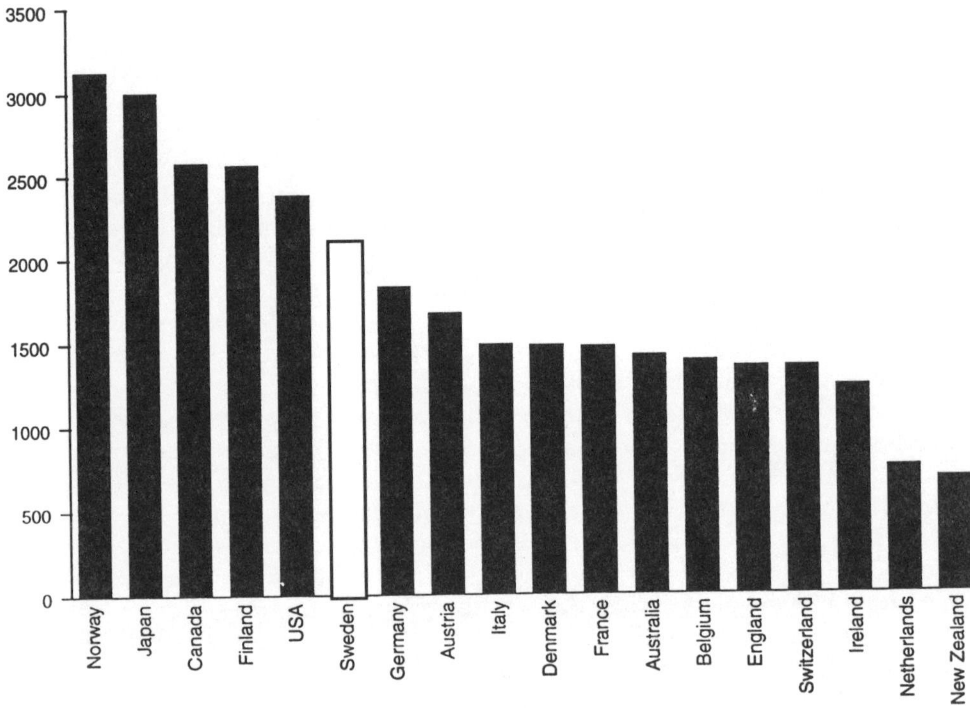

Source: Walter Korpi, 1992. *Halkar SverigeEfter: Sveriges Ekonomiska Tillväxt 1820–1990 i Jämförande Belysning* (Stockholm: Carlssons), 107.

growth, in which they supported Conservative policies, and a strong system of public welfare (Westerberg and Nordh, 1993).

THE POLITICS OF ECONOMIC THEORY

There was little debate over these issues in 1993. Indeed, Walter Korpi seemed to be virtually alone in challenging the assumptions and data of the Lindbeck Commission. Given the importance of the issues and the challenge they represented to traditional Social Democratic policies and programs, this seems surprising and in need of explanation. Why is it that national economists seemed to speak with one voice, that of the right, when the theoretical base they were operating from was not the only one nor was it the one that had been most influential in twentieth century economic thinking? Where were the Keynesians and Marxians? Given the long tradition of testing the assumptions of classical economic theory in sociology, where were the sociologists?

These questions were posed to our interview respondents, most of whom professed no answers to the questions, although most thought them "interesting." There were some exceptions, however. Bengt Mollstedt, president of the board of *Landstingsförbundet* and a Conservative politician, offered the view that centrist and leftist economists and sociologists had not "come forward" to join the debate. Implicit is the notion that they were free to make their voices heard and had no alternatives to offer. Sture Nordh, president of SKTF, offered a more sobering opinion. I asked him specifically why there was so little opposition to the just released Lindbeck Commission report. He responded, (1993–06–10),

> Walter Korpi is the only one, and I think this is very sad. We had the idea of trying to get in touch with some academics, researchers, to comment on the Lindbeck report. From their experience and knowledge stating exactly what you just said.[8] From their point of view what Lindbeck is stating is not as obviously true as he is trying to make it. It was not possible. . . . I don't know why. . . . My opinion is that the influence of how you get money, how you are financed as a researcher for your projects in Sweden is run by a couple of people, and those couple of people happen to be to quite some extent linked to Assar Lindbeck and other economists. I think quite a number of—at least younger ones—didn't dare.

While it was not possible to confirm this view, there were journalists who had reported efforts to exclude dissenting expert opinion from the debate. Per Lapins (1993) reported that in setting up commissions and expert groups there were specific instructions to exclude sociologists.[9] Sven Larsson (1993) reported on a specific case in which Lindbeck, as chief of the Institute for International Economics at Stockholm University, was said to have intervened to defund the research of Sven Grassman and to drive him from his academic appointment.

In an earlier paper drawing on published documents in the political debate (Twaddle, 1992), I noted the problem but had no answer. As summarized elsewhere (Twaddle, 1994b),

> While it was the case that the replacement of a Social Democratic government with a more right wing government made little difference in the direction or content of legislation over an eight month period, it was also clear that the proposals for change were coming from the Ministry of Health, the Federation of County Councils and the Physicians' Union, and were not supported by labor unions representing white collar or blue collar workers, or professional groups other than physicians. That paper raised questions about the absence of democratic debate, particularly the apparent abandonment of the Commission of Inquiry process and the absence of any defense of the Swedish model by the Social Democrats, who were widely believed to have created it. It also speculated about the absence of sociological input into the discussion.[10] (pp. 10–11)

The most persuasive scenario was offered by Johan Lönnroth (1993, Chapter 4), who provided a historical review of the structure of economics as a profession in which center and left positions became marginalized and excluded from the national debate. In his analysis, a "coordinated attack on the economic teachings of the new left" was organized by Lindbeck in a 1968 book which became quite influential, especially as he was then identified with the Social Democratic party. The "attack" was directed at the lack of appreciation of the market by the student movement, primarily in the United States.

Leftist viewpoints entered the universities and the representation of Marxist scholarship increased during the late 1960s and early 1970s. A debate was entered on the degree to which the market must steer economic development versus the degree to which it must be constrained, controlled, and limited. The issues crystallized in the 1970s with the Meidner proposals for "wage earner funds," which would give unions more control over investments in Swedish industry, what came to be called "fund socialism" on the right.

By the middle 1970s, there was an effort to marginalize the left in the economic debate. Neoliberals took control of the academic departments and limited employment opportunities for Keynesians and Marxists. In 1974, SNS was created as a think tank ideologically and economically linked to the SAF. From both SNS and the academic departments, now almost solidly neoliberal, came materials opposing Keynesianism. With the center and left lacking a power base, the debate became one sided. By the time the Lindbeck Commission report was issued, there was no effective opposition.[11]

What may be concluded from this is that the practice of economics in Sweden is highly ideological and the debate is one sided. Ideas put forward with no opposition are not adequately tested to be a firm foundation for public decision making. To the extent that some ideas and the data supporting them are suppressed, the debate lacks elementary integrity. Whether, or to what degree, such suppression is a fact is something we cannot judge with the evidence at hand. We can say that there is a widely held belief that such suppression exists and that center and left positions are being excluded.

There may be another dimension that may mitigate the distortions now found in Swedish economic discourse. The changes in the political/economic debate came very suddenly. The center and left were unprepared to debate issues they thought had been settled long ago. Indeed, one got a sense in interviews that those on the left were disorganized and confused and were just then, in 1993, beginning to mobilize counterarguments to the neoliberal hegemony. It was not until late spring 1993, that a group convened by the Social Democratic party issued a response to the proposed neoliberal reform of public services (SAP, 1993), and later in the year before a popular magazine published a reassertion of the relevance of Keynes—and that was written by a foreigner (Galbraith, 1993).

THE NATURE OF THE ECONOMIC CRISIS: AN ASSESSMENT

There is no dispute that Sweden had a serious short-term economic problem in 1993, the time of this study. The basic elements of that problem have been described and involved serious weaknesses in the state budget debt, the international debt, the financial institutions, and the real estate market. Nor is there dispute over the fact that the possible scope of public action was at least temporarily constrained by those problems.

There was dispute over the nature of the problem, whether it was long term, involving fundamental structural defects and requiring a change of direction, or whether it was a short-term crisis that was amenable to a more vigorous application of traditional Keynesian means. The case for a long-term structural problem was best made by the Lindbeck Commission. They contended that the collectivist approach of the Social Democratic governments in building a strong public-sector constituted "decades of mismanagement" that required reduction of public sector programs, an increase of investment in export industry, and a reduction of the scope of democratic decision making. Growth of GNP was too slow, employment levels too high. Only more "freedom of choice" and greater scope for the market could solve the problems. The strong welfare state was a mistake. Equality and security were weakening the economy and had to be reversed. This was the view of the government in power.

The center–left, represented by some labor-union economists, was skeptical, saying the economy was basically sound, although some past decisions had created serious short-term problems. The recession could be managed by stimulating demand. The bank and real estate problems were already coming under control. Unemployment would take some time to manage, but it required a reassertion of policies abandoned by the present government. As expressed by Jan Edling (1993), Head of the Political Economy Unit at LO,

> We have been trying to be a lone country for a long time while the rest of Europe has been adopting new kinds of economic policies, for example fighting inflation instead of having full employment. We kept to the full employment concept for a long time . . . through the '70s and the '80s while European countries in the EC, and also the United States, have adopted the other kind of policy. We have been doing many things trying to avoid going over to that kind of European policy. For example, in 1982 we had to devalue our crown. The reason for doing that was to make it possible to make the economy function better and to make full

employment possible and also to finance the welfare state by many people paying taxes. We did this through the '80s and we had full employment; we had over-employment, maybe. . . .

You can see that from the 1960s labor has made a better market all the time. You have improved wages; you have improved the welfare state in many ways. But something is happening after 1975, especially after 1980. Capital is gaining again from the deregulation in the work market and things like that. What's happening is that it is becoming a tougher time for government to finance the welfare state, because the money, labor costs, is what is really financing the welfare state. . . .

The parties that are running Sweden at the moment, they try to make a structural reform of the whole public sector. You have also to understand what kind of thoughts they have behind this philosophy. I think the philosophy is to make the welfare state not so big as it used to be and not supporting every situation people could come up with. Instead, they want to have a welfare state where the state provides the basic things and where people have to find their own solutions for the rest of the things. They are going down from a general welfare state to some kind of basic welfare state. The meaning is that we should get insurance or maybe more hospital fees on top of that basic level. . . . You should not have general high levels of social security; you should have low levels and if you want more, you should make your own social security system or make your employer negotiate with you about it.

LO economist Per-Olof Edin (1993) offered the following view:

There is always a level of interest rate which gives balance in total income and expenditure. The problem is that we can't come down to that level when we have deregulated the currency market and credit market and, totally international, we depend on what other countries do, in Europe especially. So you have to combine the solution with other means, but first of all you must do everything you can by monetary policy. It's a classical crisis. The problem is everyone seems to have forgotten what it looked like back in the '20s and early '30s. . . . We must use Keynesian methods to deal with it.

Earlier they said we must by law forbid the use of Keynesian policy. The fundamental solution was to . . . use monetary policy to expand the economy. It was the basic policy to divide the central bank from the political system, isolate it and give it to the professional banking system. . . . And give it only one task, fight inflation. Most economists wanted to introduce that system in Sweden. Even . . . Kjell-Olof Feldt fell for that kind of reasoning. But now, all of them have shifted, saying in this situation we have to use something that will expand the economy.

Not even Assar Lindbeck can say the reason behind this acute crisis we have today is the public sector problem. But he would claim we also have some very difficult long term problems not reflected in the deficit of the state budget or . . . the unemployment situation. Therefore we have to cut down the public sector by 10%. Then we have to strengthen the economic incentives by giving lower taxation to higher capital income, a lower level of insurance for unemployed persons and so on. I have asked him, you can't mean you do that and that will improve the state budget situation. "No, of course not," he says. There are other reasons he wants to do it. But in the political discussion in Sweden, of course, the government uses the crisis to blame it on. But I have asked Assar Lindbeck, "you prefer and reason for a cut in the level of unemployment insurance, but you can't think that will improve the money situation." "No, of course not," he says. But the government says we have to do it to better the situation in the state budget.

The acute crisis is being used to change the system. They learned that from Thatcher. Back in '88, they got balance in the state budget in Great Britain. They also came down from thirteen to eight percent unemployment and people thought now the crisis is over. Even a Conservative majority in Parliament stopped cutting social benefits in Britain. They couldn't do it. So you have to use the crisis. They have not created the crisis, but when you have this type of crisis you must take strong, hard, important, long-term decisions. . . . Therefore in the public and even some economic discussions you have a mix of this acute crisis situation and a long term problem and all economists have a common view of the reasons behind the acute crisis, what to do about it. But we have totally different views about if we have a long-term crisis and what to do about it. There you have political tensions between different economists.

I asked Edin if there was a long-term crisis. He responded as follows:

No. Most economists in Sweden are Conservative, bourgeoisie. They, of course, have . . . done all they can to prove the big public sector creates weaker growth in GDP. They have tried to prove that. They say it all the time, but, in fact they have been forced to admit that you can't prove it, but you can believe it—that it makes disincentives to work. OK, how many adults in Sweden will work if we can offer them a job? It shows that back in 1988–89 adults in Sweden worked more than in any other country in Europe. Japanese worked more and the U.S. people worked as much as in Sweden. So they can't show it. But, of course if you are bourgeois and want to reduce the public sector instead you talk about efficiency. We have always said you could improve efficiency, even in the public sector. As a whole, for example, the health and welfare system or medical care system in Sweden seems to be very efficient compared, at least, to all private systems in the world. They have to admit that. Then they say, of course you can do a privatized system very stupidly. In the U.S. you have done the most stupid system. No economist in Sweden can say the U.S. has solved the problem in a good way today. . . . No, it shows no overall sign to be good. The distribution of medical care isn't as good as in most European countries and the cost is even higher. . . . Most economists know how to solve the acute crisis. Then, we have a totally different view of whether we have a long term crisis if you have too big a public sector.

Anders Forsman (1993), head of the Department of Social and Economic Affairs for TCO, stated the case even more boldly: "I have pretty much the same view as P-O Edin. I think it's a political matter. Under this economic debate are huge differences, political views. Lindbeck will cut public spending down to 45% or something and we won't. We can afford a decent health care system. We can afford decent schools and social insurance. We are still one of the richest countries."

The short-term crisis was real. The long-term crisis seemed to have its origins in ideology and political agendas, not scientific analysis.

THE ECONOMY AND MEDICAL CARE REFORM

We now return to our core question: Is there a crisis in the Swedish economy that requires the public medical care system be reduced—made more competitive internally, exposed to market pressures, and privatized? From what we have seen so far, it would seem that if a case is to be made it must be with respect to the immediate short-term crisis. We must show that the recession and the budget deficit are generating a shortfall in the funds used to finance medical care. The other components of the crisis (inflation and the solvency of financial institutions) were generally thought by all economists to be under control (although the right said that control of inflation was only temporary). The effects of unemployment were indirect, somewhat increasing the levels of disease in the population while dramatically increasing levels of illness and sickness.[12]

Economic Pressures for Reform

Whatever economic pressures there were with respect to other parts of the welfare state, it would be hard to make a case that the medical care system had to be scaled back on economic grounds. This does not mean a case could not be made. Certainly, the rapid increase in the percentage of aged people in the population would be expected to exert strong cost pressures. Sweden had the highest percentage of elderly people of any country in the world and the proportion was increasing. Certainly, the development and introduction of new, expensive technology could also be expected to exert strong cost pressures as well. Especially in a country where the medical care system is as tied to hospitals as in the Swedish case one might expect these trends to be resulting in greatly increased expense in relation to the carrying capacity of the society.

Yet the actual cost of medical care as a percentage of GNP had been declining for a decade. In part this was a function of the strong growth of the economy during the early and middle 1980s, in part it was the result of the Dagmar Reform, which limited the private practice of medicine, and in part it was because of an expanded primary care system that shifted much medical care out of expensive hospital environments and into relatively cheaper ambulatory care settings. For the most part, these reforms reduced costs while maintaining quality.

Another reform that saved money was the Ädel Reform, which transferred responsibility for care of the aged from the counties to the municipalities. In this case, the shrinkage of expenditures and the deskilling of personnel resulted in a sharp decline in the quality of nursing home care in the large cities. While contributing to reduced medical care costs, that reform reduced the quality of the "product" as well.

It would be hard to argue that the state budget deficit did not pose short-term difficulties in funding public services, particularly if those services were themselves generating budgetary shortfalls. The fact is, however, that they were not. The funding of medical care is largely through transfer payments and the transfer budgets remained in balance throughout the crisis. The problem with the state budget was not to be found in the social service sector.

The Sufficiency of the Economic Imperative

The case that reform of medical care was made necessary by a crisis in the economy, then, could not be sustained. There was indeed a short-term crisis in the economy, but it did not directly or indirectly impinge on the capacity of the country to sustain high-quality medical services. Indeed, if all other sectors had done as well in reducing expenditures in relation to GNP, Sweden would have had a surplus sufficient to afford a large expansion of the welfare state.

The pressures for market reforms involving competition and privatization could not be made on economic grounds. As many economists told us, they were fundamentally ideological. The source of those pressures, then, must be sought in the political system, to which we turn in Chapter 6.

NOTES

1. This phrase was repeated verbatim by almost everyone who held this position.

2. The arguments among economists have been going on for several decades around neoliberal, Keynesian, and Marxian perspectives. These correspond to some degree to right, center, and left positions, but the linkage with political positions is inexact. Only the Conservative Party has been consistently neoliberal over the past several decades. The Social Democratic Party has been Keynesian and the Left Party a mix of Marxian and Keynesian perspectives. On most issues, the Liberal Party and the Center Party have been Keynesian as well. Much of the argument among economists has been technical as well as ideological. For a sampling of opinion from a technical standpoint, the reader is referred to Bergström (1993) which reprints articles from *Ekonomisk Debatt*. For a review of the ideological arguments, see Lönnroth (1993).

3. After a devaluation of the crown in 1982.

4. In measuring labor-force participation, "open" unemployment refers to those persons who are drawing unemployment compensation. It does not include those in job retraining programs, subsidized work, or on early pensions as a result of their unemployablity. Factoring these participants into the "active labor market" programs would, of course, increase the percentage of unemployed. Definitions in all countries result in underestimates of unemployment. In the United States, for example, those too discouraged to actively seek work in a given three-week period are counted as no longer in the labor force.

5. We will return to this in Chapter 6.

6. The reform in Sweden was far from unprecedented. The United States under the Reagan administration and the U.K. under the Thatcher administration had both instituted tax reforms of a similar nature. In both instances, disastrous budget deficits were the result. The apparent blindness of Swedish economists and politicians to that experience seems incredible to an outside observer.

7. The WTO and NAFTA treaties are part of the same process.

8. I had just observed, "When I read the Lindbeck Commission report, I made five or six pages just listing assertions of fact that are directly contradicted by research in my field that I know about."

9. This is a serious charge. If true, it would mean a serious breach of the norms of academic freedom and bring suspicion about the integrity of the commission and expert-group process.

10. Some interesting thoughts on the abandonment of the Swedish model by the Social Democrats are to be found in Augustsson and Hansén (1991), Gröning, Korpi, Nilsson, Ström, Wibe, Arvidsson, Bäck, Pinheiro, Åmark (1993), and Wickbom (1989).

11. This summary glosses a much more detailed and nuanced presentation. The reader is urged to read Lönnroth's fourth chapter for a more adequate review of this argument.

12. On the distinctions between disease, illness, and sickness, see Twaddle and Nordenfelt (1994).

Chapter 6

The Political Crisis

In previous chapters, we have explored two themes that have dominated the discourse in Sweden on health care reform. One was that there were structural problems in the medical care system that made it no longer possible to meet the needs of the population without a major change in organization. The charge was that the system was inefficient and needed more market-oriented processes to make it more efficient. While we found evidence of inefficiencies, particularly in the provision of elective services to the populations in need of them, major structural changes were not needed to solve the problems. Some very simple reforms had successfully eliminated long queues for elective surgery and the bed blockers in geriatric care. Indeed, there is nothing in the literature to suggest that market-oriented reforms (competition, privatization) can improve efficiency without damaging effectiveness or equity.

The other theme was that the economy had become so stagnant and the cost of services had increased so dramatically that, even while the medical care system was excellent and posed few structural problems, the nation could no longer afford to carry such an expensive program. Market mechanisms, primarily competition but also to some degree privatization, could relieve the public budget of a major source of strain, reduce the total cost of services, and manage demand better. The research literature does not provide support for this line of reasoning (although there are theoretical arguments in neoliberal economic theory that seemed to have taken precedence over the evidence). Again, there seemed to be no reason the problems could not be solved within the framework of the existing Swedish model.

If the structure of medical care and the robustness of the economy both posed problems for medical care organization, and there was no doubt that they did, they appeared to be problems that presented, at best, necessary arguments for reform. Neither alone nor together could they be argued to be sufficient. That is, while they raised issues that were plausible reasons for promoting reform, they could not explain the ideological direction that the reform debate took between 1989 and 1994: why the dialogue shifted from one framed in terms of solidarity, planning, and equity to one framed in terms of markets, competition, and privatization. To seek that explanation, we turn now from the medical care and economic systems to the political system.

We explore two trends that may be sufficient to explain the shift in discourse. The first is the demise of the Social Democrats. It is certainly the case that the Social Democratic Party (SAP) became weaker between 1975 and 1994. Since they were the party that most vigorously promoted the growth of the welfare state, including as a (if not the) major component the public system of medical care, a weakening of their political position would simultaneously weaken support for medical care as a universal system.[1]

The second trend is the rise of the right. Only partly as a corollary of the weakening of the Social Democrats, the right wing of the Swedish political spectrum had gained power. Indeed, during the period that is the focus of this study the *Moderaterna Samlingspartiet* dominated the political debate. Their agenda always had been to reduce the welfare state and organize economic activity through markets, competition, and privatization. While during the period from the 1930s through the 1980s their agenda was at the margin of Swedish politics (even during a center–right coalition government from 1976 to 1982), by the late 1980s until at least 1994 it was at the center of Swedish politics. It is that shift that we need to understand.

THE DEMISE OF THE SOCIAL DEMOCRATS

> In 1969 the Social Democrats were a majority party, with over half the electorate behind them. Few signs in the sky foretold any threat to their dominant position in the whole Swedish society.
>
> In 1969, the Social Democrats were an ideological party, which was guided by the dreams and visions of the class struggle. In 1989, pragmatism was in control.
>
> In 1969 questions of distribution stood in the foreground. Growth took care of itself. In 1989, growth was the dominant question. Distribution was taken care of by already enacted reforms and by the voracious giant of the "demand machine."
>
> In 1969 the catchword was socializing or nationalization or in any case social influence. In 1989 one talks openly of privatizing care, child care and TV. (Wickbom, 1989, 16–17)

While it would be an overstatement to say that the Swedish model of the welfare state was the creation of the Social Democratic Party (Uddhammar, 1993), it is clearly the case that the party was a major force in its development (Esping-Andersen, 1985; 1990; Hadenius, 1988). In collaboration with the labor movement, the Social Democrats actively promoted programs for job security, income protection, and worker participation in economic decision making in what has come to be known as the active labor market. Unemployment insurance, job retraining, programs for linking workers with jobs, and pensions were at the core of that development. In addition, the extensions of educational opportunity, medical care, and a variety of family support programs were promoted as investments in the future of the society (Myrdal, 1982). Particularly the pension system, support to families with children, child care, taxation policy, housing policy, redistribution at the municipal level, and foreign aid were enacted with broad support across the political spectrum (Uddhammar, 1993).

Clearly, the development and maintenance of a strong welfare state is powerfully influenced, if not determined, by strong left–labor political parties (Bäck and Möller, 1990; Esping-Andersen, 1985; 1990; Korpi, 1978; cf. Terbörn, 1978) . The weakening of such parties seems to be associated with a lessening commitment to the welfare state in one of two not mutually exclusive ways: It may reflect a lower level of public support for the welfare state or it may provide an opening for more right-of-center ideologies and programs to gain political power.

Indeed, it seemed to be the case that the Social Democratic Party had lost strength since the early 1970s. In 1976, they lost control of the government for the first time since 1932. At that time, a coalition of the Center, Liberal, and Conservative parties assumed power under the leadership of the Center Party. They returned to power from 1982 to 1991, when they were replaced by another center–right coalition, this time of the Conservative, Christian Democratic, Center, and Liberal Parties under the leadership of the Conservatives. While no frontal challenges to the socialist programs were mounted during the 1976–1982 period, the 1991–1994 government was notably interested in rolling back the welfare state by substituting markets, competition, and privatization for the principles of solidarity, planning, and equality. That is to say, there was an important ideological shift in the direction of the welfare state.

With reference to the medical care system, this shift was evident at a conference at Högberga, organized by Johan Calltorp in 1990. The rhetoric of markets and competition dominated that meeting, at which seven foreign scholars who had studied the medical care system met with leading politician, planners, researchers, and administrators from Sweden.[2] Several reforms had taken place, mostly under the Social Democrats between 1982 (the new Health and Sickness Care Law of 1982) and 1984 (the Dagmar Reform), both of which were reviewed in Chapters 1 and 4 and will be discussed again in Chapter 7.

Our task here is to explore what happened between 1982 and 1993 to cause this ideological and political shift. I argue that two major changes occurred within the Social Democratic Party that resulted in a loss of commitment to their traditional program and a weakening of ties with the labor movement (at least partially alienating its traditional constituency while failing to make gains with other sectors of the population).

First, several of the leading intellectuals within the party became increasingly concerned with the development of a centralized state bureaucracy and wrote critiques of the impact of that bureaucracy on the traditional core value of the socialist movement, democracy. Gunnar Myrdal's 1982 book, *Hur styrs landet?* provides a good illustration.

Second, when the Social Democrats returned to power in 1982, their finance minister, Kjell-Olof Feldt, and a group of national economists gathered in the finance ministry took the position that the growth of the welfare state threatened the integrity of the national economy. They pulled back from the traditional support of the welfare system and argued that it had to be made smaller and more efficient to allow the state budget to be brought under control after the "irresponsible" management of the center–right government between 1976 and 1982 (Feldt, 1991). This was seen widely as an abandonment of Keynesianism and an adoption of neoliberal economic theory. One result was that the Social Democrats were seen as moving to the right and accepting the critiques and programs of the center and right parties. Another was a feeling of abandonment by the labor movement and a large degree of working-class abstention from the 1991 election.

Gunnar Myrdal and the Critique of Centralization

In his remarkable book, Gunnar Myrdal (1982) presented a hard critique of trends in Swedish society. Myrdal, who was a labor economist, a member of the "Stockholm group" of national economists who laid the groundwork for Keynesianism, and a sometime participant in Social Democratic governments, offered the thesis that the programs initiated to promote and expand democracy had in fact produced less democratic institutions.[3] His general thesis might be glossed as follows:

- Programs were created to meet real needs of people, needs that were not being met in the private market economy or were being met in a way that provided opportunity to only a socioeconomic elite, denying equal opportunity to others. Among these, singled out only as examples, are the cooperative movement, highway construction, housing construction, medical care, and higher education. In their initial stages, those programs were small in scale, oriented toward local communities, and subject to considerable local influence structured in ways that increased the influence of middle- and low-income persons. They were much closer to being governed by "direct democracy."

- Over time, as the institutions grew in size, they became more centralized, covering larger geographic areas and promulgating a standard of service that was more uniform over those areas. The result was that decisions were made in settings more removed from local communities and ordinary people had less influence over the content of the programs and the conditions under which services were delivered. As events played out, huge national bureaucracies governed most programs. They were removed from, and increasingly insensitive to, local conditions and needs.
- As programs grew, collective discussion and consensus were replaced by decision making by designated decision makers who were specially trained for their role. In the early days, most of those who were charged with executive authority "came up through the ranks." They had begun with menial jobs and gradually assumed more responsibility. They had a first-hand knowledge in their own biographies of the problems faced by those at the grass roots level and a capacity to envision the needs their programs were addressing. More recently, people with professional training, most often with no grassroots experience, were entering decision-making levels directly from college or university programs. To them, the conditions and needs at the grass roots were abstract and second or third hand and their proposals were generalizations not grounded in experience.[4]
- Even while ideologically committed to making the society more equal, such programs were increasingly developed and governed by a large, centralized bureaucracy far removed from the everyday experience of those they are intended to serve. What is lost is not only the close connection between programs and the lives of ordinary people, but the process of collective decision making: democracy itself. The grass roots have become more passive and take less of a role in managing their own lives. The vitality of the nation is reduced.

While this analysis could be made by anarchist or neoliberal critics, and varieties of the arguments have been offered from those sectors, it is important to see that the solution Myrdal offered is a strong set of universal public programs, flexibly interpreted and adapted to local conditions by local people. Indeed, over the past two decades at least, decentralization has been the overarching Swedish program, leading Odin Andersson, the "dean" of researchers in social science research on medical care in Sweden, to observe, "I think it is important to note that Swedes tend to solve all of their problems by decentralizing."[5]

Of particular interest in the context of this project is Myrdal's (1982) discussion of the centralization of medical care in large hospitals. He began this brief discussion with a statement that he understood some of the technical advantages of the large hospital, but still had misgivings about it. He contrasted the movement in the United States to develop a more sophisticated family medicine with a move in Sweden to expand numbers but reduce sophistication: "The Board for Continuing Medical Education [*Nämnden för Läkares Vidareutbildning*] whose majority as usual consists of bureaucrats—representatives of hospital directors, the national board of medicine and Chancellery offices—has proposed a shortening of general medicine education, this in opposition to a unified physician corps of both specialists and general physicians" (p. 35). This is something he saw as a general tendency among bureaucratic decision makers, to "systematically bring all specially trained people to a lower level of training." Whatever the technical advantages of specialists, they could not deal with all of the health needs of patients. Well-trained generalists were essential: "To return to the main question, I am willing to accept our large hospitals, among other reasons because they already exist. But I do not understand the antagonism toward the small hospitals we already have or should create as a complement" (p. 35). Small hospitals have strong advantages, he wrote. They are cheap. Long term patients can remain close to home, friends, and relatives. Closing them is irrational on both economic and humanitarian grounds.

When Myrdal (1982) questioned a friend in the medical department he found that the decisions were made by bureaucrats in the hospital department: "This, that departments in our bureaucratized society often block each other, is another fact of which I have many examples" (p. 36).

Medical care provided but one example in which the growth of bureaucracy had undermined democratic process by centralizing decision making for ever larger geographic districts in the hands of decision makers who operated independently of, and sometimes in opposition to, the will of the people. It was part of a process in which grassroots democracy was seriously undermined and ordinary people no longer saw themselves as being among the decision makers.

Myrdal (1982) developed several examples in much more detail than he did the case of medical care. He devoted entire chapters to the large university, the development of municipal governments after the reforms of 1959 and 1962, and the new constitution establishing a unicameral legislature. He examined some of the history of the modern development in the Stockholm School of economists (e.g., Cassel, Heckscher, Wicksell, Lindahl, Ohlin, and Myrdal), the policy decisions of the Social Democratic party and how they might have gone differently (e.g., schools, agriculture, population policy, housing, women's issues), the centrality of Albin, Möller, and Wigforss to the development of SAP policies, and the work of various commissions in the 1940s.

This argument, in different forms, was picked up (without attribution) by the post-1982 "Chancellery House Right" of the Social Democratic government under Kjell-Olof Feldt, who led the party in a critique of social-welfare policies and an attempt to scale back the state investment in welfare. This was seen by right-wing politicians and bureaucrats as a "more realistic" group within the Social Democratic Party. For example, one professional interest group leader remarked, "He belonged to what is called in Swedish the '*kanslihushögern*.' Within the Social Democratic Party he was a more pragmatic type" (Twaddle, 1994b, 19).

It was seen by many union leaders as an abandonment of the working class. One interpretation was that the Social Democrats had capitulated to the analysis of the Conservatives. As expressed by one union president,

> The main attack on the system was an ideological attack. . . . They succeeded because people feel we do not have the kind of economic growth that we were used to . . . and for the first time there was an argument. There was a discussion. There was an alternative. Ulf Adelsohn, as the former leader of the Conservative Party, now Carl Bildt stating and all the others stating, "Hey, we've got the solution. What has to be done is reduce taxes. We have to have the market work more efficiently. We have the world's highest taxes. We have a system of public services that is extremely inefficient and the burden of that inefficiency is killing our industry, the base."
>
> This was the international wave. I mean you've seen it in your country, you've seen it in Great Britain. . . . Everyone can see that it didn't work in your countries. . . .
>
> There is a mainstream . . . of ideas about the difficulties and the problems and how they should be solved. And the room for other views in media is very very small. . . . The attitude toward the trade union movement is "Hey, we know your opinions. We know your attitudes; why should we publish your point of view?"

As we shall see further on, the argument was also picked up by the right wing of Swedish politics, which accepted the critique without accepting the goal of improving the democratic process except by the identification of "democracy" with the "market."

Kjell-Olof Feldt and the Chancellery Right Wing

After the enactment of the Supplementary Pension program in 1968, the Social Democrats lacked a single core proposal to serve as a centerpiece of their policy. Attention shifted from issues focused on distribution to the economy itself. The most important new initiative came from a "democracy at work" proposal offered by LO in its 1971 convention. That proposal was to limit the power of employers at the workplace.

Several pieces of legislation followed: the Security of Employment Act of 1974 (*Lag om anställningsskydd*; LAS), the 1974 Act Concerning Certain Employment-Promoting Measures (*Lag om vissa anstälningsfrämande åtgärder*), the 1974 Act Concerning the Status of Shop Stewards (*Lag om facklig förtroendemans ställning på arbetsplatsen*; FL), the 1977 Act on Employee Participation in Decision Making (*Lag om medbestäm-*

mande i arbetslivet; MBL), all of which were intended to enhance the power of the worker at the expense of management (Hadenius, 1988). The net effect, however, was to galvanize employers, as we will see.

At this time, when the Social Democrats had no single issue that galvanized its traditional constituency, several events weakened their public standing:

- The 1967 party congress placed emphasis on government initiatives to make business more competitive, introducing "capitalistic" arguments for state initiatives.
- In May 1968, students occupied the Student Union at Stockholm University to protest what was seen as a business-oriented higher-education reform package, attracting little public sympathy.
- The miners in northern Sweden staged a wildcat strike in 1969, starting a wave of such strikes, saying the state-owned company "was not only sucking the mine workers dry but northern Sweden as well" (Hadenius, 1988, 131). The government became just another employer and the class struggle was framed in opposition to the Social Democrats.
- The Soviet Union invaded Czechoslovakia in August 1968 in the midst of a Swedish election campaign, making many party rallies anti-Soviet protest meetings. Social Democrats were portrayed as having a weak stand on opposition to Soviet oppression (Hadenius, 1988).
- The government took foreign policy positions in opposition to the United States in Vietnam, leaving them open to criticism—on the one hand for not providing more open support for the Vietnamese guerrillas and on the other for not taking a similar stand vis-à-vis the Soviet Union in Eastern Europe.
- Between 1970 and 1973, there were new concerns about the shrinking industrial sector and the danger of an adverse balance of payments. Credit policy was tightened. Tax reforms reduced marginal income tax rates.
- In 1973, the international oil crisis hit Sweden especially hard because it had no oil reserves of its own. Rather than cut back on programs, the government and some of the opposition parties reached the "Haga agreement . . . which cut State taxes and increased employer social insurance contributions in an effort to pave the way for labor–management contracts in which pay raises would not be eaten up by taxes and inflation" (Hadenius, 1988, 135).

As the 1976 election campaign began, the Social Democrats not only lacked a core issue that would mobilize their constituency, but also were weakened by attacks coming from both the left and the right. The 1976 elections were framed around two issues that had not been on the national political agenda before: nuclear power and wage-earner funds. While much of the population was passionate about each of those issues, the Social Democrats were internally divided and had no public position on either (Hadenius, 1988). The result was a small loss at the polls for the Social Democrats and a small gain for the nonsocialist parties. It was enough to send the Social Democrats into opposition for the first time in forty-four years.

During the period between 1976 and 1982, when the Social Democrats were out of government, a bourgeois government held power, consisted initially of the Center, Liberal, and Conservative parties, with the Center holding the Prime Minster's portfolio. When that government collapsed over the nuclear power question (the Center withdrew), the Liberals formed a single-party minority government. During this period, the economy showed signs of difficulty. Unemployment rose, but even more "Was the sharply rising deficit in the budget as well as the fact that the state under bourgeois aegis had started to borrow abroad. Especially for an older generation of Social Democrats 'living on borrowing' was synonymous with a decadent and irresponsible lifestyle" (Feldt, 1991, 19).

According to Kjell-Olof Feldt's (1991) memoir, the Social Democrats formed a Crisis Group to frame a long-term policy should they return to power in 1982.[6] By 1980, they had reached two conclusions:

> One was that Swedish industry found itself in a serious structural crisis caused in part by strong increases in the cost of wages, which led to poor returns and lowered competitive power, and in part by external factors such as the energy crisis and the weak investment market in West Europe. . . .
>
> The other conclusion was that neither the Swedish economy nor a Social Democratic government would be able to survive with a budget deficit of the size that we, with considerable prudence, could forecast for 1982. Everyone agreed that the standing compromise in the coalition government would lead to a rapid growth of state expenditures at the same time the will was lacking to finance them with sufficiently high taxes. With the weak growth of the economy and growing unemployment, higher taxes would in any event have made things worse.
>
> In the Crisis Group we agreed that the key to solving Sweden's economic problem lay in shaping the conditions for a new period of industrial expansion in our country (pp. 20–21).

In 1980, according to Elmbrant (1993), Keynesians and non-Keynesians carried equal weight in the economic debates, but within a few years there had been a massive shift toward a neoliberal stance: "The great majority of Sweden's economists had capitulated to the Friedmanesque spirit of the age and offered now in all essentials the same kinds of analyses and recommendations" (p. 73). Effective debate on economic policy came to a virtual end.

Of core importance for medical care, economic opinion turned against welfare services. In an article in the labor-oriented newspaper, *Arbetet*, on February 18, 1981, six Social Democratic economists published a *debatt* article entitled, "Here is the Drastic Cure." A shift in core position was evident in the following statement: "In plain language this means, unfortunately, that one must cut back on development plans for care, child care, and education, at the same time we must drastically cut back some of the large system of transfer payments" (Elmbrant, 1993, 74).

Documents prepared for the 1982 election focused on improving the profitability of industry, introducing wage-earner funds, and reforming the tax system.[7] A campaign against inflation would be needed to return to full employment.[8] "Naturally there were proposals for increased state inputs, but they 'must be of the character that they strengthen the land's productive capacity and improve possibilities to deal with the large deficit in the economy'" (Feldt, 1991, 22). Even more to the point, the Crisis Group actively sought input on a proposal to

- restore a "waiting day" for sickness insurance.
- increase mobility in the labor market.
- institute a two-hour-longer work week over several years.
- reduce the right to leave from work with maintenance of wages.
- close unprofitable companies to make space for new, competitive ones.
- prune transfers such as pensions, child support allowances, grocery supports, and housing allowances (Elmbrant, 1993, 75–76).

This line of thinking did not become the platform of the Social Democrats in 1981. Their campaign program, *Framtid för Sverige*, was a balanced mix of Keynesian and liberal economics, and affirmed traditional party values. Indeed, Palme campaigned against neoliberal threats to the Swedish model. He promised higher support for unemployment compensation and municipal child care, reinstatement of support for the value of pensions, and removal of the waiting day in sickness insurance (Elmbrant, 1993; cf. Feldt, 1991).

Nevertheless, neoliberal policies were enacted by the new government. Among their first acts was a 16 percent devaluation of the crown (following on a 10 percent devaluation by the previous bourgeois government), which unleashed speculation, stimulated international trade, and supported the import of luxury goods. The well-off benefited. The working class did not. Wages were held down by agreement with LO and workers lost the equivalent of a month's wages. A second economic initiative, also taken from the neoliberal book, was an attempt to set norms for price increases. A third was the proposal that Sweden "work and save itself out of the crisis." Priority was placed on the budget deficit. State expenditures on social programs were cut by almost 5 percent; state investment was cut (Elmbrant, 1993; cf. Feldt, 1991). Indeed, the main thrust of the mandate period was the promotion of traditional Conservative policies, with one important exception: the wage-earner funds. These funds were to shift investment from international speculation to Swedish industry, thus generating jobs in Sweden. They were also a means of placing new economic power in the hands of representatives of working-class interests. On both counts, the funds qualified as progressive legislation. Over strong objections from the Swedish Employers' Association and the Conservative Party, they became law (Feldt, 1991; Elmbrant, 1993).

As luck would have it, the Social Democrats assumed government responsibility at the time of an international upturn. During their first mandate period, unemployment fell and inflation generated additional revenues, bringing the budget deficit under control. As preparation for the 1985 election began, Ingvar Carlsson, who would become prime minister upon Olof Palme's murder in less than two years, put forward a proposal to the party leadership that the party should run on the issue of freedom of choice, particularly in medical care, education, and child care. As the Conservatives campaigned openly on the issue of a "system shift" that would reverse the trends of the past four decades, that became the focus of the election. The Social Democrats won handily by supporting the Swedish model (Elmbrant, 1993). Yet after the election, the Social Democrats continued on the course they had set during the previous mandate period.

As presented by Feldt (1991), who held the finance portfolio in the Social Democratic government from 1982 to 1990, the party had not changed its focus. It still supported full employment and, indeed, through the wage-earner funds was expanding the economic power of workers. What had changed were the conditions. Partly as a result of the shock waves centered on the oil crisis and the international adjustments it required, partly as a result of the incompetence and mismanagement of the bourgeois coalition government, and partly as a result of long-term socioeconomic changes, the means for achieving traditional socialist goals had to change. Without sufficient growth and profitability there is no long-term possibility for high employment. Without low inflation, wage gains are ephemeral. What was needed was a "third way" between the traditional Social Democratic policies and the neoliberal policies of the Conservatives. As seen by observers from outside the party, however,

> The third way's policies were nothing less than a system change with a Social Democratic signature. The workers' party pursued openly and consistently a policy that favored commerce at the expense of the public sector, that favored stockholders at the expense of the employed and which formed an entirely new class of capitalists: Coupon clippers, real estate sharks, finance puppies and all "yuppies" who lived well on the crumbs of the transaction economy's boom-party. (Wickbom, 1989, 43)

By the time of the preparation for the 1991 elections, the transition was virtually complete. The campaign program, entitled *90-tals Programmet*, was one in which Keynesianism had all but disappeared. The core program was fighting inflation, controlling interest rates, holding taxes down, and reducing the size of the public sector. Every economic proposal was taken from core tenants of neoliberal economic theory. While there was language on the need to defend the weak and maintain a good standard of service, there were no proposals specifically to enhance the quality or extent of public services.

The proposals for health and medical care were embedded in a general critique of social services, which were seen as too centralized and undifferentiated. The general programmatic thrust was to limit politicians to setting goals and leaving to the personnel at each level to decide how those goals would be met. Decentralization of decision making would be from national to county to municipal levels of government and from politicians to the workers. A greater variety of service organization would be encouraged, giving the public more choice of settings and personnel. Particular problems noted with reference to medical care were as follows:

- Everyone can not get the care they wanted.
- There are obvious class differences in health status.
- Within medical care we find personnel shortages, queues, differences in care, and growing costs in some areas.
- Many patients have difficulty locating the right sources. They feel deserted and forgotten in a large and impersonal care system (Leijon, Feldt, Malm, Molin, Toresson, Andersson, Edin, and Eklund, 1989, 215).

Particularly in long-term care, the boundary between medical care and social services should be flexible, making a trial of decentralizing medical care of the aged from counties to municipalities desirable. Municipalities already had responsibility for social services. Further, the document advocated a trial in which the municipalities took responsibility for primary medical care, contracting with the counties for specialist and hospital services. Primary care needed expansion to provide a more humane oversight of health needs and better continuity of services.

The role of politicians should be more limited:

> The role of the central state power is to set overall and national goals of good quality and access to care and to see that possibilities and methods for assessment are shaped. The Department of Health and Welfare should have a new and important role. The local politician's duty should then be to choose which units should produce which medical care services and to make demands on hospitals and care centers to fulfill the demand for quality. (Leijon, Feldt, Malm, Molin, Toresson, Andersson, Edin, and Eklund, 1989, 216)

While flatly rejecting privatization as a solution, on the grounds that it would lead to increased class differences in quality and access, the report endorsed the introduction of market mechanisms into the public sector:

The duty of the hospital . . . is to provide the different *buyers* with good care. A single hospital can serve several *buyers*—municipalities in their own catchment areas, other municipalities, the social insurance office, local rehabilitation programs, et cetera—with different medical services. Production and finance responsibilities should be more clearly divided than today. That gives a clearer division of responsibility and better stimulus to improved care. It is also important that the municipal politicians who oversee the provision of medical services demand assessments of results from hospitals, clinics and care centers. (Leijon, Feldt, Malm, Molin, Toresson, Andersson, Edin, and Eklund, 1989, 217, emphasis added)

It is clear that by 1989, the leadership of the Social Democratic Party had bought into markets and competition as a solution to the problems of the welfare state. The only thing that distinguished them from the right in this area was that they still drew the line at privatization.

This narrative can go on, and the reader is referred to Elmbrant's (1993) remarkable book for more detail and for a fuller account of the "fall of the Swedish model." Perhaps what we have presented is enough to have made the point that however else one might look at it, the economic program of the Social Democrats had become markedly different from the one that had characterized the history of the party. Putting the priority on industrial profits and fighting inflation were traditionally hallmarks of conservative economic thinking. Socialists had always focused on full employment, equity, and job security. Socialists had worked to build public programs, not to reduce them (e.g. Elmbrant, 1993; cf. Feldt, 1991).

From outside the government, however, things looked quite different. Conservatives welcomed the "new realism" of the Finance Ministry, seeing the change as a shift from a less "ideological" to a more "neutral" and "scientific" stance. We will return this theme when we discuss the rise of the right.

Where Did My Party Go?

The left, having depended on the Social Democratic Party to manifest "socialist principles," was appalled, seeing the change as an abandonment of working-class interests in favor of a Conservative neoliberal stance. The aftermath of the 1985 election was an open breech between the Social Democratic Party and the LO, characterized as the "War of the Roses." Worker participation in the 1991 election dropped, as many Social Democrats wondered aloud where their party had gone.

After the 1982 election, LO "played ball" with the new Social Democratic government by agreeing to hold down wage demands and, indeed, accepting a short-term decline in compensation for workers. The rationale was that the government had inherited a large national debt and needed both time and some economic slack to accomplish needed restructuring. LO remained quiet, making no public protest on behalf of the Social Democrats for the 1985 campaign.

When, after the election, the government made it apparent that wage restraint and the prioritizing of inflation over unemployment was to be a long-range policy, Stig Malm, the president of LO, went public. The trigger was the budget proposal. It stated a plan for a three-million-crown reduction in state support to municipalities and an increase of twenty crowns in individual contributions to unemployment insurance. In both instances, the government adopted points from Conservative proposals the Social Democrats had opposed in the election (Elmbrant, 1993, 118). According to Elmbrant, "Stig Malm's mouth moved like the rump of a lamb. The budget was Conservative, he said, and repeated annoying slogans from the election campaign that Sweden needed a Social Democratic government. He exhorted LO's people in the parliamentary group to raise the daily compensation for unemployment. This revolutionary flag was one of the few incidents where the special interests of unions made themselves apparent" (p. 118).

Following Palme's assassination, when the budget deficit was clearly coming down, word was leaked that "everyone was thinking in the same direction" about a possible tax reduction. Kjell-Olof Feldt issued a memorandum showing what a tax reform might look like and a parliamentary Commission of Inquiry was appointed. Malm became more strident during the spring and summer of 1987. It was now he coined words such as "casino economics":

> "Feldt's policy has placed Capital in a position where they lack opposition in modern times," he said.
>
> LO's President had also stated that there was no urgency about any marginal tax reductions, but Feldt should rather take the country's finance puppies by the ear.
>
> "Finance puppies," that was Malm's inspired phrase for the Swedish money market, the hundreds of 25–30 year olds in white suits who from a number of stock brokerages in central Stockholm placed 35–40 billion crowns a day alone in trade in state paper.
>
> The modern stock and money market had gotten wind in its sails from devaluation and the budget deficit. Industry could book record profits and the stock market spiraled up. . . . The money market had gotten a kick forward by deregulation. . . . Stig Malm's phrase "finance puppies" had touched a very Swedish and Lutheran nerve. (Elmbrant, 1993, 157–58)

Very clearly, organized blue-collar labor, which had for a hundred years worked hand in hand with the Social Democratic Party to build the Swedish model, no longer saw the party as unambiguously representing its interests. A breach had formed. LO officials no longer felt they had a party representing them.[9] The feeling that the Social Democrats had moved away from socialist principles could be found among rank-and-file union members as well. At issue was whether the Social Democrats had become a bourgeois party. The official ties of the LO members to the Social Democratic Party, which had existed throughout the century, were strained. The leadership of LO still wanted to maintain collective membership in the party, but for the blue-collar union of public employees (Kommunalarbetareförbundet) things had gone too far. When the LO leadership failed to oppose a proposed wage freeze for 1990, Lillemor Arvidsson, the first female president of an LO union, resigned "collectively and individually" from the Social Democratic Party in protest (Elmbrant, 1993, 217).

Lars Åke Augustsson and Stig Hansén (1991) interviewed a number of Social Democratic leaders, labor leaders, and economists about the meaning of the concept "socialism" among those tied to a party that had made that definition problematic. There were a range of answers, with "traditional" socialists focused on justice, full employment, security, and strong public services," and "revisionists" focused on adapting to secular trends, competitiveness, internationalization, and the like. The fundamental division was best articulated by Sten Andersson, who was speaking in the context of growing class differences in Sweden:

> If our movement gives up our fundamental goals and principles for election tactics we are lost. Moreover, I am convinced that way down deep in the people, way down in the bourgeois leadership they do not like such great differences.
>
> Even if it should come to the point where Social Democrats became a 25% party or smaller, we must still be prepared to stand up for our principles and our vision of humanity. I dislike the reasoning that is put forward by our leaders, that the middle class has now grown so much that we must become a middle class party. (Augustsson and Hansén, 1991, 16–17)

There were also attempts by a number of people to enter a public debate to bring the Social Democrats back to their principles. One of these may serve to illustrate. Gröning et al. (1993) published a set of *debatt* articles dealing with the demise of the Social Democrats in the 1991 election.[10]

Gröning set forth the problem by asserting that during the 1980s the traditional Social Democratic voter could no longer "recognize the party." The SAP was "dominated by inflation, productivity, budget deficit and a strong economy. . . . The economy has played a key role and become a goal instead of a means and thereby the Social Democrats have lost the purely human" (p. 11). The conclusion of many was, "It is unimportant who holds the power of government because we no longer see any differences" (p. 11). Those advocating a return to the Right Party politics of the 1920s are "new thinkers." While the Social Democrats did need to rethink whether the state should do everything, they did not have to abandon solidarity. The party should have taken the quality of life as an ideological issue.

Walter Korpi analyzed election data to show that in 1990 the Social Democrats had held only a minority of their 1988 adherents. Most of those who failed to vote for the socialists did not move to other parties, but cast blank ballots. The 1991 election, then, was not a center–right gain as much as a Social Democratic loss. As he showed,

> The Social Democratic government was very successful when it came to reducing unemployment. But this strategy with the great devaluation and high industrial profit required that the unions should hold back their members' wage growth. When that strategy became permanent after the 1985 election this weakness began to become apparent. In a period of full employment, growing wage differences, dramatic increases in the value of stocks, deregulating the banks, and unrestrained speculation in real estate, the strategy was reinstated, cooling off and the sacrifice of wage earners. (Gröning et al., 1993, 37)

Full employment was the defining issue for the Social Democrats. When they abandoned it as a goal, their voters no longer recognized the party.

Carina Nilsson, a researcher for LO, held that the Social Democrats had withdrawn from their historic relationship with organized labor. The party was under pressure from the employers, who had withdrawn from central negotiations on wages, work environment, and occupational health, a campaign by the Conservatives and Liberals to define labor as a "selfish special interest." Economists, who had always had a strong voice in Social Democratic governments, became so dominant that others

> declined to express viewpoints on most things, seldom on grounds of knowledge, but often with a reactionary direction. With their macro perspective on life, it is difficult to see the underlying causes in work life for growing medical care costs and reductions in productivity.
>
> Social Democracy's dependence on economists has meant that economics has become the goal and not the means for improving people's lives. . . .
>
> A society with growth and high productivity is a base, but not a guarantee, for the good society. (Gröning et al., 1993, 58)

Social welfare programs, particularly with respect to working conditions, medical care and sickness insurance, were being scaled back. Instead of universal programs, many Social Democrats in government were adopting the Liberal view that such programs should be limited to the weak. That is, they should be means tested. What was needed was an affirmation of the benefits of these programs for everyone.

Martin Ström, a member of the Metal Workers' Union, noted the strong tradition of democratic decision making had been abandoned. While study groups in the labor movement were discussing the need for modification of tax policy, for example, the leaders of the Social Democrats came to an agreement with the Liberals linking their policy to the market. The democratic process in social movements, such as labor, was both a political base for the Social Democrats and an alternative to "egoism" and the free market. When the Social Democrats abandoned that process, workers became passive and withdrew from politics. The politics of protest became more dominant, leading to the defection of Social Democratic voters to the populist right-wing New Democratic Party in 1985.

The historian Klas Åmark presented a much more complex analysis of the impact of social change on the Social Democratic Party, making it much more difficult for them to identify and maintain an electoral majority with a clear and consistent ideological line. His argument may be glossed as follows:

The post–World War II economic expansion coupled with the policies of the Social Democrats transformed Sweden from a "poverty state" to a "welfare state." Between 1950 and 1970, real incomes for metal workers increased two and a half times:

> apartments became modern, spacious, equipped with bathrooms, refrigerators and freezers and with access to modern washrooms. Schools were constructed and instead of six years in a "folk school" working class children now went to 11 years of school before they entered the factories. The welfare state was constructed quickly with state health insurance (1955), Supplementary pensions (1958), municipal child care, parental leave, five weeks of vacation and 40 hour workweeks, etc. (Gröning et al., 1993, 126)

The success of the society in raising the standard of living for wage earners had several consequences that undermined the commitment of workers to the very party that generated their improved living standard. More and more they identified themselves, not as working class but as some variant of middle class. In 1950, Segerstedt and Lundquist conducted the first sociological study of *People in Industrial Society*, in which they reported that 80 percent identified themselves with the working class. A majority saw workers and white-collar wage earners as holding political power. A replication of that study in 1987–1988 showed a majority identifying with some variant of middle class, even while 75 percent expressed a preference for a "socialist party." Political power was said to be in the hands of a small elite. That elite included the leadership of the Social Democratic Party, which no longer was seen to be their representatives and spokespersons. The leadership of the party was "up there" in contrast to "we workers down here."

The growth of the welfare state expanded public-sector employment. This was where women were added to the labor force; it shifted the role of the Social Democrats in worker–employer relations, and it meant a new set of dependencies. As government, national, county, and municipal, became the major employer, the leaders of that government became cast into the role of employers, often in an adversarial relationship with workers. Further, the development of the welfare state increased the freedom of workers and

> gave them an independence that they had not had before: they became less dependent on their parents or children, they became more independent in relation to their employers, whether public or private. It is not the case that it is only the market that gives individual freedom—it is often precisely the opposite. But the welfare state creates in any event new socio-economic dependency relationships, new political constellations, and new differences in interests. (Gröning et al., 1993, 132)

Immigration changed with the economic expansion and labor shortage of the 1960s. By 1980, one in seven people in Sweden were of immigrant background. Instead of most coming from Finland, active recruitment shifted to the Third World. Multinationalism became a fact. Internally, there had been a great shift of population from rural and small-town environs to the large cities.

New divisions in the society cut across the class divisions. These included public versus private employees, men and women, generations, large city and smaller places, and native versus immigrant (including a new problem of racism). The Social Democratic Party was

> built before everything else on two bases. First was the labor movement, which mobilized a large part of the working class behind itself election after election. . . . Second, the SAP was successful in its choice of alliance partners in politics. From the 1930s until the mid 1950s the party governed in more or less organized cooperation with the Farm Alliance. The Supplementary Pension question became the departure point where the party changed alliance from the farmers to service workers. (Gröning et al., 1993, 134)

Since the 1950s, the possibilities for a unified and coherent policy had changed and worsened:

> Then the tendency toward centralization was still strong; the influence of the state over both commerce and municipalities and counties grew; a centrally steered regulation influenced ever more of life in Sweden. Then came the challenge of the 1970s crisis—that it is the large program, the strict central regulation of commerce, the labor market—and the public sector began to be seriously questioned.
>
> The politicians' solution to difficulty in directly steering the land became a combination of decentralization of decisions and a softening of the central regulations. "Frame laws" became the contemporary solution. . . . But decentralization implied as well differentiation and differences. . . .
>
> Differentiation included a spreading of the income distribution. It also meant "individual citizens more frequently have to fight for their rights," with results dependent on the power they could mobilize. Instead of a unified set of labor

interests, the constituency of the party had "split up into a string of different groups with different interests, cultures, world views, and assessment patterns." (Gröning et al., 1993, 138)

The party was faced with two conflicting tendencies, tradition or modernization. In the "War of the Roses," Kjell-Olof Feldt represented the modernization side: Social Democrats as employers and directors. Stig Malm represented the traditional side: Social Democrats as promoters of equity and solidarity. Those forces were in a standoff, with serious negative consequences for either option: loss of identity as a socialist party or an increasingly problematic relationship to a shrinking constituency.

In all this, it is important to recognize that labor was not in total opposition to changes in the Swedish Model. Indeed, many labor leaders interviewed recognized serious problems that needed new solutions, including making the public bureaucracies more responsive and efficient, improving the profitability of industry, containing the cost of public services, and the like. This appreciation extended to the rank-and-file membership, as expressed by a local youth leader who was active in SKAF:

Sweden couldn't stand up against the outside too long. We did it after the Second World War, but we can't do it now. We got into the international business in the 1980s with the Social Democratic Party's help. Now we're in the middle of it, and when you have less profit in the industry you have to do another system to increase the profit for the industry. I think this is one of the basics—to increase profit in the industry, to move money from the *transfereringsystemet*—where you pay tax and get it back in the form of transfer payments—you move money from that system to other systems, more private systems in a higher speed than before. I think that's a great motive behind this change. . . . Sweden had to change basic industries. We had an export of steel, wood. We had cars. We have a big defense industry. And all these basic industries have to change now because we haven't sold enough. And that's a crisis; that's about low profits, but that's not about the system. . . . Now you try to save the industry and don't put pressure on the industry to change. You have to—in the first place you put money in the bank. They are kaput. The banks are kaput, every Swedish bank. . . . All the Swedish money is out on the streets in Bonn and Brussels and now they want more money—the savings money is gone and they want more money from the taxpayers. . . . I think that's the wrong way, to take money from social welfare and put it in the banks, put it in industry without putting pressure on the, . . . make demands on them to do this and this. . . . You make lots of demands on us, that we are going to think in another way, that we are going to produce other things. OK, we will do it, but not the industry. We don't put the same pressure on the industry We only give them money. (Twaddle, 1994b, 96–97)

In summary, the Social Democratic Party lost power, certainly hegemony and perhaps even legitimacy, not only with the population at the center and right of the political spectrum, but more importantly, with its own constituency, the labor movement. It was seen to abandon support for the welfare state and socialist principles. Perhaps more important, it was seen as changing without meaningful involvement of labor interests. The analysis of events by organized labor organizations was not considered in moving toward a more neoliberal policy. Instead, the party relied for information on economists and other analysts who were traditionally tied to the right of the political spectrum. Labor not only failed to dominate, it was no longer at the table. In adopting a more conservative stance in this way, the Social Democrats alienated their constituency, leaving no opposition to a sharp swing to the right.

This, however, accounts for only part of the changing political climate. Another important element was the impressive growth of ever more conservative and even extreme right-wing points of view in political debates.

THE RISE OF THE RIGHT

During the 1940s, 1950s, and 1960s, the Conservative Party was an active cooperating participant in the development of the welfare state. Even while the Social Democrats took a leading role in making proposals, it is nevertheless the case that they worked across party lines and developed a consensus. On questions of pensions (both the basic pension in 1948 and the supplementary pensions in 1960), support for families for children (1947), child care (1943),[11] tax redistribution among municipalities (1957 and 1961), foreign aid (1952), a progressive income tax (1947), social planning and construction (1947), and state ownership of key infrastructure (1949 and later), the Conservative party entered into negotiations with the Social Democrats, reached compromises, and voted for the legislation (Uddhammar, 1993).

By the 1970s, there had been a change, and the Conservative Party increasingly took a line in opposition to the welfare state, seeking not only to limit its growth, but to reverse the trends toward increased regulation of commerce, expansion of worker rights, and the expansion of planned public services. The new line was that a less-regulated market was more "efficient" and would provide greater economic growth and better ensure the high Swedish standard of living.

We will explore three types of activity: an offensive launched by the Swedish Employers Association to create an ideological shift in the debate, the activity of the center-dominated nonsocialist government of 1976–1982 and the election campaign of 1991, and the activity of the conservative-dominated nonsocialist government of 1992–1994.

The Employers' Offensive

The 1970s was the time, according to Hadenius (1988), of the "Directors Revolt," which "assembled more and more power oriented against government policies, against fundamental Social Democratic values, and against the right of the social movements to decide the conditions of social debate." The revolt had two slogans: "freedom and growth," which in the 1960s had been labeled "profit and selfishness" (Wickbom, 1989, 37).

According to Wickbom and to informants in the labor movement, the shift came at the initiative of SAF. They entered into a long-term strategy to change the mind-set of Swedish culture by framing the public debate, preparing "educational materials," and distributing them to teachers in the compulsory schools.[12] The debate was framed as "Profits are needed for our prosperity! It is just to be competent! Take care of yourself! Creative Sweden!" (Wickbom, 1989, 37). The materials consisted of stories designed to teach neoliberal economic theory and celebrate the values of free-market ideology. This became the center of a massive public-relations effort about "economic realities." In the words of a local SKAF official,

> I think the Swedish employers, SAF, learned their lessons from American capitalists in the late 1960s and the beginning of the 1970s. They were out . . . in universities to teach how to tackle mass media. They were out in Switzerland for courses on how to tackle the trade unions. They have had 20 years of preparation in . . . *problemformuleringsinitiativ*. . . . The party that first puts out the question will always win. And they did it in 1971 and they hit the schools—*grundskolan*—with massive material and I think they are only cashing in the profit now in the 1990s, from what they did in the 70s. . . . And that's . . . one of the reasons that all of us think, "Yes, we're in a crisis. We have to dress differently, We have to save money . . . and so on." Twenty years of indoctrination. (Twaddle, 1994, 97–98)

Wickbom (1989) also called the "70s offensive . . . broader and deeper" than earlier collaborative efforts of industrial leaders. A "Director's Club, consisting of the heads of the five largest Swedish corporations,[13] had been formed in 1973 and had provided discrete support to non-socialist parties." They were the nucleus of a much more active political role in which they mobilized the Swedish Employers Association. "It was broader in its use of such American propaganda instruments that the parties had not yet learned to use. It was deeper in its ideological ties to the stream that would be called Reaganomics and Thatcherism" (p. 38). The Directors Club/SAF initiative provided the platform "for the propaganda apparatus that today to a great extent shapes the Swedish debate and which strongly influenced the bourgeois governing policy" (Bresky, Scherman, and Schmid, cited in Wickbom, 1989, 38).

One important development was the creation of an organization called the "New Welfare" (*Den Nya Välfärden*) by Patrik Engellau, a business consultant, and Rune Berggren, former head of the state auditor's office. It was financed by the SAF-owned Fund for Commerce (*Näringslivets Fond*). This think tank, while officially independent, was a promoter of neoliberal arguments for reduced public welfare programs and lower taxes (Engellau, 1987; Elmbrant, 1993, 256–57). The work of this group became important in the 1991 election, as we will see.

We may presume that "20 years of indoctrination" must have had an effect on public consciousness, serving to both undermine socialist constructions of reality and to legitimate those of the business community. Of critical importance was the unilateral withdrawal of the employers from the Saltsjöbaden accord, regarded as the core of the Swedish model. In 1938, the peak organizations of employers and workers had worked out a system where they came to "central agreements" on the general level of wage increases for the year. The employers and unions were then obligated to negotiate within those limits. The 1938 agreement had come about to avoid the threat of legislative solutions to labor market problems.

In 1990, the workers' organizations (LO and TCO) proposed a two-year agreement as a contribution to stabilization:

> The Swedish Employers' Association flatly said no. SAF was against all forms of central negotiations. Wage negotiations belonged in the factories, they said. . . . Then Ulf Laurin of SAF phoned back to Prime Minister Carlsson and proposed, surprisingly, a legislated wage freeze. In exchange SAF would accept a price freeze and a freeze on stock dividends.
>
> The proposal was in many ways very strange coming from the employers. SAF wanted to decentralize wage negotiations. Can one think of a more centralized model than a wage freeze? (Elmbrant, 1993, 215)

According to Feldt (1991),

> The central question was if the parties were prepared to quickly sign an agreement for both 1990 and 1991 which stated that wages would not be raised in 1990 because of the tax reform's effects on prices and that the negotiations for 1991 would "take full account of the tax reform's effects on wage earners' disposable incomes."
>
> As far as I knew, the Swedish Employers' Association would say no because their most influential organization, the Manufacturing Association, now always declined to be subservient to SAF's negotiators and wanted to negotiate on their own. (p. 455)

With this change, the key to the Swedish model was destroyed. Without central wage negations, the policy of wage solidarity was undermined. The employers divided the labor movement into the discrete unions, which had less power independently than they did collectively. They were able to exploit the weakness of the socialists and drove a wedge between the Social Democratic party and the blue-collar unions.

The Centrist NonSocialist Government of 1976–1982

Through the 1960s, the bourgeois parties were not only in opposition to the Social Democrats, but also sharply divided among themselves. As all were small by comparison to the Social Democrats, they had no credibility with the electorate as possible heads of government. That changed in the early 1970s, as the parties directly addressed their capacity to govern: "The non-socialist parties had not agreed in advance on any government program, but had considered it sufficient to declare that they were prepared to take responsibility to govern together. The so-called middle parties—Center and Liberals—stated that they could accept sharing power with the Moderates because the middle parties would dominate the Government and their program would provide the guidelines for Government policy (Hadenius, 1988, 145).

At least two new issues were found in the 1976 campaign, one of which, nuclear energy, did not fit the old left–right divisions. Sweden had built several nuclear power plants and another was soon scheduled to come on line. Here, the Center Party, and its leader, Thorbjörn Fälldin, took its stand: "Fälldin linked his opposition to nuclear power with other ecological issues. He depicted the Social Democrats as advocates of an unwieldy, inhuman society which posed major hazards to ordinary people and accorded higher priority to growth and profitability than to quality of life" (Hadenius, 1988, 144). Fälldin pledged that he would never sit in a government that fueled a new atomic plant.

Another major new issue was wage-earner funds, which was more a traditional left–right issue. It was one not developed by the Social Democrats at the time of the campaign, however. LO had proposed a form of "excess profits" tax on large corporations to be managed by labor representatives for investment in Swedish industry. The idea was to increase investment in Swedish industry and at the same time enhance the power of workers in the economy. The Social Democrats took no position on the proposal, in part because it came shortly before the campaign and they had not had time to study it.

Nevertheless, a campaign against "fund socialism" was mounted by the Conservatives and to some degree the Liberals as an attack on economic freedom. They portrayed it as a Social Democratic program. Since neither the socialists nor worker organizations other than LO had studied the issue, and even LO did not mount a campaign on its behalf, the attacks went unanswered.

There were other issues in the campaign, including some minor scandals involving government officials. Olof Palme took a rather strident ideological stand which alienated many voters and which undermined the cooperation that characterized the political process in Sweden. The Social Democrats were thought to be arrogant, seeing themselves as having a mandate to govern that was assumed rather than sought, and they were portrayed successfully as an inflexible "concrete party" (Wickbom, 1989).

In the 1976 election, a three-party nonsocialist coalition assumed control of the government under the leadership of the Center Party. Coalition partners were the Liberals and the Conservatives. The Social Democrats went into opposition for the first time since 1932. As the Liberals and Center Party were generally in favor of a strong welfare state, differing from the Social Democrats primarily on the way in which it should be structured, and they were the strong partners in the coalition, the government did not mount a frontal challenge to the Swedish model. The Conservatives, who may have been willing to offer such a challenge, lacked the clout to make a serious effort at implementing their program. The result was that the government tinkered with health and welfare programs, making few substantive changes. Another way of looking at this is that the middle parties, the Center and Liberals, were anxious to counter the Social Democratic charge that they would dismantle social welfare by protecting social programs and distancing themselves from the right-wing Conservative Party.

In any event, the government pursued an essentially Social Democratic economic policy, trying to deal with industries in crisis. Unemployment was rising. Many of the traditional basic industries were being undercut by foreign competition or lost their markets for other reasons, leading to a perception that fundamental restructuring was urgent. As expressed by Wickbom (1989), "the ship had sprung a leak. All that could be done was to pump and plug the worst holes" (p. 41). There was no time to forge a new, bourgeois-oriented policy.

The new government was divided on the nuclear power issue. The Center Party had positioned itself as an antinuclear party, which would not participate in a government that authorized the fueling of any new atomic energy plant. While they initially waffled on that issue when the next plant came on line, they ultimately resigned from the cabinet. The Liberals refused to go into coalition with the Conservatives and formed a minority government. The Three Mile Island catastrophe in the United States threw the Social Democrats into confusion. A decision was taken to have a public referendum after the next election.

The core issue in the 1979 election, once the nuclear power issue was removed, was the wage-earner funds. This time, the Social Democrats supported them. In addition, the Conservatives campaigned aggressively for a reduction in marginal tax rates. Both the Social Democrats and the Conservatives gained in the election, but the left–right split still favored the bourgeois bloc. A three-party nonsocialist government was formed again after the 1979 elections, with the Center party again in the leadership position (Hadenius, 1988).

The main activity of the government was coping with the recession. Government revenues fell, but expenditures did not. Large budget deficits were financed by borrowing abroad. The governing parties were divided among themselves, with the Conservative Economic Affairs minister favoring tax reductions and the middle parties seeking a broader accommodation, including the nongoverning parties.

Against all expectations, the government and the Social Democrats did manage to agree on a three-stage cut in marginal tax rates in exchange for partial elimination of income tax deductions on the interest paid for home mortgages and the like: "This put the Moderates in a precarious situation. Should they accept the agreement and thereby give in on an issue that was perhaps their most important one in maintaining their political image? Or should they resign from the Cabinet in protest, thereby once again demonstrating that the three non-socialist parties were incapable of reaching agreements within a Government?" (Hadenius, 1988, 154). They chose to resign, creating the third governing combination in five years.

The only initiative in the health arena was an effort to enact a *husläkare* bill (SOU, 1978, 74). A commission of inquiry was formed with a directive to propose means of countering the trend toward high technology and highly specialized hospital care by shifting the emphasis in medical care toward ambulatory care. These were widely acknowledged needs, going back at least to the Höjer Commission report in 1948. That commission proposed "that ambulatory care outside the hospitals be built up step by step to a point-of-service primary care physician system in accordance with the Commission's proposed models." The models included the development of care centers (*vårdcentraler*), expansion of training opportunities for general physicians, retraining programs for other specialists to change to general medicine, and studies directed at expanding primary care as a proportion of all care (SOU, 1978, 74). Prior to that report, decisions had already been taken administratively to cap specialty training outside of general practice, geriatrics, and psychiatry while expanding the size of medical school classes. The intent was that a much larger proportion of medical students would be forced into general practice.

The proposal did not have the full support of the governing parties. The Conservatives, perhaps reflecting the opposition of the Swedish Medical Association, opposed it. The Center Party supported the existing system and saw no need for changes. The Liberals stood alone and their proposal was never acted upon. With the return of the Social Democrats to power in 1982, it went onto the back burner.

The Social Democrats entered the 1991 election seriously weakened. Their policies seemed to follow traditional bourgeois proposals. The 1991 election campaign was framed to make it seem the Social Democrats had become a bourgeois party on economic issues, even to the right of the Liberals. Their historic constituency felt abandoned and a large proportion cast blank ballots. It would be more accurate to say the Social Democrats lost the 1991 election than to say the bourgeois coalition won it.

The Right-Wing Nonsocialist Government of 1992–1994

A coalition of the Conservative, Christian Democratic, Center, and Liberal parties took power after the 1991 election. There was a vast difference in their stance as compared to the 1976–1982 government, where the Conservatives were the smallest party, ideologically differentiated from their coalition partners and marginalized within the government. This time they were the largest party and it was their program that the new government promoted. The coalition partners were given support in one or more of their "questions of the heart," but the new government was otherwise hard line and right wing.

Important groundwork for the new government had been laid in the 1985 election, when Conservative Party leader Adelsohn campaigned for a "jump start" (*rivstart*), a very quick implementation of right-wing programs. Adelsohn had used the campaign to profile the Conservatives as opponents of the Swedish model, which was a significant hardening of the Conservative line.

> It was literally Ulf Adelsohn's old jump start from 1985 that was now reworked by Carl Bildt.
>
> The six year old Conservative planning folder, containing what one should do if one won a system change election, was dusted off and freshened up. Now ideas were put forth which had been written down then: to divide finances into expenditure and income departments, to have only one office of coordination, to have organized comradely time together among ministers, to have group leaders take part in the government's preparations, and to take symbolic decisions swiftly at the start. The latter was something that directors in commerce go to courses to learn ("that which one doesn't do in the first three months never gets done"). (Elmbrant, 1993, 278)

Another important development was the emergence of a new political party, the New Democrats (*Ny Demokraterna*) under the leadership of Count Ian Wachmeister and record promoter Bert Karlsson. Wachmeister had been an active participant in the New Welfare organization and had made an effort to convert the organization into an antitax, antiwelfare political party. That effort failed, but Wachmeister and Karlsson, when they founded the New Democrats, simply took the New Welfare program as their platform, with the addition of an anti-immigrant stance (Elmbrant, 1993).

The election, in one view of things, was one that nobody won. The four bourgeois parties together did not have a majority, nor did the socialist bloc. The New Democrats, while just over the threshold for entry into Parliament, and with only twenty-five seats, held the balance of power. They could not, however, be brought into the government, as the Liberal leader, Bengt Westerberg, had committed his party to stay out of any government that included the New Democrats. Hence a new four-party minority government was dependent on the support of either the New Democrats or the socialists to enact programs.

While the Conservatives were the largest bourgeois party and they had support from the Liberals on economic issues, there were important differences as well. The Center and Liberal Parties supported strong public welfare programs, although they differed from the Social Democrats and each other on how they should be shaped. The Conservatives were set in opposition to the Social Democrats in principle.[14] This was a line that had to be dealt with carefully. Most often, the middle parties compromised to ensure that a nonsocialist government could hold together for a whole mandate period (Elmbrant, 1993).

The new government took a strong neoliberal line.

- They took two immediate symbolic decisions: to compensate an automobile dealer a million crowns in damages for excess taxation, and to approve 3.6 billion crowns in new shares for Nordbanken.
- They moved to privatize the bank, holding that the bank crisis was an example of the evils of state ownership. This was in spite of the fact that "The bank crisis, to the contrary, showed that the liberal doctrine in its purest form could not stand. An unbounded capitalism was not necessarily creative. . . . On the contrary, an unbounded capitalism could be self destructive, resulting in stagnation and a need for larger public support" (Elmbrant, 1993, 282).
- They reduced taxes during their first year on working capital in industry, rented property, property, capital gains, inheritances, gifts, profits from sales, securities, and private pensions. In addition, they lifted the limits on deductions for interest.
- They moved to abolish closed-shop unions in the hope of undermining labor power in political decision making at a time when the demand for labor was weak.
- They moved aggressively to bring Sweden into the European Union, described as Prime Minister Bildt's "question of the heart" (Elmbrant, 1993).

In the face of the bank crisis, the state budget deficit following the tax reform of 1991, and rising unemployment, these moves served to aggravate the economic situation. Further, they contributed to a massive reallocation of resources from the middle and lower classes to the rich and powerful. There was considerable conflict between the Conservatives and particularly the Liberals within the government, and worsening economic conditions by 1993 were forcing a moderation of the Conservative stand.

In Elmbrant's (1993) analysis, this government accomplished the "fall of the Swedish model."[15] The economic crisis deepened, finally resulting in the government seeking an agreement with the Social Democrats on a "crisis package" that stopped lowering of taxes in exchange for an agreement to make cuts in some workers' benefits. That the Social Democrats agreed to those terms perhaps speaks louder than anything else of the rise of the right in Swedish politics.

In health policy, the government took a much more moderate stance than in economic policy. In part this was because the Ministry of Social Affairs, where medical care concerns fall, was held by the Liberals, who supported strong public services. With one exception, the initiatives taken by the Minister of Health, a Deputy Social Minister, were pragmatic attempts to solve real problems rather than an ideologically driven program. Two had actually been enacted under the previous government, but implemented after the bourgeois coalition came into power: the Ädel Reform and the care guarantee. The remaining initiative was the "heart question" of the Liberal Party, the point-of-service primary care physician. Medical care was, then, one area in which the hard-right new line was somewhat mitigated.

THE POLITICAL "SYSTEM SHIFT"

The political crisis, then, was the main source of the changes in Swedish medical care policy noted during the final years of the 1980s and into the early 1990s. A badly weakened Social Democratic Party drew back from its long-term commitments to equality, solidarity, and planning. In so doing, they alienated their traditional core constituency, the labor movement, and were voted out of office. This weakness, along with a long-term campaign to "educate" the Swedish public on the superiority of market economies for problem solving, allowed the right wing to step forward with their commitments to markets, competition, and privatization. Knowing that they had little time to institute their policies, they acted quickly to dismantle as many of the Social Democratic programs as possible and to change the structure of decision making so as to make their changes as permanent as possible. The Conservatives had built the roadbed, but the socialists had greased the rails. With the 1991 election, a new, aggressive, anti-welfare-state set of policies could be implemented with no more than token opposition. Indeed, in a very real sense, the new right-wing dominated government was only accelerating a trend that had been put in place by the opposition. It is in this context that the reforms in medical care can best be understood.

NOTES

1. The Liberal and Center Parties supported a strong public medical care system, but favored a residual, rather than universal, form of entitlement.

2. Conservative politicians at that meeting vigorously denied that privatization was a part of their agenda. They were solely concerned, they said, with introducing market competition into the public sector. The work of Saltman and von Otter was held as an exemplar.

3. It should be emphasized that Myrdal (1982) was not presenting a critique of Social Democracy per se. In his introductory chapter, he described himself as an "arch-Socialist" (*ärkesosse*) (p. 11) and goes on to state, "Science is critical and social science becomes a critique of the social order" (p. 21). Indeed, he affirms the values traditionally associated with social democracy: equity, full participation in decision making by all sectors of the society, access to services unaffected

by economic power, and so forth. His critique focused on the unintended consequences of programs that mostly developed under Social Democratic leadership: a reduction in the degree of direct participation in decision making and a decline in grassroots democratic processes.

4. With reference to the preceding chapter's thesis, Myrdal (1982) noted the same trends in academic work. He particularly faulted his own discipline, national economics, for taking an increasingly short-term view divorced from social institutions. Marshall and Adam Smith, he held, were more institutional economists than were those currently dominating the discipline in Sweden and the "Anglo-Saxon" world. The current leaders were "more removed from a true grasp of reality. In their fundamental work in high theory they write for each other within a sect isolated from all other social science, which must make their research less realistic and relevant" (p. 17).

5. This comment was made in response to a draft of a paper in 1985 (Twaddle and Hessler, 1986).

6. Members were said to include Ingvar Carlsson, Rune Molin from LO, Leni Björklund from Stockholm County, and Feldt (Feldt, 1991, 15).

7. Generally seen as the brainchild of Rudolf Meidner, wage-earner funds were a form of excess profits tax on large corporations. Monies collected would be placed into funds managed for investment by the unions. The rationale for the funds varied from time to time, but generally they were promoted with the idea that labor interests would be more likely to invest in Sweden, rather than abroad, and the money would be used to generate Swedish jobs. To Conservatives, the funds were anathema and generally described as "fund socialism," allowing workers to purchase controlling interests in Swedish industry. To counter this, the legislation, when proposed, placed a limit on the percentage of stock any fund could hold in a single company.

8. It should be noted that unemployment, while high by Swedish standards, was still below the historic low for the United States. When it reached 3 percent, the coalition government fell. At that time, there was still an effort in the United States to define 4 percent as a "full employment" goal.

9. By 1993, interviews with LO officials and Social Democratic members of Parliament suggested an important division within the Social Democratic Party. The Parliamentary group was much more committed to traditional socialist values. The party leadership was following a much more conservative line.

10. Here we review only those chapters that attempted some explanation of the weakening of the Social Democratic party.

11. This is the date of the first legislation. Child care grew incrementally from 1943–1990.

12. Compulsory school consists of nine years, begining at the age of seven.

13. Asea, LM Ericsson, Electrolux, SKF, and Separator (Alfa-Laval).

14. Elmbrant (1993) described the Conservative policy as standing against the Social Democrats and had diffculty with their partners, who "supported welfare, security and material equality" (p. 281).

15. He defined that model as having seven components: (1) a struggle for collective solutions and class cooperation; (2) a struggle for democratically achieved decisions; (3) powerful and equal organizations in the labor market solve conflicts with free means (with collective bargaining, not legislation); (4) export in-

dustries are privileged, but required to participate in a common building of society; (5) high taxes, but production and growth are favored; (6) unemployment is a scourge and is combatted with active market policies; and (7) welfare is a public duty, with justice and equality as principles (not care of the poor, but a concern for everyone).

CHAPTER 7

Socioeconomic Trends, Ideology, and Medical Care Reform

In the previous chapters, we have reviewed the various efforts to reform medical care in Sweden between 1980 and 1994 and identified the sources of those efforts in the organization of medical services, the state of the Swedish economy, and the changing political climate in the country. In this chapter, we try to summarize where we have been, assess the models that have guided our investigation, and offer an explanation of the reforms based on the materials at hand.

SOCIOECONOMIC TRENDS AND MEDICAL CARE REFORM IN SWEDEN

Those proposing a reform of medical care to make it more responsive to a putative market portrayed a need for reform couched in changing socioeconomic conditions that made such reform necessary. In the various documents reviewed and in interviews with a variety of participants in health policy formation, it was evident that not only were there a number of trends that made continuation of the "traditional" system more difficult, but those trends were widely acknowledged and understood across the political spectrum. The most important ones are summarized here.

Problems with Increasing Health Care Costs

Population Aging

This was a major factor creating stresses in the medical care system. Sweden had the oldest population in the world, with 17 percent over the age of sixty-five in 1992. Projected trends were for well over 20 percent of the population to fall into the over-sixty-five category with increasing proportions over seventy-five years of age. Increasing age carries with it a larger burden of chronic disease and a larger demand for medical care. Further, larger proportions of the population were in need of residential support and assisted-living arrangements. Increased cost pressures were expected to increase even further.

Advances in Medical Technology

The technological capacity of medicine was expanding rapidly in Sweden as in the rest of the developed world. New technology is often costly. With the abandonment of central rationing of technology, high technology had diffused downward from regional to county and sometimes even to local hospitals, increasing the duplication of services at the local level, driving up the capital intensiveness of medicine, and pushing up costs.

Declining "Productivity"

It is very difficult to define and measure productivity in human services because the "product" is so variable. How does one compare, for example, the time/cost ratio of two surgical procedures, one of which is technically difficult, requiring a slow, deliberate course of action, and the other a very simple one that can be accomplished quickly (say a mitral valve replacement and reduction of an umbilical hernia)? Or, how does one compare a diagnosis of a common condition with a distinctive presentation with a diagnosis of a rare condition with a subtle presentation? Production in the sense of the number of units delivered makes little sense as a concept under these circumstances.

Nevertheless, a productivity decline was widely taken to be a fact. Physicians were seeing fewer patients per capita than they had in the past for two reasons. First, they were bargaining with their employers for more time off instead of higher salaries. They worked less overtime. Hence, fewer hours were spent by each physician at work. Second, the job descriptions of physicians were changing to include more administration, more teaching, and more research. This meant less time per physician in direct patient care. To maintain capacity, the system would have to employ more physicians. This also increased costs, even when physicians were working as hard as ever during their working hours.

Increasing Insurance Costs

Insurance costs for both medical care delivery and income replacement for the sick were increasing rapidly as a result of greater per capita use of increasingly expensive medical services.

Problems in Medical Care Organization

Declining Quality of Care

Some, who were promoting market changes, asserted that the quality of care had deteriorated along four dimensions: increased waiting times, growing impersonality, problems with continuity, and, for the aged, a decline in technical quality. Except for the last, none of these seemed to be compelling as of 1993, although they had been serious problems in the recent past.

Waiting Times. In the large cities, waiting lists for some procedures, mostly elective surgery, had grown quite long. Indeed, these had been the target of the care guarantee reform discussed in Chapters 1 and 4. That reform had been quite successful, and at the time of the study waiting lists had been shortened considerably. That the lists developed at all may have been the result of a perverse incentive for physicians, who could argue for larger budgets on the grounds that the lists demonstrated an inadequate capacity to meet demand.[1] What amounted to a change in the incentive system, making it possible for patients to leave their county for care, seemed to solve the problem even when very few people actually took advantage of that opportunity.

Impersonality. It was held that the public system was cold and bureaucratic and patients often felt like objects being acted upon by uncaring providers. To some degree this was undoubtedly the case, as the public system was concentrated in large hospitals and the specialty clinics associated with them. In any system, public or private, care in the large-hospital sector tends to be experienced as impersonal by patients. There was no reason to hold that impersonality of the Swedish system was more problematic than in other countries or that it was in any way associated with the public organization of the system.

Continuity. Patients were often shunted from one physician to another for the same condition, seeing different people on different visits. They saw different physicians for different conditions. Given the identity of the situation in the United States in hospital clinics, this would seem to be a function of reliance on the hospital specialty clinic for care and the corresponding underdevelopment of primary care.[2]

Technical Quality in Care of the Aged. When the municipalities took over care of the aged, the incidence of denial of needed services and attendant morbidity increased sharply. In part this was because the transfer of funds from counties to municipalities was inadequate to sustain the level of services. In part it was because the municipalities did not have any experience with running medical care services.

Declining Equality

This is a complaint that seemed to come from the left of Swedish politics and was associated with the frame law reform of 1982 and the Ädel

Reform of 1992. The first decentralized responsibility for medical care from the national government to the counties and removed the national mandate to control the distribution of personnel and technology. The second decentralized care for the aged from the counties to the municipalities. The loss of capacity to control distribution across political units meant that the standard of service from one locality to another became more variable, making the volume and quality of service dependent on where one lived.

Lack of Integration with Social Services

Coming from the reformers, this was a concern that medical care was organized by counties and social services by municipalities. Since the two interpenetrate, especially in the management of chronic disease, it was seen as organizationally inefficient to have this division. Closer cooperation, it was argued, could be managed if medical and social care were placed within the same political unit. Indeed, this was the case made for the Ädel Reform, which at least initially could not be seen as a success, except in reducing expenditures. If adequately resourced, that reform would show fewer, perhaps negative, savings and less of a decline in effectiveness.

Organizational Rigidity

Nobody argued against the position that the medical care system lacked flexibility. It was rigid in that it lacked a capacity to adapt to differences in local conditions. The sources of that rigidity were multiple. Many decisions were being taken too high up in the system, too far removed from the needs of particular patients or local populations. Many decisions were being taken by people who neither had to administer them nor deliver services. Most were taken with little to no consultation with people who worked in the system.[3]

Bed Blockers. Many patients, disproportionately among the elderly, were treated in hospitals and needed to be discharged to a setting where they could receive continued care. The hospital had done what it could do and an assisted-living or nursing care facility was needed. Hospitals were run by counties, assisted-living and nursing homes by municipalities which had no incentive to take over the care. In the meantime, the patients were held in the hospitals, blocking beds so that other patients could not be admitted. This was a factor in the waiting lists discussed.

As part of the Ädel Reform, municipalities were charged for these bed blockers after being notified the patient was ready to be discharged. As it was more expensive to keep the patient in the hospital, the municipalities now had an incentive to find an appropriate placement. As a result, this seemed to be a solved problem in 1993.

Units Too Large. Increasingly, medical care was being concentrated in large hospitals. Small hospitals were being closed. Large hospitals are more inflexible in responding to patient needs. It had also been shown that beyond a certain point (around 500 beds), economies of scale could not be realized and often reversed. It was argued in many quarters that reducing the number of large hospitals and increasing the number of smaller ones would improve efficiency and effectiveness. That argument was seemingly ignored by policy makers.

Alienation of Health Workers. This complaint came from everyone in the system other than physicians and even from some physicians. In essence, it was that the lower in the system the worker the less likely that his or her perspectives will be taken into account in planning. Blue-collar workers and nurses, for example, held that they could identify many places where the system could be more efficient and effective, but they were not consulted. Instead, reforms threatened their jobs and the effectiveness of care while missing the changes that would increase efficiency or equity. Those running the system seemingly ignored these opportunities to increase flexibility and made those working in the system more resistant to reform.

Over and Under Capacity

Dependence on Hospitals and Specialists. Compared with any other country, Sweden's medical care system was built more around large hospitals and specialized medicine. Sweden, among developed countries, had the highest admission rates to hospitals, the longest durations of admissions, and the lowest proportion of medical care delivered by primary care physicians. Whereas there was considerable evidence that cost could be cut considerably simply by shifting the locus of care to the cheapest effective setting, Sweden had a systemic bias toward providing care in the most expensive possible setting. If high-technology hospitals were limited to cases requiring that level of technology—and if the allocation of technology to hospitals could be carefully controlled and primary care physicians covered all the cases within their level of competence—the cost of care could be markedly reduced.

Changes in the early 1990s had resulted in a new phenomenon, unemployment among physicians. The point-of-service reform, since repealed, made provision for retraining many of these as primary care physicians.

Shortages in Primary Care. The proportion of physicians in primary care in Sweden was the lowest in the developed world, even while their numbers had been increased during the 1980s. A reform in the mid-1970s which capped residency opportunities in the medical and surgical specialties had increased the supply of primary care physicians. While the supply was still inadequate, the trend line was toward increasing numbers that, over time, would solve the problem.

Problems in the Larger Economy

While there were many problems with the organization of medical services, many of them had been solved or were on their way toward solution. The remainder could be solved within the existing system. They were matters of adjusting the system, not fundamentally changing it. Indeed, almost nobody claimed there was a crisis—or anything remotely resembling a crisis—in the organization of medical care.

Instead, they pointed to what may be regarded as the infrastructure of medical care, the economy in general. It was widely held that the medical care system was excellent, even exemplary, but the economy could no longer support it. Medical care would have to be scaled back to a level that could be sustained financially. The condition of the economy was seen as problematic as a result of the almost total entry of women into the labor force, an economic recession–depression, a changing international climate, and the results of economic policy decisions during the late 1980s and early 1990s.

Increasing Employment of Women

Women entered the labor force earlier than in most other countries and in larger numbers. Very few women between the ages of twenty and sixty were at home caring for families. In the past, as in other countries, Sweden had been able to rely on the unpaid labor of women to care for men, children, and each other. It was they who raised children, tended the sick, helped needy neighbors, and the like. When they entered the paid labor force, those services were still needed and had to be provided through other means. Indeed, much of the activity of the welfare state was to provide services once provided by women outside the cash economy: education, health care, nursing care, day care, and so forth. The more women entered the labor force, the more need there was for the state to provide services (or see that they were provided).[4]

Economic Recession–Depression

Sweden had seen its economy destabilized by a series of events beginning in the 1970s and developing into the 1990s.

Oil Shock. The oil crisis of 1973–1974 permanently increased the price of petroleum products. Sweden had no oil reserves of its own and had not developed alternatives to dependence on oil sufficient to offset dependence on the international market. Atomic power had been developed, but was not seen as safe after Three Mile Island in the United States and the Chernobyl disaster in the USSR. A referendum in 1979 mandated the elimination of nuclear power plants within twenty-five years.

Hydroelectric power was well developed, but not adequate to cover needs. Solar and wind power were at an early experimental stage.

Overheating and Inflation. A stimulus package in 1982, coupled with wage pressures, resulted in a sharp increase in inflation. In retrospect, labor economists said they should not have pushed so hard for wage increases. Policies targeted at curbing inflation took over, creating pressures for savings in the public sector and a climate that encouraged cuts in public services, including medical care.

Real Estate and Banking Crisis. Part of the inflation-fighting mentality was deregulation of the banking and real estate sectors at a time when real estate values were inflated. Swedish banks invested heavily in real estate, much of it outside of Sweden. When the real estate market crashed, the banks found themselves holding mortgages larger than the values of the properties mortgaged. The government moved to "bail out" the banks in order to protect depositors. A vast amount of public money was committed to this end, making the funding of public services much more difficult.

Unemployment. The focus on fighting inflation coupled with the abandonment or reduction in active labor market practices resulted in what could only be described as an explosion of unemployment in 1992 and 1993. Even in the worldwide depression of the 1930s, unemployment in Sweden had never exceeded 7 percent. Since then, open unemployment had stayed under 3 percent. The Liberal coalition government had fallen in 1982 with unemployment as an issue when the level reached almost 3 percent. In 1991, open unemployment crossed that line, reaching 13 percent in the late summer of 1993, a level unprecedented in the life experience of most Swedes.[5] Unemployment placed greater demands on public services, further straining the capacity of the public sector to meet its obligations.

International Competition Pressures

Particularly after the deregulation of investment outside of Sweden during the 1980s, the sector of the Swedish economy exposed to foreign trade grew rapidly in both relative and absolute terms. Swedish corporations increased their investments in Europe by opening branch operations, acquiring subsidiary firms, and merging with continental companies. Increasingly, the Swedish economy was becoming tied to the economies of Europe. This, indeed, was the major reason the international sector pushed for Swedish entry into the European Community.

The level of economic development in Europe was quite diverse, ranging from weak economies in the South (e.g., Portugal, Spain, Greece) to the very powerful German economy in the North. Internationally exposed Swedish industry found itself increasingly in competition with countries that had lower wages, weaker workplace safety requirements, weaker environmental regulation, and substantially lower standards of living. It was difficult to compete under circumstances where other firms had lower costs of production.[6]

One result was increasing pressure on the state to remove requirements that increased production costs, focusing mainly on the Swedish model of the welfare state: the active labor market, environmental regulations, and job-security provisions. Another result was a decision on the part of employers to unilaterally withdraw from the collective bargaining agreements, in force for over half a century, in which peak labor organizations and the employers' association negotiated a general framework within which unions and management negotiated labor contracts. A campaign was developed to undermine the ideology of collective agreements and to "decentralize" labor negotiations to the firm level, thus undermining the policies of labor solidarity. By a "divide and conquer" approach, the idea was to hold back wages, working conditions, and environmental protection in order to reduce production costs.

Economic Policy

Other strains on the ability of Sweden to maintain its level of social welfare could be found in political decisions about the economy. Most important among these were the 1991 tax reform and the state budget deficit it created, and the decision to enter the European Community (which in 1994 became the European Union). In terms of the greatest immediate stain on the Swedish model, these seemed the strongest pressures.

Tax Reform and Budget Deficit. The tax reform was similar in form and impact to the earlier tax reforms in the United States and the U.K. As in those cases, taxes on the wealthy were reduced sharply. The working population saw very little tax reduction and in some instances tax increases. The effect was similar: Tax revenues fell suddenly, creating a budgetary shortfall. State debt exploded. The state had to borrow to meet its obligations and an increasing percentage of state revenue had to be diverted toward servicing the debt.

The reform was initiated with the claim that declining taxes would increase investment and thus increase tax collections. This was the same claim that had been put forward in the United States under the Reagan administration and in the U.K. under the Thatcher government. It worked in Sweden even less well than it had in the countries Sweden imitated.[7] As a proportion of the economy or the state budget, the debt in Sweden far exceeded the American or British experience.

European Union. Europe was far behind Sweden in its development of the welfare state. It did not have the degree of job security, workplace safety regulation, or environmental regulations found in Scandinavia. No country in Europe had as large a public sector or the range and quality of social support services enjoyed by the Swedes.

A decision to join the Europeans in a common economic market in which there would be free movement of labor, capital, goods, and services meant Sweden would have to make large adjustments. All restrictions on immigration from other member countries would have to be removed. Foreign investment in Sweden would have to be opened. Border control to keep out unsafe products would have to be curtailed. And fundamental constitutional rights of citizens, particularly for free access to information, would come under serious challenge.[8]

One consequence was a concern that there would be a migration of population from Southern Europe—where development was weak, jobs were scarce, wages were low, and social services were weak to nonexistent—to Northern Europe—where development was strong, wages were higher, and social support services were stronger. Under such circumstances, the Swedish model would become a liability, as the EU offered no defense against extending benefits to the poor of other countries. Moreover, the European Union could mandate conditions for economic integration, limiting the ability of the state to raise taxes, regulate the workplace, ensure workers' rights, control public health and safety, and regulate the environment.

Clearly, to be part of the EU made it very difficult to maintain the welfare state apparatus that had come to be known as the Swedish model. The state budget had to be reduced. Taxes had to be brought in line with those in the rest of Europe. Health, safety, environmental, and labor legislation had to be adjusted in line with the continent. What this would involve was a decline in the standard and level of living to which Swedes were accustomed.

IDEOLOGY AND MEDICAL CARE REFORM IN SWEDEN

There can be no doubt that there were some important structural problems with medical care in Sweden, most strikingly the underdevelopment of primary care and the heavy reliance on specialized hospital-based care. Nor can there be any doubt that there was a short-term economic problem that strained the capacity of the country to provide a range of social services, the most expensive of which was medical care.

Nevertheless, there is reason to conclude that the pressures for market-oriented reform were fundamentally located in ideological differences rather than structural problems with medicine or difficult economic conditions.

First, the existing medical care system had already taken effective steps to reduce costs. As a percentage of gross domestic or national product, expenditures on medical care had fallen by almost one-third between 1982 and 1992. Much of this was associated with an increasing emphasis on primary care. The problem of waiting lists was moving toward solution. The solutions were being accomplished in a budget-driven system without market reforms.

Second, the argument over the economy, which was focused on whether there was a long-term crisis consisting of over expansion of the public sector, was divided along traditional bourgeois–socialist lines. The national economists at Stockholm University, the Swedish Employers Association, and the right-wing political parties all held that the welfare state was fundamentally flawed and in principle was a form of economic mismanagement. The labor unions, the Social Democrats in Parliament, and the institutional economists held the crisis was short term and had no causal relation to the principals of the welfare state. In this context, there was an apparent effort on the part of the national economists to silence their more centrist and leftist colleagues and to discredit other social sciences that did not support their analysis.

Third, there were important distortions of evidence by those supporting reforms. For example, an international team of economists reviewed the medical care system at the behest of the employer backed SNS. They concluded that while there were tensions in the system and always would be, the system functioned quite well and would not benefit from market reforms (Cuyer, 1991). That report was never referred to in the debates except by those skeptical of the reform effort. For another example, the economic analyses put forth in support of the reform effort (Ekonomikommissionen, 1993) presented evidence selectively and reached conclusions not supported by either their data or their arguments. For yet another example, there was a repeated assertion that the public was increasingly dissatisfied with the medical care system and that there was a demand for more patient choice of providers. No evidence was presented in support of those positions. When a poll demonstrated that the public had little interest in greater choice, the assertions continued.

It appeared likely that what was happening was that the right wing of Swedish politics was taking advantage of an economic downturn and internal divisions within the dominant Social Democratic Party to promote policy objectives that had been central to their concerns for decades. For at least twenty years, the Swedish Employers Association had been supplying the schools with "educational" materials for the study of economics. Those materials promoted an unregulated market economy. They created a generation who had been exposed to only one model of the economy, one that discredited Keynesian and leftist approaches to economic analysis.

The Social Democrats had been debating the problems of centralization for some time, so the party did not have a coherent position on the form of the welfare state, although they had met every problem in the organization of state services by decentralizing for at least two decades. In the 1980s, the Social Democratic government brought academic economists from the Stockholm school into the Finance Ministry, marginalizing the labor economists who had traditionally been used to formulate government policy. This, coupled with a need to prioritize fighting inflation after the 1976–1982 bourgeois government's management of the aftermath of the oil shock, the economic policies of the Social Democratic government shifted to the right and followed what had up to then been regarded as right-wing programs. A split appeared between the Social Democrats in the government (who wanted to redefine the party to capture more of the middle-class vote) and the Social Democrats in the Parliament (who wanted to maintain close relations with their traditional labor constituency).

The Labor constituency of the Social Democratic Party felt abandoned by the party leadership and broke the close ties that had traditionally characterized the labor–Social Democratic relationship. Almost 40 percent of those who voted for Social Democrats in 1986 cast blank ballots in 1991, creating a vacuum into which the Conservative Party moved.

In the 1991 election, a coalition of right and center parties took the government and the Social Democrats went into opposition. This time the government was dominated by the Conservatives rather than the center parties, leaving the field open for a hard-line assault on the welfare state. It was this that provided the context for attempts at market-oriented reform of medical care. Those attempts were quite modest in scope, with the exception of allowing private physicians to freely establish as point-of-service primary care physicians, because the Ministry of Social Affairs, that housed the Ministry of Health, was held by the more centrist Liberal Party.

OUR MODELS FOR THE STUDY OF MEDICAL CARE REFORM AND THE SWEDISH CASE

Using the models described in Chapter 2 as a guideline, we have looked at health care reforms and proposals for further reform in Sweden during the 1980s and early 1990s. In seeking an explanation for why the direction of reform had shifted from one based on improving effectiveness and equity to one focused on improving efficiency, we have systematically explored the sufficiency of three arguments: that the medical care system itself was structurally flawed, that the medical care system was effective but too expensive for the faltering Swedish economy, and that the shift was fundamentally ideological.

In this section, we look first at what the application of those models allows us to conclude about the change in direction of health policy in Sweden in the late 1980s and early 1990s. Second, we look at what our conclusions have to say about the models.

The Theoretical Models as Heuristic Tools

As has been reviewed, we reached several conclusions. With regard to the medical care system itself, we found the following:

1. There were structural problems with the medical care system that required changes. These included overreliance on tertiary care and underdevelopment of primary care, longer than acceptable waiting lists for elective procedures, a lack of incentives for municipalities to find placements for hospital patients who needed nursing care or assisted living arrangements, and bureaucratic rigidities.
2. These problems were being successfully addressed without violating the principles of the public welfare system. They could be "fixed" within the Swedish model. Indeed, Sweden had been more successful than any other country in containing and reducing the cost of the medical care system during the 1980s.
3. The rapid expansion of the elderly population posed a serious challenge to the capacity of the system. This was not a structural problem of the system, however.

In answer to our first research question, the medical care system clearly had developed some problems and needed some changes, but those problems were not sufficient to explain the change in direction of the reform effort.

With regard to the economy, we concluded as follows:

4. The Swedish economy had been strained by the oil shock of the 1970s and by the worldwide recession–depression of the late 1980s and early 1990s. The cost of living for both individuals and institutions had risen, most likely permanently, making it more difficult to sustain the world's highest level of social services.
5. A series of political decisions—the failure of the government during the boom period of the 1980s to realize sufficient savings, the deregulation of real estate and banking that led to the collapse of the banking institution, and the tax reform of 1991 that led to an astronomical budget deficit—seriously aggravated an already difficult economic situation.
6. A focus on fighting inflation, made necessary by circumstances and by the aftermath of earlier decisions, led to a massive increase of unemployment, further increasing a need for services and weakening economic demand.

Clearly, the economy was in a state that made support of a large public-sector welfare system more difficult. Equally clearly, the economic argument was a much more compelling one than was the argument that the medical care system itself required market-oriented changes. Yet on reviewing the evidence, it does not seem possible to conclude that privatization, competition, and markets would provide a remedy. Indeed, there is reason to hold that strengthening public control of the system and improving the planning and administrative apparatus would be a more promising avenue toward solutions to the problems of the Swedish welfare state.

The reasons for this conclusion are as follows. First, while a market mode of organization can clearly increase the profitability of the system for entrepreneurs and for large corporate interests, there is no example in the literature of a market reform improving efficiency (the overall cost of the system or units of service within the system). Second, market organization has generally resulted in a reduction of quality and equity. Access becomes more segmented and unequal, resulting in a multitiered system. Third, deregulation of services has generally increased costs and damaged access. Fourth, the economic problems in Sweden in the past three decades arose or worsened during periods when deregulation and competition were the government program and mitigated when regulation and planning were the government program.

There is another fact that seems compelling. The percentage of the Swedish economy devoted to medical care and related services had dropped during the previous decade. If anything, the system was successfully containing costs.

So in answer to our second research question, the economy posed serious problems. Like the structural problems in the medical care system, understanding these problems is a necessary component to understanding the direction of reform. It was not sufficient with regard to the public-sector services in general. It failed with specific reference to medical care, which could have been taken as a model of how to bring costs under control for the rest of the economy.

With regard to the political explanation, we found the following:

7. The shaping of public services during the 1950s and 1960s with an emphasis on providing security and uniformity of service throughout the country had created a process of centralization. Public services became more bureaucratic, with decision making removed from those ultimately affected by the decisions. An internal debate within the Social Democratic Party led to a program of decentralization in the 1970s and 1980s. The welfare-state apparatus was seen to pose some dangers as well as benefits.
8. The Finance Ministry in the 1982–1991 Social Democratic government adopted a neoliberal economic policy which prioritized fighting inflation, placed limits on the development of the public sector, and enhanced the environment for business. Internally, the party was divided on the issue of whether to remain a party of the working class, which was shrinking as a percentage of the electorate, or to directly appeal to the middle class.
9. Government support of wage containment, pricing norms, and programs to enhance profits led to an open break with the labor movement. The blue-collar unions broke their traditional membership in the Social Democratic Party. A very large percentage of blue-collar voters withdrew support from the Social Democrats in the 1991 election, many casting blank ballots and many others supporting the populist right-wing party, the New Democrats.
10. In the meantime, the employers launched a propaganda campaign aimed at school children, in which they provided "educational" materials that promoted as "scientific fact" the view that only the market could create an effi-

cient economy and that economic and social planning undermined social welfare. The long-term objective was to change the cultural climate.

11. As part of the "employers offensive," the Swedish Employers Association withdrew from the collective bargaining framework that they had agreed to in the 1930s. This meant a decentralization of wage negotiations to the level of the local firm and the undermining of the wage solidarity norms that had traded greater wage equity and worker security for labor peace. The effect was to undermine the power of the union movement.
12. In the 1991 election, the right-wing Conservative Party came to power, dominating a four-party nonsocialist government. Instead of working gradually to develop a program, they had a plan to "jump start" with a very aggressive ideologically hard-line program to destabilize the welfare state, discredit the Swedish model, and redesign the state along the lines of neoliberal economic theory.

With respect to our third research question, then, we concluded that there had been a very important political shift that was sufficient to explain the changes in medical care policy.

In helping to organize our thinking about health policy reforms in Sweden, then, it would be fair to conclude that the theoretical models we started with were quite useful in generating fruitful questions, guiding data-collection procedures, and interpreting findings. Having heuristic value may be sufficient for the applied problem we have addressed. Another question is whether those models are in need of refinement based on the experience with the Swedish case.

Theoretical Models and the Swedish Case

The trends in the development of medical care in Sweden seemed to be those that characterized the rest of the developed world (see Figure 2.1). Solving the problem of technical competence in the early part of the twentieth century had contributed to the explosion of technical capacity, leading to a centralization of medical care, increased specialization, increased fragmentation of care, and increased costs. Clearly, the focus had shifted to problems of organization and financing. What an analysis of Swedish medicine seems to offer in comparison with the United States is another set of mechanisms by which these trends can develop. In both the least-developed welfare system in the developed world and in the most-developed welfare state, the general trends seem to be parallel. Nothing in the present analysis would seem to call for modification of our model of the trends in development of Western medicine. At the same time, it calls attention to the need for closer analysis to understand developments in specific sociohistorical contexts.

The main differences seem to be in how different countries manage changes (see Table 4.1). While the United States left medical care relatively unregulated beyond requiring the licensing of practitioners—and even there provided more latitude for alternatives to mainstream medicine than did Sweden or the rest of Europe—Sweden early on organized the delivery of services as a public, more democratically controlled system. The difference is not trivial, as Sweden achieved a much greater degree of equity and, at the micro level, more efficiency than did the United States. At the same time, the trends that the model called into focus were evident.

One conclusion is that the model of trends in medicine affecting the physician–patient relationship can stand without modification based on our analysis of the Swedish case. At the same time, it must be recognized that the model is not sufficient to understand any specific national system. It must be augmented with historical detail. Its value is in indicating what kinds of historical information might be most useful in generating data amenable to crossnational comparisons.

The Swedish system was created with a significant public component as early as the seventeenth century, when provincial physicians were mandated by national law. Groundwork was hence laid for a substantial role for the state in the delivery of medical care by providing for public resources to make medicine available to the general population. As the political system became more democratic in the twentieth century and as public services expanded, particularly in the period following World War II, medical care became a cornerstone of the welfare state. The state took a leading role in seeing that medical services were available and accessible to the whole citizenry. Public authorities, mostly at the county level with substantial state oversight, financed medical care and provided for its organization and delivery. At the same time, clinical decisions remained the province of qualified medical practitioners. No public authority took any role in diagnostic procedures or treatment decisions. While decisions regarding organization and financing were public and under the control of democratically elected representatives, clinical decisions were the prerogative of the medical profession.

The major changes introduced by the reform movements were to decentralize the administration of medical care from the national to the county and local levels. In these domains, decision making moved from a democratic toward a market mode of organization. Clearly, this shift made some important differences. Public authorities relinquished control of two elements that seem essential for controlling the cost of medical care: the distribution of personnel and technology. There was a downward diffusion of expensive technology from regional to county to local hospitals. New private clinics opened to provide high-technology care to those who could afford it, often the elites from Third World countries. The medical care system was infused with new energy. At the same time, the quality of health care for the aged deteriorated sharply. Physicians shifted locations into populations that tended to be adequately served and away from areas of need. Regional differences increased. The costs of primary care exploded. Medical care became less equal, for weaker populations markedly less effective, and perhaps less efficient with a shift from democratic toward market forms of control.

The market, professional, and democratic modes of decision making described in Tables 2.1 and 2.2 called attention to an important dimension of medical care reforms: the gains and losses to be experienced by different segments of the population and the tradeoffs among values to be realized by the system—equity, effectiveness, and efficiency. The Swedish case suggests strongly that these models focused questions of importance to understanding the dynamics and outcomes of medical care reforms. At the same time, it must be acknowledged that this study is the first empirical case to make use of the models and that some of the tradeoffs may be quite subtle and complex. As with the trends in medicine, the modes of organization model should be treated as a guideline for focusing questions for sociohistorical analysis. Historical detail is needed. With a number of case studies, it may be possible to elaborate and refine the model.

Finally, models of the internationalization of the economy, in either the global post-Fordist or the world-systems versions, call attention to the growing domination of transnational corporations located in the First World. Those corporations have been able to forge new international economic conventions that integrate national economic activities and simplify international commerce, most notably WTO, NAFTA, and, most important for the Swedish case, the European Union. These developments create substantial international pressures for removing economic decisions from the political process. They are a force for limiting democracy and increasing the domain of the market.

The impact of this development on Swedish medical care has been largely indirect, but nevertheless powerful. It was the framework for decisions on the economy that included the deregulation of banking and real estate and the tax reform of 1991, all of which relinquished democratic control of economic policy and all of which seriously destabilized the economy in ways that made support of the welfare state more difficult, which may have been the intent.

The models of internationalization called attention to the embeddedness of specific welfare programs in the economy at the national level and the embeddedness of the national economy in an international or transnational economic system dominated by companies that have taken on much of the core role of states. The Swedish case underlines the importance of understanding these developments and raises questions about the sustainability of a sophisticated system of public medicine. The equity of the system seems endangered, its effectiveness threatened, and its efficiency (but not its profitability) compromised. The potency of the state in addressing these issues seems more limited.

Continued observation of the Swedish system seems warranted. The commissions that have worked on medical care seem to be staking out a position that the professional control of clinical decisions based on ethical principles is vital and that a publicly financed and organized system is vital. If any country can resist the trends of international economy with respect to medical care, it will be Sweden. How much national autonomy they can retain seems to be the key.

Again, the models of internationalization seem to have something important to say about medical care. They focus questions on issues to be addressed without saying much about how they will be addressed in different national contexts. In either the short or the long run, those national contexts may or may not be important. That they need to be monitored and investigated seems beyond dispute.

SOME IMPLICATIONS FOR THE STUDY OF REFORM IN OTHER COUNTRIES

As we have suggested here and in Chapter 1, the Swedish case, while unique in detail, reflects a trend that is widespread in the world. A sizable literature has grown with regard to medical care "reform" efforts in the U.K. under the Thatcher government and the so-called "crisis" in the financing of Medicaid and Medicare and the failure of the Clinton health plan. In both of these cases there were pressures to shift toward market forms of organization that were substantially similar in direction, if not detailed content, to the Swedish experience described in this volume.

In the U.K., the Conservative government under the leadership of Margaret Thatcher took steps to make the National Health Service more efficient by (1) sharply reducing the role of the Ministry of Health and transferring responsibility for the delivery of medical services to more local authorities, and (2) introducing "market discipline" by separating the "purchasers" and "sellers" of medical services. Local authorities, which differed for ambulatory and hospital care, would contract for services with providers who were nominally outside the arena of public ownership.[9] As we have noted, the latter reform especially was a model for the Swedish reform effort. In addition, the U.K. undertook a tax reform on the premise that reducing taxes would stimulate economic activity and hence generate increased state revenues. The tax cut failed to meet its expectations and created a massive budget deficit which was then used to justify cutbacks in public services, including the National Health Service.

In the United States, the medical care system had always been nongovernmental, with the exception of the military, the Veterans Administration system, and the Indian Health Service, all targeted at limited and well-defined populations. The dominant system was always private, financed largely through private health insurance. Special programs provided minimal services for the poor and for the aged.[10] There was no substantial public system of medical care to be reformed.

At the same time, the cost of Medicare, the national insurance plan for the aged, was increasing rapidly, even with much of the increase being passed to the aged in larger copayments and reduced benefits. Some projections pointed toward the bankruptcy of the program. With the recession of the 1980s, in which more than 80 percent of the families in the United States lost real income, the welfare rolls expanded and the cost of Medicaid, insurance for the poor, increased, mostly to be met by changes in eligibility standards and reductions in services. The worsening economic condition of families also meant that for the first time since World War II the percentage of people with private health insurance began to decline. This combination created a climate in which public concern about health insurance increased and health care reform became a political issue.[11]

The 1992 presidential election was won by the Democratic Party candidate largely because he advocated national health insurance. A more conservative Congress spurred by an aggressive campaign conducted by the insurance industry opposed insurance reforms and the powerful corporations, who very much wanted a national program that would remove the cost of health insurance from their budgets, balked when the proposed bill kept an "employer mandate" to provide insurance and merely tried to level the playing field by requiring all employers to participate.[12]

When the national reform failed, the private insurance industry moved aggressively to undertake reforms on their own. They virtually took over the medical care system by creating managed care plans in which the insurer could control the source of primary care, the use of expensive diagnostic tests, referrals to specialists, and the use of treatment modalities. In our terms, the core clinical decisions were constrained and controlled by the market rather than the profession.[13]

As in Sweden, the United States deregulated the real estate market by removing restrictions on the holdings of savings and loan associations (S&Ls) at a time when the market was seriously inflated. When the real estate market collapsed, the S&Ls were left holding mortgages for more than the value of the properties they held. A number of institutions went into receivership, necessitating a massive expenditure of national funds to protect depositors.

As in the U.K., the United States undertook a tax reform that substantially cut federal revenues and failed to provide a stimulus to the economy. The resulting budget deficit seriously constrained public programs of all kinds. In the case of the United States, we have evidence that this outcome was known in advance and was part of a plan to undermine the welfare state, weak as it has been in that country.

In both the U.K. and the United States, there were similar trends with respect to specialization, technology, and the growing cost of the system (much more attenuated in the U.K. than in the United States). Even with vast differences in the level of public services in those countries, there was a similarity in that both shifted toward a market as the solution to their problems. In the case of the U.K., it was a shift from democratic to market organization, and in the United States from professional to market organization. Facing similar economic trends, both undertook similar tax reforms with identical results.

There is reason to hold that something is going on here that transcends the level of the nation state. Health care reform may be something that needs to be addressed transnationally. This conclusion is underlined by the observation that market-oriented reforms seem to be almost universal.[14] They are found not only in the developed world—Canada,[15] Chile,[16] Germany,[17] and Japan[18]—but in the developing world as well—China,[19] India,[20] Ireland,[21] Mexico,[22] Russia,[23] South Africa,[24] and other countries of Africa[25] and Latin America.[26] To date, the data are spotty and developed on a country-by-country basis without a common research agenda. However, in every instance there is a shift from democratic modes of organization toward a market or from professional modes toward market modes.

To further understand these developments at the national level, then, would require a different research strategy, one that focuses on the transnational socioeconomic system. It is important to understand the international trends as contexts for national reforms in several ways. One important contribution would be to develop case studies of countries selected to represent a range of levels of socioeconomic development and a range of medical care systems, all with an eye on the dimensions identified here. Particularly important would be a good description of the medical care system with emphasis on technological capacity and distribution, specialization, costs, and financing, along with attention to the historical context in which the system developed. Attention needs to be paid to trends in the organization of medical care, particularly in recent decades, with special notice of the locus of control in the system. It would seem important to focus on the shifts among professional, democratic, and market modes of organization and the consequences of those shifts. Further, it is important to keep an eye on the international context, particularly the pressures from international agencies, regional trade associations, and transnational corporations, operating on their own or through national and international agencies, on the socioeconomic infrastructure of medical care or more directly on medical care itself.

With a series of case studies that all focus on similar dimensions, it would be possible to make comparisons, delineate trends, and discern the transnational structures that are weakening the nation state's capacity to provide services to its citizens. Such data would help make it possible to design a project that could more directly study and begin to place medical care in a transnational context. That task, as we have argued, is essential to understanding the modern context of medicine.

The case study of Sweden, then, can be no more than a first step in a much larger project that will require the efforts of health and medical social scientists from around the world. What we have provided is, hopefully, a meaningful contribution. There is much to be done.

NOTES

1. In 1978–1979, there were statements made by Conservative respondents to the effect that some people had to wait eighteen months or more for elective cartilage repair. We were unable to find a case where a patient had waited more than three months. Private physicians believed that much of their work was generated by patients who did not want to wait their turn in the public system (Twaddle, 1988).

2. A caveat seems in order. With the advent of managed care offered by HMOs in the United States, the problem of continuity seems to be growing in American primary care. This is in a situation where every patient nominally has a primary care physician who provides point-of-service care.

3. Indeed, in 1978–1979, it was observed that much planning took place by carefully identifying all interested organized parties and giving them a seat at the table. When plans were made, there was no recognition of diversity in the population to be serviced and all services took a singular form.

4. On economic grounds, the erosion of real wages meant that two incomes were necessary to manage a household economy. For most women the stay-at-home option was no longer tenable. For working class women, it never had been.

5. As of mid-1996, the problem had still not been solved. *Svenska Dagbladet* reported on July 15 that unemployment was at 14.1 percent, of which 9.9 percent was open unemployment.

6. These would, of course, be partly offset by the greater technological sophistication of Swedish industry, its greater capital intensiveness, and its lower labor intensiveness.

7. In the United States, David Stockman revealed that the administration fully understood that a tax cut for the wealthy would not improve collections and, indeed, it was the policy to create a debt precisely in order to undermine the capacity of the state to fund social services. Clearly, Swedish policy makers had to have known the effects of tax cuts in the United States and the U.K. While they have never acknowledged, as far as I know, a cynical manipulation of the public, it is hard to believe they did not know what they were doing.

8. The Swedish "ground laws" provided that, with a few exceptions, any document generated by a public agency was in the public domain and any citizen could see it on demand. The governing document of the European Union held that any document generated by a public agency was secret unless specific steps were taken to make it public.

9. This is not the place to undertake detailed documentation of health care reforms in other countries. Some of the recent literature on the U.K. reforms includes Vall-Spinosa (1991); Mellor (1994); Ham (1994; 1996a); Glennerster and Matsaganis (1994); Hughes, Jost, Griffiths, and McHale (1995); Ruggie (1996); Batchelor, West, and Plamping (1995); Ben-Shlomo and Chaturveda (1995); Buchan (1992); Calvert-Simms (1993); Dickson and Garside (1995); D'Sousa (1995); Foster, Norman, and Sheaff (1994); Inglis (1995); Klein (1995); McCallion, Stout, Harvey, and Rose (1991); O'Neill and Pearson (1995); Richmond (1996); Söderlund (1994); and Toon (1994).

10. The situation is more complex, of course, but only in detail.

11. Again, this is not the place for a documented argument. The reader is referred to Brown (1996); Blendon, Donelan, Leitman, Epstein, Cantor, Cohen, Morrison, Mahoney, and Koeck (1993); Bazzoli (1986); Dor (1994); Friedman and Shortell (1988); Gist (1996); Greenlick (1995); Greenlund and Elling (1995); Helms (1993); Holahan (1991); Lee and Estes (1994); Miller (1996); Navarro (1989).

12. Health insurance in the United States grew as a workplace benefit in lieu of wage increases during World War II and immediately afterward. For a description of the reform effort, the reader is referred to Albritton (1992); Brown (1996); Fuller (1994); Greenberg and Raymond (1994); Henderson (1995); Himmelstein (1994); Holahan (1991); Institute of Medicine, Committee on Assessing Health Care Reform Proposals (1993); Leyerli (1994); Miller (1996); and especially Kelly (1998).

13. See, for example, Brown (1996); Emanuel and Dubler (1995); Freeborn (1994); Fuller (1994); Greenlick (1995); Lee and Estes (1994); Leyerli (1994); Morreim (1995); Owens (1995); Shactman (1995), Schreter, Sharfstein, and Schreter (1994); and Traska (1995).

14. Some of the recent literature showing parallel reforms in different parts of the world includes "Health in 'Crisis?'" (1991); Arnould (1993); Blendon (1993); Burton (1994); Cassels (1995); Catley-Carlson (1992); Chernichovsky (1995); Ham (1994); Mechanic (1996); Murray, Kruser, and Whang (1994); Ruggie (1996); Sharpe and Faden (1996); U.S. Senate (1991); Vågerö (1994); and Wilsford (1995).

15. See, e.g., Barnett and Shystack (1994); Cairney (1995); Evans, Barer, Hartzman, Snderson, Pulcins, and Lomas (1989); Spasoff (1995); Sullivan (1995); Swartz (1993); and Wedge (1994).

16. See, e.g., Chanfreau (1979); Kritzner (1983); Scarpaci (1987); and Viveros-Long (1986).

17. See, e.g., Burchardi, Schuster, and Zielman (1994); Graf von der Schulenburg (1994); Heinrichs (1995); Kirkman-Liff and Neubauer (1992); Roy (1993); and U.S. General Accounting Office (1993).

18. See, e.g., Kawamura, Gotoda, and Yoshikura (1985); Tajimi, Shimada, Nishimura, and Sirio (1994); and Toguchi (1995).

19. See, e.g., Bloom, Sheng-lan, and Xing-yuan (1995); Grogan (1995); Ho (1998); Huang (1988); Liu, Hsiao, Li, Lui, and Rea (1995); Shi (1993); Yang, Lin, and Lawson (1991); and Zheng and Hiller (1995).

20. See, e.g., Banerji (1992); Devgan (1992); and Jyothi (1993).

21. See, e.g., Brugha (1991); and Butler (1986).

22. See, e.g., Cardoso (1993); Frenk, Gomez-Dantes, Cruz, Chacon, Hernandez, and Freeman (1994); Selwyn and Ruiz de Chavez (1985); Soberón, Frenk, Sepulveda (1986); and Stebbins (1986).

23. See, e.g., Elioutina and Tarasov (1995).

24. See, e.g., Brock and Grace (1993); and Naylor (1987; 1988).

25. See, e.g., Asenso-Okyere (1995); Banda and Walt (1995); Litviak and Bodart (1993); Monekosso (1993); Møgedal, Steen, and Mpelumbe (1995); and Ogbu and Gallagher (1992).

26. See, e.g., Alleyne (1995); Donahue (1986); Fiedler (1985); Garfield (1984); Kraudy, Liberati, Asioli, Saracena, and Tognomi (1987); Lane (1995); Rosero-Bixby (1991); and Ugalde (1984).

CHAPTER 8

Afterword

The study reported in this book covered a period from 1980 until 1994, a period containing a number of reforms and developments that led to some moderate market-oriented shifts in the organization of medical services. The push toward markets was much more pronounced in other areas of the society during this same period, but those developments lay outside the focus of this work except when they intruded into the medical care domain.

It is of course the case that the beginning and end of any analysis of social change is somewhat arbitrary. Changes continued after the end of the study period. Some of the more important ones are noted in Table 8.1. Early in 1994, the bourgeois coalition government continued to press for "reforms." They transferred money from the wage-earner funds to education and research, with emphasis on natural science and engineering. They limited the Health and Sickness Care Commission of Inquiry to altering financing of medical care, causing the Social Democratic members of the Commission to resign. Psychiatric care was transferred to the municipalities.

Clearly, the most important development during this period was the return of the Social Democrats to power under the leadership of former Finance Minister Göran Persson. They had less than a majority and depended upon the Center Party for support of the budget. A referendum to join the European Community passed narrowly. At about the time of the election, the long-term economic forecast projected a slow improvement in the economy over several years. The new government enacted an austere budget that prioritized inflation over unemployment while setting up a Commission of Inquiry to study the unemployment prob-

Table 8.1
Changes in Medical Care, the Economy, and Political Arrangements: Sweden, 1994–1998

Date	Medical Care	Economy	Politics
1994	Social Democrats resign from HSU (Feb.). State support for occupational health withdrawn (Apr.). Cost of psychiatric care transferred to municipalities (June). Commission of Inquiry recommends patients be compensated by state for injuries in medical care (Aug.). HSU 2000 subcommittee report says market reforms in other countries failed (SOU 1994:115). Prop. 1994/95:109 makes it harder to become a point-of-service physician.	Money from Löntagerfönder transferred to education and research. 500 EU rules take effect on 1 July. Austerity program instituted by new government to rationalize the state budget. Continued prioritizing of inflation over employment (Sept.). Commission set to study unemployment problem (Sept.).	Labor returns to Social Democrats to minimize damage from right-wing government. National election: Social Democrats return to power (with support of Center Party) with Ingvar Karlsson as Prime Minister (Sept.). Referendum to join EU passes 52/47/1 (Nov.).
1995	HSU gets altered directive—no longer to look at financing alternatives; will look at pharmaceutical prices and ways to increase choice of physicians (Feb.). Repeal of point-of-service law and care guarantee law (June).	Longtidsutredningen projects slow improvement in economy (Feb.). 1991 tax reform deepened depression, was not properly financed, increased income differences, but was "necessary" (SOU 1995:104).	
1996	Early pensions and sickness payments reduced (Jan. 1). Reduction of access to personal assistants for handicapped (Jan.). Parliament reports decline in quality of care for elderly. Marginalization of physicians (Oct.). Queues for medical care growing (Nov.). HSU reports gap between medical care need and resources—of crisis proportions in care of the aged (SOU 1996:163).	Proposal to set ceiling on expenditures by sector in state budget. "Calmfors Commission" proposes Sweden stay out of the European Monetary Union at the beginning (SOU 1996:158). Occupational Sickness and Injury Commission proposes replacing early pensions and income replacement for sickness with "monthly compensation plan" (SOU 1996:113).	Finance Minister Göran Persson replaces Ingvar Karlsson as Prime Minister (Mar.).

Table 8.1 (*continued*)

Date	Medical Care	Economy	Politics
	Parliament decides those who can do any work will not get early pensions or sickness payments (Dec.).		
	14 percent drop in number of private physicians reported in past year (SOU 1996:175).		
1997	Sickness insurance reduced. Responsibility for sickness payment for first four weeks transferred to employers. Counties and municipalities given responsibility for medical research (1 Jan.).	"Kalmar model" applied to nation; unemployed can be put to work to improve quality of state services (June).	
	Review of policy on sterilization between 1930 and 1976 ordered (Sept.).	Government commits to 50 percent reduction in unemployment by 2000 (Sept.).	
	Committee on Children proposal for minimum standard for school health and student health services (SOU 1997:116).	Municipal "savings" said to injure children in violation of UN Convention (SOU 1997:116).	
	HSU 2000 proposes more emphasis on preventive activities (SOU 1997:119).	Tax increase for high incomes (Sept.).	
	HSU 2000 proposes that patients have more choice of physicians and treatment (SOU 1997:154).	Unemployment heading for European levels; segregation increasing social differences (SOU 1997:118).	
	Class differences in health status growing (Nov.).	State insurance company proposed to handle pension funds (SOU 1997:131).	
		National bank directors more independent (SOU 1997:50; Prop. 1997/98:40).	
		Proposal to reduce income replacement for sickness (SOU 1997:85).	
		Directive issued to study dismantling of local support administration (Nov.).	

Table 8.1 (*continued*)

Date	Medical Care	Economy	Politics
1998	New laws take effect: Care support for parents of sick and handicapped children increased; Nursing homes to be dismantled by 1999; Income replacement for sick raised to 80 percent of wage. Proposal to shift dental care toward prevention with more cost sharing by patient for expensive restorative treatment (SOU 1998:2). Care guarantee to be reinstated in 1999 as general guarantee, not just for certain conditions (Jan.). Commission on cooperation between public and private sectors directed to review process for counties to contract with private health care providers (Mar.). Counties empowered to sponsor physicians for specialty training (July).	New laws take effect: Parental support increased to 80 percent of wage; Widow's pension to be means tested; Child support allowance increased; Employer contributions to social insurance decreased. Budget process in effect since 1996 said to result in more short-term view (Jan.). State transfers to counties will be more long term (Jan.). Increased funding for care of the aged (Apr.). Municipalities get more of value-added tax for care in retirement, service homes, and nursing homes. Budget surplus achieved.	Conservatives criticize government for abolishing care guarantee (Jan.). National election: Social Democrats returned to power with support of Left and Environmental Parties (Sept.).

lem. In 1996, Prime Minister Ingvar Carlsson resigned and was replaced by Finance Minister Göran Persson. The government then proposed setting a ceiling on expenditures in the state budget by sector. In 1997, they made a number of additional economic decisions:

- The Kalmar model was adopted nationally. Unemployed people could be put to work to improve the quality of state services.
- The government committed itself to cutting unemployment in half by 2000.
- Taxes were increased for high income people.
- A directive was issued to study dismantling the national commission on administration of local support systems.

In 1998, a number of new laws took effect to return the level of parental support to 80 percent of wages, to institute a means test for widow's pensions, to increase child support allowances, and to decrease employer contributions to social insurance. Decisions were taken to make state transfers to counties more long term. Further proposals were made to increase funding for the care of the aged, and increase the share of the value-added tax returned to municipalities for care of the aged.

In 1998, the state budget was back in balance for the first time in many years. Problems in the economy continued, however. Commission of Inquiry reports in 1997 showed that the savings in municipal budgets were reducing services to children, with the result that children were being injured. Unemployment seemed to be headed for European levels and the increased segregation caused by unemployment was increasing inequality. Commissions in 1998 reported that the budget process was creating an increasingly short-term view of economic policy, and that management costs in social insurance had increased dramatically during the 1990s. Proposals were made to create a state insurance company to handle pension funds, to make bank directors more independent (and remove decisions from the political process), to reduce income replacement for the sick, to merge budgets of counties and municipalities, and to limit early pensions to people over thirty, creating a new allowance system for handicapped people between nineteen and twenty-nine.

Commissions active during the previous government began to report in:

- A subcommittee of HSU 2000 that had studied market reforms in other countries concluded that those reforms were not successful in improving efficiency or effectiveness in medical care. Further, such reforms created greater inequality.
- An Occupational Sickness and Injury Commission proposed replacing early pensions and income replacement during sickness with a unified "monthly compensation plan."
- A Commission that studied the 1991 tax reform concluded that the reform had deepened the depression and increased income differences. While not properly financed, the reform was still said to be necessary to ensure competitiveness in Europe.
- A Commission proposed that Sweden stay out of the European Monetary Union until other countries had a chance to test it.

In 1998, a new election returned the Social Democrats to power, this time with support from the Left and Environmental Parties.

On the medical care side, in 1994, the government proposed that there be more restrictions on becoming a point-of-service physician. In 1995, a new directive was given to HSU 2000 which removed the mandate to look at financing alternatives and added mandates to study pharmaceutical prices and ways of increasing patient choice of physicians. The point-of-service law and the care guarantee law passed by the previous government were repealed.

In 1996, HSU 2000 reported that there was a growing gap between the medical care needs of the population and the resources that were being allocated to medical care. This gap was particularly critical with reference to care of the aged. Other reports noted a decline in the quality of care for the aged and the marginalization of physicians in care of the aged, queues for medical care were again increasing, and there was a 14-percent decline in private physicians in the past year.

Decisions were taken to reduce early pensions and income replacement for sickness, to reduce access to assistants for the handicapped, and to require anyone who was able to work instead of getting pensions or sickness payments.

In 1997, it was reported that class differences in health were growing. Proposals were entered to reduce sickness insurance, to transfer responsibility for sickness payments to employers for the first four weeks of each sickness episode, to make counties and municipalities responsible for medical research, to set minimum standards for school health and student health services, to put greater emphasis on prevention, and to increase choice of physician and treatment modalities.

In 1998, it was reported that long-term sickness was increasing. Several new laws took effect to provide support for parents of sick and handicapped children, to dismantle nursing homes, and to raise income replacement for the sick to 80 percent of wages. A Commission on Cooperation between Public and Private Sectors was created and directed to review the process for counties to contract with private health care providers. Several other decisions were taken: to shift dental care insurance toward prevention by requiring larger copayments for restorative work; to reinstate the care guarantee in 1999, this time as a general guarantee not limited to a list of conditions; to empower counties to sponsor physicians for specialty training; to amend the health and sickness care law to limit patients to free choice of physician within their geographic area and to increase the right to choose a physician within that area; and to allow second opinions and greater choice of treatment modalities. This is the point where our narrative ends, bringing us to the beginning of November 1998.

The changes since the end of the study in 1993 seemed to be quite mixed. On the economic side, the state budget was rationalized and greater attention could be turned toward unemployment. The economic outlook was brighter, but still with some concern about effects of external developments, primarily in the EU.

On the political side, the Social Democrats were returned to power and managed to run a minority government, for the first time actively involving the Left Party in 1998.

Medical care policy seemed unsettled. Except for repealing bourgeois reforms, there seemed to be little that suggested a traditional Social Democratic thrust. Increasing freedom of choice and reducing health insurance benefits seemed fully in accord with the policies of the right. Decentralization seemed also to support the weakening of the counties and continued transfer of authority and responsibility to the municipalities, a Conservative Party platform. Only the increase of funding for programs where people had been shown to be injured by cuts could be seen as consistent with the old Social Democratic Party.

The play continues.

Appendix A

The Health and Sickness Care Law of 1982 (as of January 1, 1994)

Preliminary Decisions

1 § As health and sickness care in this law, we include means for medical prevention, diagnosis and treatment of diseases and injuries. Transportation of the sick is part of health and sickness care.

On the issue of dental care there are separate decisions. *Law 1992:567.*

The Goal for Health and Sickness Care

2 § The goal of health and sickness care is good health and care on equal terms for the whole population.

Demand for Health and Sickness Care

2a § Health and sickness care shall be managed so that it fulfills the demand for good care. That means that it will especially

1. be of good quality and satisfy the patients' need for security in care and treatment,
2. be easily accessible,
3. build on respect for the patients' independence and integrity,
4. foster good contacts between patients and health and sickness care personnel.

Care and treatment shall, as much as possible, be designed and implemented in consultation with the patient.

The patient shall be given information about his/her health status and on the methods of treatment that are under consideration. If the information can not be given to the patient it shall instead be given to a close relative. Information may not be given to the patient or any relative if there is an impediment provided in 7 Chap 3 § or 6 § of the law on privacy (1980:100) or in 6 § paragraph two or 6a paragraph one of the law (1990:11) on supervision of health and sickness care personnel etc. *Law 1985:560.*

2b § Health and sickness care shall work to prevent health problems. Those who turn to health and sickness care shall, whenever possible, be given information on methods of preventing disease or injury. *Law 1985:560.*

2c § When someone has died the duties of health and sickness care are completed with reference to the deceased. The survivors shall be shown consideration and solicitude. *Law 1992:567.*

The County Health and Sickness Care

The responsibility of county government

3 § Every county will offer good health and sickness care to those who are resident within the county. It will also work in other ways for good health for the whole population. Everything said in this law about county governments applies as well to municipalities that are not part of a county unless otherwise provided in 17 §. What is stated here does not prevent another agency from running health and sickness care.

The responsibilities of counties do not include such health and sickness care that a municipality within the county has responsibility for according to 18 § first and third paragraphs.

A county may conclude negotiations with another entity in order to carry out the duties the county is responsible for according to this law. A duty that requires the activity of a public authority may not with support of this decision be turned over to a company, an association, . . . a foundation, or a single individual. *Law 1992:1382.*

3a § The county shall offer those resident in the county

1. health promotion [*habitering*] and rehabilitation
2. aids for disabilities and
3. translation services for congenital deafness, deaf-blindness, adult deafness, and speech impairments.

The county's responsibility does not include treatment, rehabilitation and health promotion that a municipality within the county has responsibility for under 18a §. The county's responsibility does not imply any reduction in the duties an employer or others may have under other laws.

Health promotion or rehabilitation along with supplies of therapeutic goods [*hjälpmedel*] shall be planned in cooperation with the individual. The proposed and decided items in the plan shall be clear. *Law 1993:91.*

4 § If someone who is visiting in the county without being a resident there needs urgent care, the county will offer such care.

A county may also, in other instances, offer health and sickness care to those resident in another county if the counties agree on that. *Law 1992:567.*

5 § For health and sickness care that requires admission to a care institution there shall be hospitals. Care given under such admissions is called inpatient care [*sluten vård*]. Other health and sickness care is called ambulatory care [*öppen vård*].

The county shall organize ambulatory care so that everyone has access to and can choose a point-of-service primary care physician [*husläkare*]. Decisions on such physicians are found in the law (1993:588) on point-of-service primary care physicians. *Law 1993:587.*

6 § The county is responsible for having in the county a suitable organization for transporting persons to and from the hospital or physician which support requires that the transportation be done with vehicles that are specially equipped for the purpose.

7 § The county shall plan health and sickness care beginning with the population's need for such care. Planning will include health and sickness care provided by agencies other than the county and municipalities within the county.

8 § In the planning and development of health and sickness care the county will cooperate with social institutions, organizations, and individuals. *Law 1992:567.*

9 § The national government may prescribe that the nation be divided into regions for health and sickness care that consist of several counties.

Counties will work together on issues that influence health and sickness care. *Law 1992:567.*

Boards [Nämnder]

10 § The governance of health and sickness care is exercised by one or more boards. For such a board everything applies as written on boards in the Municipality Law [*Kommunallagen*] (1977:179).

The counties may create a special board of health and sickness care or empower another board to be the health and sickness care board. If this is not done, the administrative committee is the health and sickness care board.

11 § repealed by Law 1991:909

12 § repealed by Law 1991:903.

Personnel

13 § Within health and sickness care shall be found the personnel needed to provide good care. For a unit as provided in 14 § a patient-responsible licensed physician shall be identified for every patient.

On the duties of health and sickness care personnel on supervision over that personnel there are separate decisions. *Law 1990:601.*

14 § For units for diagnosis or care and treatment other than the point-of-service primary care physician there shall, with reference to patient safety, be found a special physician with specialist certification who answers for the collective leadership of the work activity. Such a physician shall be called chief physician [*chefsöverläkare*]. In the carrying out of that leadership that person shall follow the directives of the county in matters not directly involving diagnosis or care and treatment of individual patients or supervision of the attending physician.

The chief physician may find that those holding positions in the unit who have the appropriate credentials and experience may perform specific duties of leadership. *Law 1993:587.*

15 § Physicians in general practice or specialty residency training according to the law (1984:542) on qualification to work in health and sickness care shall be appointed for set terms.

The national government may provide that physicians in specialty training according to the above law who have completed medical school may be appointed for limited terms. *Law 1991:1971.*

16 § The national government is authorized to issue regulations on qualifications for positions in health and sickness care and on appointments. The national government may delegate the issuance of such regulations to the Ministry of Health and Welfare.

On the question of units within health and sickness care which have been put at the disposal of basic college training of physicians there are separate decisions.

Municipalities' Health and Sickness Care

17 § Decisions in 18–25 §§ apply to municipalities which are part of a county as well as, in the case where it is specially provided, the municipalities that are not part of a county.

Responsibility of Municipalities

18 § Every municipality shall offer good health and sickness care to those who live in a residence [*bondeform*] or house such as defined in 20 § second paragraph and 21 § third paragraph of the social service law

(1980:620). Every municipality shall also, in conjunction with the day care [*dagersamhet*] as defined in 10 § of the social service law, offer good health and sickness care to those who stay there.

A municipality may also offer those who reside in the municipality health and sickness care in the home (*hemsjukvård*).

The county may turn over responsibility for offering such care to a municipality within the county, as stated in the second paragraph, if the county and the municipality come to an agreement on it and the national government approves.

The municipalities' responsibility in accord with the first and third paragraph and the municipalities' authority in accord with the second paragraph does not include such health and sickness care as furnished by a physician.

A municipality may enter negotiations with another entity if that furthers the duties the municipality is responsible for under this law. A duty that requires governance by an authority may not with the support of this decision be turned over to a company, an association, . . . a foundation, or a single individual. *Law 1992:1382.*

18a § Municipalities shall, in conjunction with such health and sickness care as defined in 18 § first through third paragraphs, also offer, . . . rehabilitation and appliances for the functionally handicapped.

The county may also without coordination with transfer of responsibility for health and sickness care as provided in 18 § come to agreement with a municipality that the county will have responsibility for functionally handicapped who are attended by a municipality. *Law 1993:391.*

19 § If a transfer has occurred according to 18 § third paragraph, the county may give the appropriate economic support to the municipality as motivated by the transfer. *Law 1992:567.*

20 § The municipality shall plan its health and sickness care from the starting point of the population's need for such care.

Planning will also take into account the health and sickness care offered by other than the municipality and county. *Law 1992:567.*

21 § In the planning and development of health and sickness care, the municipality shall coordinate with social organs, organizations, and individuals. *Law 1990:1465.*

Boards

22 § Governance of a municipality's health and sickness care shall be practiced by the board or boards the municipal council decides upon in accordance with 4 § of the social service law (1980:620).

In a municipality that is not part of a county governance of health and sickness care shall be practiced as provided in 18 § first or second paragraph in accord with 10 §. *Law 1992:567*

Personnel

23 § The health and sickness care personnel needed to provide good care shall be found in a municipality.

On the duties of health and sickness care personnel and on the supervision of such personnel there are separate decisions. *Law 1992:567.*

24 § Within the work area decided upon by the municipality there shall be a nurse who is responsible

1. that there are routines for making contact with a physician or some other health and sickness care personnel when required by a patient's condition.
2. that decisions on delegation of responsibility for care duties are consistent with the safety of the patients.
3. that the reports go to the board that governs health and sickness care activity if a patient, in connection with care or treatment is injured or placed at risk of serious injury or disease.

If a work activity mainly involves rehabilitation a physical therapist or occupational therapist has the responsibility stated in the first paragraph.

Decisions in the first and second paragraph apply as well to municipalities that are not part of counties if in such health and sickness care activities as provided in 18 § first or second paragraph there are no physicians. *Law 1992:567.*

25 § The national government is empowered to issue regulations on qualifications for service in municipal health and sickness care and on appointments. The national government may delegate to the Ministry of Health the issuance of such regulations. *Law 1992:567.*

Common Decisions on Counties and Municipalities Health and Sickness Care

Payment for Care

26 § Payment for services may be taken from patients on grounds decided upon by the counties or municipalities if nothing else is specially directed. Patients resident within the county or municipality will all be treated alike.

The municipality may only take out the treatment fees for such care as they are responsible for paying according to 2 § of the law (1990:1404) on the municipalities' responsibility for paying for certain health and sickness care. The same applies to the question of such psychiatric long-term care with primarily personal care content for which the municipality has responsibility for paying according to 9 § of the same law.

Fees for care provided for in 18 § or for such long-term medical care that a municipality has responsibility for paying under 2 or 9 § or the law (1990:1404) on the municipalities' responsibility for paying for certain health and sickness care may not, together with fees as provided in 35 § third paragraph of the law on social service (1980:60), be at such a level that the individual has inadequate means for his or her personal needs. *Law 1993:48.*

27 § The Ministry of Health has supervision of the counties and municipalities health and sickness care. The Ministry shall thereby follow and support work activities. With the delegation of supervision, the Ministry has the right to conduct inspections. *Law 1992:567.*

Further directives

28 § The national government is authorized in questions of county and municipal health and sickness care to issue further regulations for the protection of individuals or concerning the direction of work activities in general.

The national government may delegate to the Ministry of Health and Welfare the task of issuing directives for the protection of individuals. *Law 1992:567.*

Health and Sickness Care in War, etc.

29 § The national government is empowered to issue special directives on health and sickness care in war, under threat of war, or under such extraordinary circumstances which give rise to the nation finding itself in war outside of Sweden or threat of war. *Law 1992:1423.*

Appendix B

Sample Elements: Organizations and Individuals Interviewed

Based on information on hand at the beginning of this study, the then-current national and county governments were the ones pushing reforms. Much experimentation was underway at the county level. Further, the physicians' union was taking an active and leading role in the reform effort. We had information that there were important sources of resistance in the nurses' union and the blue-collar public employees' union (Twaddle, 1992). What remained was to search for other organizations active in the debates, but which had not yet come to our attention. It seemed likely that occupational groups in health care (e.g., physical therapists, medical social workers) might be active, but a check with those unions produced no position papers or spokespersons addressing the issues. Since all the unions are organized into peak organizations (LO on the part of blue-collar unions, TCO on the part of white-collar unions, and SACO on the part of academic unions), arrangements were made to interview officers of the peak organizations and for them to identify unions within their organizations that were actively engaging the debates. SACO headquarters reported that the only active union was the physicians and that SACO took its lead from them, taking no independent role in the debate. LO reported that SKAF was the only interested union in their organization, but LO itself was developing materials germane to the debate. TCO reported that SKTF was very actively engaged in the controversy and that TCO was developing materials. In addition, there were some individuals who were very actively involved in the debates, but in a manner that did not represent particular organizations in an official capacity. We included them whenever possible.

Our sample, then, consisted of the following organizations, within which we identified our primary points of contact, individuals who were the subjects of interviews and who provided us with the documents to understand their positions and roles in the debates. Since the persons interviewed were all publicly identified already in the debates, there is no reason to disguise their identities. Their organizations were well known and they were well known as spokespersons, so any such attempt would fail in any event.

The National Government: Department of Social Welfare (Socialstyrelsen)

The Deputy Minister of Social Welfare and the Minister of Health was Bo Könberg. He was fully responsible for the health care policy of the government. Assistant Minister of Health Ingrid Petersson was the one who drafted the legislative proposals of the ministry.

Könberg was a politician with the *Folkpartiet Liberalerna* and had a special interest in health policy and social insurance issues. He had been linked with the proposal for a point-of-service physician plan since the mid-1970s. I had met Könberg on two previous occasions. In 1990, we had been seated next to one another for three days at a conference on health policy in Stockholm. In 1992, we met again at a conference on Swedish health policy at Emory University, organized by Richard Saltzman. Ms. Pettersson was a bright young politician whom I had also met at Emory.

The Health and Welfare Committee of Parliament (Socialutskottet)

This was the committee that considered all bills relating to medical care and health. It also had a consultative role in consideration of social insurance issues. The political parties with positions on health care would have those positions articulated on the committee. In consultation with committee chairman Bo Holmberg, we selected one member of each political party to interview.

Interviews were completed with the following: Bo Holmberg, representing the Social Democratic Party, which had taken a leading role in the development of the modern Swedish welfare state; Leif Bergdahl of the New Democratic Party, a populist, anti-immigrant party that was newly formed for the previous election; Leif Carlsson, Conservative Party, the leading opponents of the Social Democrats; Jerzy Einhorn, an oncologist who represented the Christian Democratic Party; Ulla Orring of the Liberal Party; Rosa Östh of the Center Party; and Eva Zetterberg of the Left (formerly Left Communist) Party. All interviews were conducted at the Parliament in the Health and Welfare Committee Chamber, with the exception of Dr. Bergdahl, who was interviewed in the Committee Library.

Federation of County Councils

The Federation was a leading sponsor of the reform effort. Their report, *Crossroads*, was the major document laying forth a position in favor of reform and in defining the issues. Two interviews were done to clarify their position. One was with Bengt Mollstedt, president of the board of directors. He was a Conservative Party politician who had held positions as city counselor and director of the Department of Health and Hospitals in Göteborg and who then chaired the Health Policy Committee of the Council of Europe. I had known him since 1978, when he had been very helpful in facilitating my research on primary care. I consider him a friend. The other interview was with Olof Eliasson, Director of the Department of Health Care Services. He was the top staff person in charge of the county governments' coordinated efforts to manage health care. Hence, he was the key operational person in the Federation with regard to this issue.

Physicians' Union

As noted, the physicians' union was a leading proponent of reform, having taken steps to initiate the debate in collaboration with the Federation of County Councils. The secretary general of that union was Anders Milton, whom I had met both at the conference in Stockholm and at the conference at Emory University.

Nurses Union

Inger Ohlsson was president of *Vårdförbundet SHSTF*. I had met her at the Stockholm conference. Lena Sundström was the secretary general. The nurses had taken a leading role in questioning the reform effort, and during the study period had launched a major public-relations campaign attacking the ideology of the reformers.

Landsorganizationen I Sverige (LO)

This was the peak organization of blue-collar unions. In the years of close association with the Social Democratic Party, LO had taken an important role in the development of the welfare state. Two persons were interviewed after having been identified by the President as the ones who could best represent the LO position on medical care reform. Per-Olof Edin was an economist with the Political Economy Unit who had earlier served in the Ministry of Finance under the previous Social Democratic government. Jan Edling was head of the Political Economy Unit.

Union of Municipal Employees

On the recommendation of Liljemor Arvidsson, president of the union representing blue collar public employees including all those employed in health care, an interview was done with Per Rudin at the national headquarters. Rudin was a former nurse assistant who dealt with health and welfare issues for the union. In addition, I visited the union local in Linköping, where I interviewed Tommy Pettersson, a youth worker who was playing an active role in union activities.

Swedish Service Workers Union (TCO)

This is the peak organization of white-collar unions. Anders Forsman, head of the Socioeconomic Analysis Unit, was interviewed. He was an economic historian by training and assumed responsibility for all social and economic analysis for the organization.

Union of Municipal Employees (SKTF)

This is the union that represented virtually all of the white-collar workers in the public sector. Sture Nordh, president of the union, was interviewed. He was very much in the debate on social welfare, having coauthored a book with the head of the Liberal Party defending the principles of the welfare state against neoliberal reform efforts.

Others

Several others were interviewed, not so much for their organizational affiliations but because they had taken a role in the debates presenting viewpoints not otherwise represented. These included the following.

Gunlog Bratt was a Liberal Party representative to the County Council of Östergötland. She was interviewed at the suggestion of Lennart Nordenfelt, Professor at Tema H, University of Linköping. Östergötland was one of the counties experimenting with health care reforms and had implemented a point-of-service reform well in advance of the national government.

Johannes Vang was a physician employed by the World Health Organization in Denmark, but who kept an apartment in Linköping and took an active role in the Swedish reform debates. He was the principal author of the Federation of County Council's *Crossroads* report, perhaps the most influential document in the reform effort.

Gösta Tibblin was Professor of General Medicine at Uppsala University, the first person to hold such a post in the country. He had a distinguished career as a cardiologist and epidemiologist before assuming that post. He was interviewed as a person well positioned to speak to the impact of reforms on primary care, where much of the effort was focused.

Johan Calltorp was Associate Professor of Social Medicine at the Karolinska Institut in Huddinge. He was a prominent researcher in social medicine who had studied issues central to the debates on medical care reform, especially the implications of economic incentives for the efficiency and effectiveness of medical intervention.

Glossary

Allmanläkare General practitioners of medicine.
Ansvarsnämden See Hälso- och Sjukvårdsansvarsnämden.
Avgift Fee.
Barnavårdscentraler Child health centers. Staffed by pediatric nurses and visited weekly by pediatricians. Provide medical surveilance of children from birth until entry into the school health system. See skolhälsovård.
Barnmöterska Nurse midwife. All but the complicated pregnancies and deliveries are managed by nurses.
C See Centerpartiet.
Centerpartiet (c) The Center Party, formerly the Farmer's Party, which absorbed and then lost the green wave movement in the 1970s and early 1980s when they compromised on the nuclear power issue. Now reclaiming the environmental vote. Traditionally close to the Social Democrats on economic issues, but recently dominated by a conservative wing.
Distriktssköterska District nurse who works independently in her own reception.
Folkhemmet Literally, the people's home, a core Social Democratic image of a sociey in which the population is like a family, taking care of one another in times of need.
Folkpartiet liberalerna (fp) Literally, the Folk Party or People's Party, usually translated as the Liberal Party. Strongest among white-collar, middle-management workers. Policy is supportive of a strong welfare state in a market economy. At the time of these interviews, the head of the Folkpartiet was the Minister of Social Welfare and the member responsible for health policy was the Minister of Health.
Folkpension The pension guaranteed to all through social insurance.
Folkrörelsen Literally, peoples' movement. Refers to a variety of mass movements that were historically important in extending the franchise and developing political parties that represented the interests of common people,

including temperance, mental health, and unions. In more recent times, a strong environmental movement has grown.

Fortidspension Early retirement pension.

Fp See Folkpartiet.

Färdigbehandlade Literally, completely treated. Refers, in this context, to people, primarily the elderly, who are in the hospital only because a suitable alternative placement has not been arranged. These people block beds in acute care that should be otherwise used, according to the hospital. They are sometimes called "bed blockers."

Företagshälsovård Occupational or industrial health care.

Försakring Insurance.

Förslag Proposal.

Färdigbehandlade Literally, completely treated. Patients whose hospital treatment is completed and who need another form of treatment organization.

Grundskolan Primary school. The first three years of compulsory schooling.

Grundtrygghet Literally, basic safety. In the debates on social insurance (income replacement from unemployment, sickness, etc.) a position calling for the same basic allowance to everyone. See also, inkomsbortfall.

HSAN See Hälso-och Sjukvårdsansvarsnämden

HSU or HSU 2000 See Hälso-och Sjukvårds Utredningen.

Husläkare Literally, house doctor. The name for a family practitioner who provides primary medical care services. The development of the *husläkare* has been a political goal of the Folkpartiet since the mid 1970s. A bill was enacted in the spring of 1993 to have individual registration with a family practitioner a universal feature. The bill allows for private physicians to be included in the system, which is a major change in the system.

Hälso-och Sjukvårdsansvarsnämden (HSAN) National Board of Health Care Responsibility with authority to hear complaints about medical care and to discipline health professionals.

Hälso-och Sjukvårds Utredning(en) (HSU 2000) A commission of inquiry investigating options for medical care organization.

Inkomsbortfall Literally, income loss. In the debate on social insurance, the principle that the programs should replace a percentage of the income lost from unemployment, sickness, or the like. See also, grundtrygghet.

Kanslihushöger, Kanslihushögern Members of the Social Democratic government of 1982–1990, centered on the Minister of Finance, Kjell-Olof Feldt, who adopted neoliberal economic policies.

Kds See Kristendemokraterna Samlingspartiet.

Kommun Municipality. Regional government in Sweden is organized at three levels, the national *(Stat)*, the county (*Län*), and the municipality (*Kommun*). These do not form a hierarchy, but are independent, each with special responsibilities. The *Kommun* is usually an area larger than a town or city with responsibility for schools, roads, and since the Ädel Reform in 1992, care of the aged.

Kommunalarbetareförbundet (SKAF), Svenska Kommunal Arbetares Förbundet Literally, the Municipal Workers Union, which represents the blue-collar workers who are employed by the governmental organization known as *Kommun.* It is the union within LO that represents almost all of those employed in health and medical care.

Kommunaltjänstmänsförbundet (SKTF), Svenska Kommunal Tjänstemannens Förbundet Literally, the Union of Municipal Service Workers, which represents almost all of the whitecollar workers in health and medical care, most of whom work for a *Län.*

Konkurrens Competition.

Kontinuiteten Continuity.

Kristendemokraterna Samlingspartiet (Kds) The Christian Democratic Party, moderately conservative on economic issues, progressive on social security, and antifeminist. Membership tends to come from socially conservative church activists.

Köp–Sälj Purchase–Sale. A form of organization pioneered in the U.K. by which the financing and delivery of medical services are separated. Public entities contract competitively with service providers. Not generally regarded as a successful experiment.

Landsorganisation i Sverige See LO.

Landsting County Council.

Landstingsförbundet The Federation of County Councils. Each *Län* is governed by an elected body known as a *Landsting*, or county council. This is the county council's national organization.

LO Landsorganisation i Sverige, usually translated as the Swedish Federation of Swedish Labor Unions. It is always referred to by its initials. This is a peak organization of blue-collar unions.

Läkarförbundet Literally, Sveriges Läkarförbund, the Swedish Medical Association, which functions as a union for physicians. It publishes the influential *Läkartidningen*, which translates as the *Physicians' Journal,* It has within it constituent organizations representing specialty groups (e.g., *distriktsläkare*) or groups with special employment circumstances (e.g., house physicians). See also, Läkarsällskap.

Läkarsällskap The professional organization of physicians promoting the knowledge base of clinical medicine.

Län Literally, county. Counties are responsible for medical care and college, as opposed to university, education. See also, Kommun.

Länsjukhus County hospital.

M See Moderaterna Samlingspartiet.

Miljöpartiet The Environmental Party. Built in the late 1970s primarily to oppose nuclear power generation after the Center Party compromised on the issue. Held seats in parliament after the 1982 elections, but lost them in the 1990 election.

Moderaterna Samlingspartiet (m) Literally the Moderate Assembly Party, but generally translated as Conservative Party. They represent the economic elites and coporate interests. Inspired by the Reagan–Bush administrations in the United States and the Thatcher government in the U.K., they are aggressively neoliberal.

Moderates Conservatives. See Moderaterna Samlingspartiet.

Modravårdcentral Maternal health center.

Nyd See Nydemokraterna.

Nydemokraterna (Nyd) The New Democratic Party or members of the New Democratic Party. This is a new party formed for the 1992 election and voted out in the 1994 election. They are neoliberal on economic issues, anti-immigrant, and favor progressive taxation. Their voters tended to be young, unemployed Social Democrats disaffected by their party's turn to the right.

Nyliberaler Neoliberals, an economic school associated with Milton Freeman in the United States and Assar Lindbeck in Sweden, who influenced the economic policies of the Pinochet, Reagan, Bush, Thatcher, and Bildt governments.

Open Care See Öppen vård.

Öppen vård Ambulatory care outside of hospitals.

Politiker Politicians.

Primarvårdcentraler Primary care centers.

Privatläkare Private physicians.

Ramlag A "frame law" that sets broad parameters within which other governmental units must legislate.

Remiss A process by which proposed legislation is circulated for public comment before being introduced to the legislature.

Riksdag The national parliament, consisting, since 1971, of a single chamber with representatives, or *ledamoter*.

Riksförsäkringsverket Social Insurance Administration.

S See Socialdemokraterna.

SACO Centralorganisation SACO/SR, the peak federation of academic unions combining the Swedish Union of Academics and the State Civil Service Union.

SAF Sveriges Arbetsgivareförening, the Swedish Employers Association.

Samma för alla Literally, the same for everybody. A phrase often used to describe equality and justice, particularly on the left.

SAP See Socialdemokraterna.

SBU Statens Beredning för Medicinsk Utvädering, Swedish Council on Technology Assessment in Health Care.

SHSTF Vådfördundet Sveriges Hälso-och Sjukvårds Tjäanstemäns Förbundet, the Swedish Association of Health Professionals, representing nurses and laboratory technicians.

Sjukhem Nursing home.

Sjukvård Literally, sick care, but better translated as medical care.

Sjukvårdsminister Minister of Health, who is also the Deputy Minister of Welfare.

SKAF See Kommunalarbetareförbundet.

Skolhälsovård School health care. A system in which a pediatric nurse staffs a full-time school clinic with support from weekly visits of a pediatrician.

SKTF See Kommunaltjänstmänsförbundet

Socialdemokraterna (SAP or S) The dominant Social Democratic Party, closely tied historically to the labor movement, particularly LO. They are seen as the architects of the welfare state whose political direction is currently under attack.

Socialstyrelsen National Board of Health and Welfare.

Socialuttskottet The parliamentary Committee on Health and Social Services. This is the committee that reviews most of the legislation in the area of health and medical care and makes recommendations to the *Riksdag* on the passage or nonpassaage of bills.

Stadsläkare A city physician employed by the department of public health to provide, among other things, clinical services to businesses too small to have their own occupational health units.

Stat Literally, the state, refering to the national government. The national government provides a legal framework within which the counties and municipalities must work, but leaving them free to organize how they do that work. See also, Kommun, Län.

Studieförbundet för Näringsliv och Sämhälle (SNS) Research Company for Commerce and Society. A right-wing think tank allied with SAF.

Styrelse Board

TCO Tjänstemännans Centralorganisation, usually translated as the Federation of Public Service Workers. This is a peak union organization representing white-collar workers. It is always referred to by its initials.

Tjänstemännans Centralorganisation See TCO.

Undersköterskor Assistant nurses.

Utredning(ar) Commission or committee set up to do investigations and make policy recommendations. When set up by Parliament we refer to them as Commissions of Inquiry, analogous in many ways to the Royal Commissions in the U.K. In Sweden, these have been a routine instrument of policy formation until the 1991–1999 government, which preferred relying on expert groups.

V See Vänsterpartiet.

Valfrihet Freedom of Choice. The slogan of the right in the current debates.

Verklighet Reality.

Vård Care, usually referring to nursing care, or ward, as in a hospital ward.

Vårdbidrader Nurse assistants, similar in training to the American licensed practical nurse.

Vårdcentral A primary health care center staffed by specialists in general medicine, pediatrics, maternal health, community nursing, social work, and, depending on the size of the area, other occupations.

Vårdgaranti Care guarantee. A law saying that if your county fails to treat you within a period of time you can get care from any other county and yours will pay for it.

Vårdkö Waiting list for care.

Vårdlag Medical care team.

Vårdnadbidrag Care allowance covering family support, child care, and sickness care, proposed by Center Party.

Vänsterpartiet (v) The Left Party, former the Left Communist Party. Their tradition was Eurocommunist; that is, not tied to either the Soviet Union, the People's Republic of China, or any other external power. Pursued socialism within a democratic context. Pursuing a closer approximation to direct democracy.

References

We follow the Swedish alphabet. Letters appear in the same order as in the English alphabet with the addition of three letters following Z: Åå, Ää, and Öö.

Abbott, Andrew. 1988. *The System of Professions.* Chicago: University of Chicago Press.

Agrell, Wilhelm. 1992. "Farväll till svensk neutralitet." In EG/EU—Till Vilket Pris? Edited by Stockholm: Lts Förlag, 12–20.

Agrell, Wilhelm, Jörgen Bengtson, Per Olov Enquist, Per Gahrton, Per Jensen, Karl-Erik Lagerlöf, Gudrun Schyman, Ronny Svensson, Gunilla Thorngren, Marita Ulvskog, Sören Wibe, Michael Williams. 1992. *EG/EU—Till Vilket Pris?* Stockholm: LTs Förlag.

Albritton Frankie P. 1992. *Health Care Insurance Reform in the United States: A Market Approach with Application from the Federal Republic of Germany.* Lanham, Md: University Press of America.

Alford, R. R. 1975. *Health Care Politics.* Chicago: University of Chicago Press.

Alleyne, G. 1995. "Prospects and Challenges for Health in the Americas." *Bulletin of the Pan American Health Organization,* 29:264–71.

Almström, Bjarne. 1991. "Socialförsäkringen—och EG." In *Den sociala dimensionen in Europasamarbetet: Rapport från ett seminarium in februari 1991.* Stockholm: Utrikesdepartment, 55–56.

Andersson, Sivert. 1991. "Arbetarskyddet i ett Europaperspektiv." In *Den sociala dimensionen* in *Europasamarbetet: Rapport från ett seminarium in februari 1991,* Stockholm: Utrikesdepartment, 19–20.

Andersson, Sten. 1993. *I De Lugnaste Vattnen.* Stockholm: Tiden.

Antonio, Robert, and Douglas Kellner. 1992. "Communication, Modernity, and Democracy in Havermas and Dewey." *Symbolic Interaction* 15:277–97.

Arnould, Richard, Robert Rich, and William White, eds. 1993. *Competitive Approaches to Health Care Reform.* Washington, D.C.: Urban Institute Press.

Arvidsson, Lillemor. 1990. *Vård på Lika Vilkor*. Stockholm: LO 90.07 2.00, Art. nr.566-0936-1.

———. 1992. *Synpunkter på Förslag Angånde Husläkarsystem*. Stockholm: Svenska Kommunalarbetareförbundet (mimeo).

Arvius, Chister. 1989. "Europastandardiseringens Betydelse för Sverige och för Integrationen i Västeuropa." *Fakta Europa*. Stockholm: Utrikesdepartmentet.

Asenso-Okyere, W. K. 1995. "Financing Health Care in Ghana." *World Health Forum* 16:86–91.

Augustsson, Lars-Åke, and Stig Hansén. 1991. *På Spaning Efter Socialismen*. Stockholm: Ordfronts Förlag.

Banda, Ellias Ngalande, and Gill Walt. 1995. "The Private Health Sector in Malawi: Opening Pandora's Box." *J. International Development* 7:403–21.

Banerji, D. 1992. "Report of the Commission on Health Research for Development and the Countries of the South." *International J. Health Services* 22:169–77.

Barnett, R., and A. Shustack. 1994. "Cost Containment: The Americas: Canada." *New Horizons* 2:332–35.

Batchelor, P. A., R. G. West, and D. Plamping. 1995. "The NHS Reform Programme: Implications for Dental Public Health and the Community Dental Services." *Community Dental Health* 12:171–74.

Bazzoli, G. J. 1986. "Health Care for the Indigent: Overview of Critical Issues." *Health Services Research* 21:3:353–93.

Bengtson, Jörgen. 1992. "Statsförbundet Norden—ett alternativ till Europiska unionen." In *EG/EU—Till VilketPris*, edited by W. Agrell. Stockholm: LT. Förlag, 159–77.

Ben-Shlomo, Y., and N. Chaturveda. 1995. "Assessing Equity in Access to Health Care Provision in the U.K.: Does Where You Live Affect Your Chances of Getting a Coronary Artery Bypass Graft?" *J. Epidemiology and Community Health* 49:200–204.

Bergqvist, Roland. 1991. "LO, EG och arbetsrätten," In *Den sociala dimensionen in Europasamarbetet:Rapport från ett seminarium in februari 1991*. Stockholm: Utrikesdepartment, 37–38.

Bergroth, Alf. 1992. *Försäkringskassan i form för framtiden: Brygga mellan teori och praktik*. Stockholm: Folksam.

Bergström, Hans. 1992. "Pressures behind the Swedish Health Reforms." In *Viewpoint Sweden*, Bulletin no. 12. New York: Swedish Information Service.

Bergström, Villy. 1992. "Party Program and Economic Policy: The Social Democrats in Government." In *Creating Social Democracy*, edited by K. Misgeld, K. Molin, and K. Åmark. University Park: Pennsylvania State University Press, 131–174.

———. 1993. *Varför Överge den Svenska Modellen: 12 Uppsatser om Arbetslöshet och Stabiliseringspolitik*. Stockholm: Tiden.

Bergström, Villy, and Karl-Gustaf Löfgren. 1993. "Arbetsmarknadspolitiken Under Krisen." In *Varför Överge den Svenska Modellen*, edited by V. Bergström. Stockholm: Tiden, 58–68.

Berleen, Göran, Stefan Håkansson, et al. 1992. *The Reform of Health Care in Sweden*. Stockholm: Swedish Planning and Rationalization Institute.

Bildt, Carl. 1992. "Sverige Halkar Efter Ekonomiskt." in *Halkar Srerige Efter*, Edited by W. Korpi. Stockholm, Carlssons, 220–24.

Bion, J. 1994. "Cost Containment: Europe: The United Kingdom." *New Horizon* 2:341–44.

Blendon, R. J., K. Donelan, R. Leitman, A. Epstein, J. Cantor, A. Cohen, I. Morrison, T. Mahoney, and C. Koeck. 1993. "Health Reform Lessons Learned from Physicians in Three Nations." *Health Affairs* 12:194–203.

Bloom, Gerald, T. Sheng-lan, and G. Xing-yuan. 1995. "Financing Rural Health Services in China in the Context of Economic Reform." *J. International Development* 7:423–41.

Bloom, Samuel. 1963. *The Doctor and His Patient.* New York: Free Press.

Bloor, M. and Gordon Horobin. 1975. "Conflict and Conflict Resolution in Doctor–Patient Interactions." In *A Sociology of Medical Practice*, edited by C. Cox and A. Mead. London: Collier MacMillan.

Boden, Ann Carlin. 1992. *Strukturomvandling I Hälso- och Sjukvården.* Stockholm: Vårdförbundet SHSTF (mimeo).

Bonanno, Alessandro, and Doug Constance. 1997. *Caught in the Net: The Global Tuna Industry, Environmentalism, and the State.* Lawrence: University Press of Kansas.

Bonanno, Alessandro. 1994. *From Columbus to ConAgra: The Globalization of Agriculture and Food.* Lawrence: University Press of Kansas.

Borrego, John. 1981. "Metanational Capitalist Accumulation and the Emerging Paradigm of Revolutionist Accumulation." *Review* 4:713–77.

Brante, Thomas. 1988. "Sociological Approaches to the Professions." *Acta Sociologica* 31:119–42.

———. 1992. "Expert Society: The Origins and Development of Professions in Sweden." *Studies in Higher Education* 1992:2.

———. "Authorities, Conflicts, and Institutions." Sociologiska Institutionen, Göteborgs Universitet.

Brock, R. M., and H. K. Grace. 1993. "Community Partnerships: Toward a New South African Health Care System." *Academic Medicine*, 68:828–30.

Brown, E. Richard. 1979. *Rockefeller Medicine Men: Medicine and Capitalism in America.* Berkeley and Los Angeles: University of California Press.

Brown, Phil. 1996. *Perspectives in Medical Sociology.* Prospect Heights, Il.: Waveland Press.

Brugha, C. M. 1991. "Better Management of Irish Hospitals." *Irish J. Medical Science* 160:239–42.

Buchan, J. 1992. "Cost-Effective Caring." *International Nursing Review*, 39:117–20.

Burchardi, H., H. P. Schuster, and S. Zielman. 1994. "Cost Containment: Europe: Germany." *New Horizons* 2:364–74.

Burton, R. I. 1994. "Discovering the Right Questions—Our Call to Action—Who Will Define Health Care Rationing, and How?" *J. Hand Surgery* 19:169–80.

Butler, B. 1986. "Changing Health Policy." *World Irish Nursing*, 15:508.

Bäck, Mats, and Tommy Möller. 1990. *Partier och Organizationer*, Stockholm: Publica.

Bäckström, Anders. 1991. "Vissa risker för sysselsättningen." In *Den sociala dimensionen in Europasamarbetet: Rapport från ett seminarium in februari 1991.* Stockholm: Utrikesdepartment, 44–45.

Cairney, R. 1995. "Health Care Reform Comes to Alberta: 'We're Making This Up as We Go Along,'" *Canadian Medical Association J.* 152:1861–163.

Calltorp, Johan. 1989a. *Prioritering och beslutsprocess i sjukvårdsfrågor*. Uppsala: Institutionen för Socialmedicin.

———. 1989b. "The 'Swedish Model' Under Pressure: How to Maintain Equity and Develop Quality." *Quality Assurance in Health Care* 1:13–22.

Calmfors, Lars. 1993a. "De Institutionella Systemen på Arbetsmarknaden och Arbetslösheten." *Ekonomikommissionen*, Bilaga 4, Bilagadel 1, 109–76.

———. 1993b. "Löner, Sysselsättning och den Ekonomiska Politiken." In *Varför Överge den Svenska Modellen,* edited by V. Bergström, Stockholm: Tiden. 34–57.

Calvert-Simms, D. 1993. "Changing Realities: An Analysis of the British Health Care System and its Implications for Nursing." *Canadian J. Nursing Administration* 6:24–28.

Cardoso, J. M. 1993. "The Impact of the Free Trade Agreement on Mexican Medicine and Radiology." *Invest Radiol* 28 suppl. 3:S31.

Carlqvist, Knut. 1993. *Åt Envar efter Arbete: Fackets Förlorade Rötter*. Stockholm: Timbro.

Carniero, Robert L., ed. 1967. *The Evolution of Society: Selections from Herbert Spencer*. Chicago: University of Chicago Press.

Carnoy, Martin, and Derek Shearer. 1980. *Economic Democracy: The Challenge of the 1980s*. White Plains, N.Y.: M. E. Sharpe.

Carr-Saunders, A. M., and P. A. Wilson. 1933. *The Professions*. Oxford: Clarendon Press.

Cassels, Andrew. 1995. "Health Sector Reform: Key Issues in Less Developed Countries." *J. International Development* 7:329–47.

Catley-Carlson, M. 1992. "Global Considerations Affecting the Health Agenda of the 1990s." *Academic Medicine* 67:409–24.

Chanfreau, D. 1979. "Professional Ideology and the Health Care System in Chile." *International J. Health Services* 9:87–105.

Chaston, I. 1994. "A Comparative Study of Internal Customer Management Practices within Service Sector Firms and the National Health Service." *J. Advanced Nursing* 19:299–308.

Chernichovsky, Dov. 1995. "Health System Reforms in Industrial Democracies: An Emerging Paradigm." *Milbank Quarterly* 73.

Clarke, Simon. 1990. "The Crisis of Fordism or the Crisis of Social Democracy." *Telos* 83:71–98.

Constance, Douglas, and William Heffernan. 1991. "The Global Poultry Agro/Food Complex." *International J. Sociology of Agriculture and Food* 1:126–142.

Cuyer, A. J. 1991. *Health Care and Health Care Finance in Sweden: The Crisis That Never Was; the Tensions That Ever Will Be*. Stockholm: Studieförbundet Näringsliv och Samhâlle, No. 33.

Cuyer, A. J., Robert Evans, J. Matthies Graf von der Schulenberg, Wynand van de Ven, and Burton Weisbrod. 1991. *International Review of the Swedish Health Care System*. Stockholm: Studieförbundet Näringsliv och Samhälle, No. 34.

Dahlin, Ann. 1994. "Husläkarna togs bort med en rösts övervikt." *Från Riksdag och Departmentet* 15 (29 April): 12.

Denzin, Norman. 1968. "Incomplete Professionalization: The Case of Pharmacy." *Social Forces*, 46:375–82.

Deurell, Mats. 1998. "Politikerföraktet: Ett hot mot domokratin eller ett tecken på ifrågasättande, kritiska medborgare?" *Från Riksdag och Departmentet* 24:3–4.

Devgan, A. K. 1992. "Strengthening Primary Care—A Move Toward Privatization." *Nursing J. India* 83:283–84.

Dickson, J. L., and M. Garside. 1995. "Resource Management Progress of the Program in the NHS in England." *Medinfo* 8:1634.

Donahue, J. M. 1986. "Planning for Primary Health Care in Nicaragua: A Study in Revolutionary Change." *Social Science and Medicine* 23:149–57.

Dor, Avi. 1994. *Are Contract-Managed Hospitals More Efficient?* Rockville, Md.: Center for General Health Services.

D'Sousa, M. F. 1995. "The Multifund and Outcome Research." *International J. Epidemiology* 24 suppl. 1:S113–18.

Dubos, René. 1959. *Mirage of Health*. Garden City, N.Y.: Doubleday.

Duffy, Diane. 1989. "The Effect of Sweden's Corporatist Structure on Health Policy and Outcomes," *Scandinavian Studies* 61:128–45.

Edgren, Jan. 1973. *Med Växlande Framgång—ett Försök till Förnyelse av Lönesystem och Arbetsformer*. Stockholm: Svenska Arbetsgivareföreningen.

Edin, Per-Olof. 1993. Interview with author, 26 April, Stockholm.

Edling, J. 1992a. *Finns det alternativ till karensdagar?* Stockholm: LO Bakgrund och Fakta.

———. 1992b. *Utredningen om församrad arbetsskadeförsakring—ett hafsverk av regeringen!* Stockholm: LO Bakgrund och Fakta.

———. n.d. *Sanningen om karensdagar och sjukfrånvaro*. Stockholm: LO Bakgrund och Fakta.

———. 1993. Interview with the author, 4 June, Stockholm.

Edström-Fors, Eva. 1991. "Kommun får nytt utvidgat ansvar för äldreomsorgen: Ädelreformen genomförs." *Vård* 3:8–13.

Ekdahl, Åke. 1993. "Ökad borgerligt EU-motstånd: 26 procent för och 45 emot enlight SCB." *Dagens Nyheter*, 10 December, p. A10.

Ekonomikommissionen. 1993. *Nya Villkor för Ekonomi och Politik*, Stockholm Finansdepartmentet, SOU 1993:16.

Eliasson, Olof. 1993. Personal communication.

Elioutina, S., and V. Tarasov. 1995. "Current State and Perspectives of Healthcare Informatics in Russia." *International J. Biomed Comput*, 39:163–67.

Elmbrant, Björn. 1993. *Så föll den svenska modellen*. Stockholm: T. Fischer.

Emaneul, E. J. and N. N. Dubler. 1995. "Preserving the Physician–Patient Relationship in the Era of Managed Care." *J. American Medical Association* 273:323–29.

Engellau, Patrik. 1987. *På Spanning efter moder Sveas själ*. Stockholm: Timbro.

Engman, Eva. 1998. "Ökning av långtidssjukskrivna oroar regeringen." *Från Riksdag och Departmentet* 29:14.

Engström, Odd. 1994. "Därför säger vi ja." *VI* 11:44.

Enquist, Per Olov. 1992. "Efter den europeiska tystnaden." In *EG/EU—Till Vilket Pris?* edited by W. Agrell. Stockholm: Lts Förlag, 4–11.

Enthoven, A. C. 1980. *Health Plan*. Reading, Mass.: Addison-Wesley.

———. 1986. "Managed Competition in Health Care and the Unfinished Agenda," *Health Care Financing Review* Annual Supplement: 105–19.

Enthoven, A. C. and R. Kronick. 1989. "A Consumer Choice Health Plan for the 1990s." *New England J. Medicine*, 320:29–37, 94–101.

Esping-Anderson, G. 1985. *Politics Against Markets.* Princeton, N.J.: Princeton University Press.

———. 1990. *The Three Worlds of Welfare Capitalism.* Princeton, N.J.: Princeton University Press.

Evans, R. G., M. L. Barer, C. Hertzman, G. M. Anderson, I. R. Pulcins, and J. Lomas. 1989. "The Long Goodby: The Great Transformation of the British Columbia Hospital System." *Health Services Research* 24:435–59.

Fairfield, Roy P., ed. 1961. *The Federalist Papers.* Garden City, N.Y.: Doubleday.

Feldt, Kjell-Olaf. 1991. *Alla Dessa Dagar—I Regeringen 1982–1990.* Stockholm: Norstedts.

Fiedler, J. L. 1985. "Latin American Health Policy and Additive Reform: The Case of Guatemala." *International J. Health Services*, 15:275–99.

Flexner, Abraham. 1910. *Medical Education in the United States and Canada.* New York: Carnegie Foundation for the Advancement of Teaching.

Fogelberg, Boo. 1991. "EG och de handicappades rättigheter." In *Den sociala dimensionen in Europasamarbetet: Rapport från ett seminarium in februari 1991.* Stockholm: Utrikesdepartment, 57–58.

Forsman, Anders. 1993. Interview with author, 25 May.

Foster, S., C. Norman, and R. Sheaff. 1994. "Health Care Reforms: The Issues and the Role of Doctors." *Lancet* 344:175–77.

Freeborn, Donald. 1994. *Promise and Performance in Managed Care: The Prepaid Group Practice Model.* Baltimore: Johns Hopkins University Press.

Frenk, J., O. Gomez-Dantes, C. Cruz, F. Chacon, P. Hernandez, P. Freeman. 1994. "Consequences of the North American Free Trade Agreement for Health Services: A Perspective from Mexico." *American J. Public Health* 84:1591–97.

Friedland, William. 1991. "The Transnationalization of Agricultural Production: Palimpsest of the Transnational State." *International J. Sociology of Agriculture and Food* 1:48–58.

Friedman, B., and S. Shortell. 1988. "The Financial Performance of Selected Investor-Owned and Not-for-Profit Hospitals Before and After Medicare Prospective Payment." *Health Services Research* 23:237–67.

Freidson, Eliot. 1970. *Profession of Medicine.* New York: Dodd-Mead.

Freidson, Eliot, and Judith Lorber, eds. 1972. *Medical Men and Their Work.* Chicago: Aldine.

Fuller, Benjamin F. 1994. *American Health Care: Rebirth or Suicide?* Springfield, Il.: Charles C. Thomas.

Gahrton, Per. 1992. "När ekonomin styr miljöarbetet." In *EG/EU—Till Vilket Pris?* edited by W. Agrell. Stockholm: Lts Förlag, 101–22.

Galbraith, J. Kenneth. 1993. "Den Keynesianska Revolution." *Ordfront Magasin* 19, no. 4:40–43.

Gallagher, Eugene, ed. 1976. *The Doctor—Patient Relationship in the Changing Health Scene.* Washington, D.C.: DHEW (publication no. NIH 78–183).

Garfield, R. M. 1984. "Health Services Reforms in Revolutionary Nicaragua." *American J. Public Health* 74:1138–44.

Garpenby, Peter. 1989. *The State and the Medical Profession: A Cross-National Comparison of the Health Policy Arena in the United Kingdom and Sweden*, Linköping: Linköpings Universitet.

Gerdtham, Ulf G, and Bengt Jönsson. 1992. *Sjukvårdskostnader i de Nordiska Länderna*: Stockholm: Handelshögskolan, Ekonomiska Forksningsinstitut.

Ginsberg, E. 1996. "The Health Care Market: Theory and Reality." *Journal of the American Medical Association* 276:777.

Gist, John. 1996. "Entitlements and the Federal Budget: Facts, Folklore, and Future." *Milbank Quarterly* 74:3.

Glennerster, H., and M. Matsaganis. 1994. "The English and Swedish Health Care Reforms." *International J. Health Services* 24:231–51.

Graf von der Schulenburg, J. M. 1994. "Forming and Reforming the Market for Third-Party Purchasing of Health Care: A German Perspective." *Social Science and Medicine*, 39:1473–81.

Gramsci, Antonio. 1971. *Selection from Prison Notebooks*. New York: International Publishers.

Greenberg, Henry M., and Susan U. Raymond. 1994. *Beyond the Crisis: Preserving the Capacity for Excellence in Health Care and Medical Science*. New York: New York Academy of Sciences.

Greenlick, M. R. 1995. "Educating Physicians for the Twenty-First Century." *Academic Medicine* 70:179–85.

Greenlund, K. J., and R. H. Elling. 1995. "Capital Sectors and Workers' Health and Safety in the United States" *International J. Health Services* 25:101–16.

Grogan, C. M. 1995. "Urban Economic Reform and Access to Health Care Coverage in the People's Republic of China." *Social Science and Medicine* 41:1073–84.

Gröning, Lotta, Walter Korpi, Carina Nilsson, Mårten Ström, Sören Wibe, Lillemor Arvidsson, Kerstin Bäck, Mona Hillman Pinheiro, Klas Åmark. 1993. *I Mörkret Blir Alla Katter Grå*. Stockholm: Tiden.

Hadenius, Stig. 1988. *Swedish Politics During the 20th Century*, Stockholm: Swedish Institute.

Ham, C. 1994. "Health Care Reform in the Netherlands, Sweden and the United Kingdom." *Health Affairs*. 13:106–19.

———. 1996a. "Learning from Tigers: Stakeholder Health Care." *Lancet* 347:951–53.

———. 1996b. "Population Centered and Patient Focused Purchasing: The U.K. Experience." *Milbank Quarterly* 74:191–214.

Hamilton, Carl, and Dag Rolander. 1993. *Att Leda Sverige in i Krisen*. Stockholm: Norstedts.

Harrison, Bennett, and Barry Bluestone. 1988. *The Great U-Turn: Corporate Restructuring and the Polarization of America*. New York: Basic Books.

Harvy, David. 1990. *The Condition of Postmodernity*. Oxford: Basil Blackwell.

Hasselius, Inge. 1991. *Valfrihet och Effectivitet I Vården, En Idékiss*, Stockholm: Sveriges Läkarförbundet (mimeo).

"Health in 'Crisis'? Critical Problems in Health and Health Care." 1991. *Social Science and Medicine* 32:359–324.

Hedin, Bernt. 1991. *ÄDEL-reformen: Framtidens Äldre- och Handikappomsorg*. Stockholm: Socialstyrelsen and Handikappinstitutet.

Henderson, J. W. 1995. "The Politics of Health Care Reform." *J. Medical Association of Georgia* 84:35–37.
Heidenheimer, Arnold, and Nils Elvander, eds. 1980. *The Shaping of the Swedish Health System*. New York: St. Martin's Press.
Heinrichs, K. 1995. "The Impact of German Health Insurance Reforms on Redistribution and the Culture of Solidarity." *J. Health Politics, Policy and Law* 20:653–87, 689–94.
Helms, Robert B. 1993. *American Health Policy: Critical Issues for Reform*. Washington, D.C.: AEI Press.
Hernbäck, Eva. 1993. "Ädelvård blev billigare: Stockholm sparade 392 miljoner under 1992." *Dagens Nyheter*, 22 June, p. D5.
Hessler, Richard M., and Andrew C. Twaddle. 1982. "Sweden's Crisis in Medical Care: Political and Legal Changes." *J. Health Politics, Policy and Law* 7:440–59. Reprinted in R. Rist, ed. 1985. *Policy Studies Review Annual*. New Brunswick, N.J.: Transaction Books.
———. 1986. "Power and Change: Primary Care at the Crossroads in Sweden." *Human Organization* 45:134–47.
Hicks, Alexander, and Lane Kenworthy. 1998. "Cooperation and Political Economic Performance in Affluent Democratic Capitalism." *American J. Sociology*, 103:1631–72.
Hicks, Alexander, and Joya Misra. 1993. "Political Resources and the Growth of Welfare in Affluent Capitalist Democracies, 1960–1982." *American J. Sociology* 99:668–710.
Himmelstein, David U. 1994. *The National Health Program Book: A Source Guide for Advocates*. Monroe, Maine: Common Courage Press.
Hirschman, Albert. 1992. "Firms and Markets." *Contemporary Society* 21:741–44.
Ho, L. S. 1998. "Market Reforms and China's Health Care System." *Social Science and Medicine* 41:1065–72.
Holahan, John, ed. 1991. *Balancing Access, Costs, and Politics: The American Context for Health System Reform*. Washington, D.C.: Urban Institute Press.
Hollingsworth, J. Rogers, Jerald Hage, and Robert Hanneman. 1990. *State Intervention in Medical Care: Consequences for Britain, France, Sweden, and the United States, 1890–1970*. Ithaca and London: Cornell University Press.
Holmlund, Bertil. 1993. "Arbetslöshetskrisen—Kunjunturfemonen eller Systemfel?" *Ekonomikommissionen* 12:397–454.
Huang, S. M. 1988. "Transforming China's Collective Health Care System: A Village Study." *Social Science and Medicine* 27:879–88.
Huber, Evelyne, Charles Ragin, and John D. Stephens. 1993. "Social Democracy, Christian Democracy, Constitutional Structure, and the Welfare State." *American J. Sociology* 99:711–49.
Hughes, David, T. S. Jost, L. Griffiths, and J. V. McHale. 1995. "Health Care Contracts in Britain and the United States: A Case for Technology Transfer?" *J. Nursing Management* 3:287–93.
Hulstrand, Lars. 1982. *Hälso och sjukvårdslagen mm*. Stockholm: Publica.
Härnqvist, Margarita. 1978. Interview by author, in Göteburg.
———. 1983. Interview by author, in Göteburg.

Ibo, Hirobumi. 1980. "Health Insurance and Medical Services in Sweden and Denmark 1850–1950." In *The Shaping of the Swedish Health System*, edited by A. Heidenheimer and N. Elvander. New York: St. Martin's Press, 44–67.

Immergut, Ellen. 1989. "Procedures for Conciliation: The Institutional Basis of Swedish National Health Insurance, 1930–70." *Scandinavian Studies* 61:146–68.

Ingebritsen, Christine. 1992. "The Swedish Welfare State and Europe, 1992: Politics Against Markets?" Paper presented at the annual meeting of the Society for the Advancement of Scandinavian Studies, Minneapolis, May 1.

Inglis, A. L., J. Coast, S. F. Gray, T. S. Peters, and S. J. Frankel. 1995. "Appropriateness of Hospital Utilization: The Validity and Reliability of the Intensity–Severity–Discharge Review System in a United Kingdom Acute Hospital Setting." *Medical Care* 33:952–57.

Institute of Medicine, Committee on Assessing Health Care Reform Proposals. 1993. *Assessing Health Care Reform*. Washington, D.C.: National Academy Press.

Isaksson, A. 1985. *Per Albin: I. I vägen mot folkhemmet*. Stockholm: Wahlström & Widstrand.

Jameson, Frederic. 1991. *Postmodernism, or the Cultural Logic of Late Capitalism*. Durham, N.C.: Duke University Press.

Jensson, Per. 1992. "Sverige, EG, djurhållningen och maten." In *EG/EU—Till Vilket Pris?* edited by W. Agrell. Stockholm: Lts Försberg, 123–37.

Jessop, Bob. 1991. *State Theory*. State College: Pennsylvania State University Press.

Johansson, Astrid. 1993a. "Ädelreformen gav sämre äldrevård." *Dagens Nyheter*, 20 September, p. A7.

———. 1993b. "Äldre får sämre vård: Personnel på sjukhem kritisk mot Ädelreform." *Dagens Nyheter*, 18 September, p. A14.

———. 1993c. "Ombonat men ont om läkare: Tribblehemmet har levt snart två år med Ädelreformen—känslorna är blandade." *Dagens Nyheter*, 17 September, p. A6.

———. 1993d. "Skillnaden stor mellan sjukhem: Första utvärderingen av Ädelreformen antyder att vården blivit sämre i storstäderna." *Dagens Nyheter*, 19 September, p. A6.

———. 1993e. "Svårt värdera Ädel-effekten," *Dagens Nyheter*, 16 October, p. A6.

———. 1993f. "Vårdgarantin krymper köer." *Dagens Nyheter*, 16 October, p. A14.

Johansson, George. 1994. "Ja eller nej: Snabbbguide till EU valet—nu är det du som bestämmer." *Vi*, 17 March.

Jonung, Lars. 1989. *Inflationen och ekonomisk politik i Sverige*. Stockholm: Dialogos Economics.

Jyothi, K. 1993. "Health for All by 2000 a.d.: The Role of MCH Services." *Nursing J. India* 84:155–58, 168.

Järnebeck, Gunnar, and Ingrid Laxhed. 1990. *Den Svenska Hälso- och Sjukvården*. Stockholm: Riksdagens Revisorer (Report 1990/91:4).

Jönsson, Bengt, and Clas Rhenberg. 1985. *Effectivare Sjukvård Genom Bättre Ekonomistyrning*. Linköping: Tema Hälso- och Sjukvården i Samhället. Universitet i Linköping.

Kaplow, Abraham. 1964. *The Conduct of Inquiry*. San Francisco: Chandler.
Karlsson, Börje. 1993. "Ädelreformen: Könberg ryter till." *Dagens Nyheter*, 29 September, p. A7.
Kassirer, J. 1995. "Managed Care and the Morality of the Marketplace." *New England Journal of Medicine* 333:50.
Kawamura, N., Y. Gotoda, and H. Yoshikura. 1985. "The Rise in Medical Care Expenditures in Japan: Trends in Disease Patterns: 1977–81." *American J. Public Health* 75:1442–44.
Kelly, Shawn. 1998. "A Socio-Historical Analysis of the Role of Interest Groups in Shaping the National Health Insurance Reform." Ph.D. diss., University of Missouri, Columbia.
Kett, J. 1968. *The Formation of the American Medical Profession*. New Haven: Yale University Press.
Kirkman-Liff, B., and G. Neubauer. 1992. "The Development of Quality Assurance in the German Health Care System." *QRB Quality Review Bulletin*, 18:266–74.
Klein, Rudolf. 1995. "Big Bang Health Care Reform—Does It Work? The Case of Britain's 1991 National Health Service Reforms." *Milbank Quarterly* 73:299–337.
Koblik, Steven. 1975. *Sweden's Development from Poverty to Affluence, 1750–1970*. Minneapolis: University of Minnesota Press.
Kolk, Jaan, Gunn Franzén Lung, Roger Mörtvik, Ingemar Lindberg, Jan Edling. 1991. *Är Svensken Latast och Sjukast i Världen?*, Stockholm: LO.
Kopparbergs Läns Landsting. 1990. *Strategirapport avseende informations- och styrsystem inom hälsovården*. Lund: Cenergo Consultants ab.
Korpi, Walter. 1978. *The Working Class in Welfare Capitalism: Work, Unions and Politics in Sweden*, London: Routledge.
Korpi, Walter. 1992. *Halkar Sverige Efter: Sveriges Ekonomiska Tillväxt 1820–1990 i Jämförande Belysning*. Stockholm: Carlssons.
Kraudy, E., A. Liberati, F. Asioli, B. Saraceno, and G. Tognomi. 1987. "Organization of Services and Pattern of Psychiatric Care in Nicaragua: Result of a Survey in 1986." *Acta Psychiatr Scand* 76:545–51.
Kritzner, B. E. 1983. "Chile Changes Its Health Care System." *Social Security Bulletin* 46:16–18.
Könberg, Bo, and Ingrid Petersson. 1993. Interview, March 9.
Lagerlöf, Karl Erik. 1992. "Vara med och bestämma." In *EG/EU—Till Vilket Pris?* Edited by W. Agrell. Stockholm: Lts Förlag 21–31.
Lambert, John. 1991. "Europe: The Nation State Dies Hard." *Capital and Class* 43:9–23.
Landstinget Dalarna. 1990. *Varför göra en bra sjukvård bättret*. Falun: Landstinget Dalarna.
Landstingsförbundet. 1982. *Den nya hälso-och sjukvårds lagen*. Stockholm: Landstingsförbundet.
———. 1990. *Some Innovative Projects of Swedish County Councils*. Stockholm: Landstingsförbundet.
———. 1991a. *Crossroads: Future Options for Swedish Medical Care*. Stockholm, Landstingsförbundet.

———. 1991b. *Landsting i förändring: Några exampel.* Stockholm: Landstingsförbundet.
———. 1993a. *Framtidens Primärvård: Slutrapport.* Stockholm: Landstingsförbundet.
———. 1993b. *Landstingens Ekonomi.* Stockholm: Landstingsförbundet.
———. 1993c. *Vägval.* Stockholm: Landstingsförbundet.
———. 1995. *Vad ska man kalla det som händer I Mora?—och andra frågor om styrmodeller*, Stockholm: Landstingsförbundet.
Lane, P. 1995. "Economic Hardship has Put Nicaragua's Health Care System on the Sick List." *Canadian Medical Association J.*, 152:580–82.
Lane, Robert. 1991. *The Market Experience.* Cambridge, Cambridge University Press.
Langby, Elisabeth. 1983. *Vinter i Välfärdslandet.* Stockholm: Brombergs.
Lapins, Per. 1993. "Lobbygruppen mot Välfärden." *Fack Journalen* 2:11–17.
Larsson, Håkan. 1992. "Visst finns det alternativ!" In *EG/EU—Till Vilket Pris?* Edited by W. Agrell. Stockholm: Förlag, 178–86.
Larsson, Sven I. R. 1993. "Lindbeck vs. Grassman: Historian om hur Assar Lindbeck Manöverade ut Sven Grassman in Kylan och Ströp in Fri Debatt om den Svenska Ekonomin." *Ordfront Magasin* 19, no.3:22–28.
Lee, Philip, and Carroll Estes, eds. 1994. *The Nation's Health.* Boston: Jones and Bartlett.
Leijon, Anna-Greta, Kjell-Olof Feldt, Stig Malm, Rune Molin, Bo Toresson, Dan Andersson, Per-Olof Edin, and Klas Eklund. 1989. *90-tals Programmet: En debattbok om arbetsrörelsens viktigaste frågor under 90-talet*, Stockholm: Tidens Förlag.
Leyerli, Betty. 1994. *The Private Regulation of American Health Care.* Armonk, N.Y.: M. E. Sharpe.
Lidal, Bengt. 1991. "EG har ingen gemensam sociapolitik." In *Den sociala dimensionen I Europasamarbetet: Rapport från ett seminarium in februari 1991.* Stockholm: Utrikesdepartment, 50–51.
Lifton, R. J. 1988. *The Nazi Doctors: Medical Killing and the Psychology of Genocide.* New York: Basic Books.
Light, Donald W. 1991. "Effectiveness and Efficiency Under Competition: The Cochrane Test." *British J. Medicine*, 303:1253–54.
———. 1992a. "Equity and Efficiency in Health Care." *Social Science and Medicine* 35:465–69.
———. 1992b. "The Radical Experiment: Transforming Britain's National Health System to Interlocking Markets." *J. Public Health Policy* 13:146–55.
Lindbeck, Assar. 1968. *The Political Economy of the New Left.*
Lindholm, Ann-Marie. 1983. "Sjuk patient blev boende." *Dagens Nyheter*, 14 August, p. D4.
Lindholm, Nalle. 1978. Interview with the author, in Göteburg.
Lindqvist, Hans, and Eva-Britt Svensson. 1994. "Därför säger vi nej." *VI* 11:44.
Lipietz, Alain. 1992. *Towards a New Economic Order: Postfordism, Ecology and Democracy.* New York: Oxford University Press.
Litviak, J. I. and C. Bodart. 1993. "User Fees Plus Quality Equals Improved Access to Health Care: Results of a Field Experiment in Cameroon." *Social Science and Medicine* 37:369–83.
Liu, Y., W. C. Hsiao, Q. Li, X. Lui, and M. Rea. 1995. "Transformation of China's Rural Health Care Financing." *Social Science and Medicine* 41:1085–93.

LO (Landsorganizationen i Sverige). 1986. *Fackföreningsrörelsen och Välfärdsstate: Rapport till 1986 Ars LO-kongress Från LOs Utredning om den Offentliga Sektorn*. Stockholm: LO.

———. 1991. *LO-Medlemmar I Välfärden: Om Hälsar*, Facket på din sida, Rapport 10, Stockholm: LO 91.02 10.000.

———. 1993. *Om viljan Finns. . . : LOs Program mot arbetslöhet*. Stockholm: LO.

Lovén, John. 1992. *Välfärd i Blåsväder?* Stockholm: Socialstyrelsen.

Långtidsutredningen. 1990. *Långtidsutredningen 1990*. SOU 1990:14, Stockholm: Finansdepartmentet.

Lönnroth, Johan. 1993. *Shamanerna: Om ekonomi som förgylld vardag*. Stockholm: Arena.

Lööf, Hans, and Roland Spånt. 1993a. "Vad Beror den Svenska Krisen På?" *Välfärdfakta* 4:3–4.

———. 1993b. "Vi Håller Europeisk Tillväxttakt—Och Riskerar Samma Arbetslöshet." *Välfärdfakta* 4:1–2.

Madison, James. 1961. "Federalist Paper No. 10." In *The Federal Papers*, edited by Roy P. Fairfield. Garden City, N.J.: Doubleday.

Marx, Karl. 1973. *Grundrisse*. New York: Vintage.

———. 1974. *Economic and Philosophic Manuscripts of 1844*. Moscow: Progress.

Maryott, E. Edgar. 1906. *The New Medical World: A Book for Reference and Consultation Containing a Thorough Description of Disease with the Latest and Best Methods for Its Treatment, Also Popular and Practical Discussions on Medical Progress, Health, Marriage, Maternity, the Care of Children, Nursing the Sick and Many Other Topics of World Wide Interest. The Most Complete Nurses' Guide Published*. Springfield, Mass.: Hampton Publishing.

Mburu, F. M. 1994. "Health Delivery Standards: Vested Interests in Health Planning." *Social Science and Medicine* 39:1357–84.

McCallion, G. M., R. W. Stout, S. P. Harvey, and D. Rose. 1991. "The Development of a Programme of Care for Elderly People in Northern Ireland." *Aging* 3:337–42.

McKinlay, John. 1976. "The Changing Political and Economic Context of the Patient–Physician Encounter." In *The Doctor-Patient Relationship in the Changing Health Scene*, edited by E. Gallagher. Washington, D.C.: DHEW (publication no. NIH 78-183) 155–188.

Mechanic, David. 1996. "Changing Medical Organization and the Erosion of Trust." *Milbank Quarterly* 74:171–89.

Medicinsk Ekonomi + Teknik. 1994. "Inget huvudbettänkande från HSU 2000 före valet." *Medicinsk Ekonomi + Teknik* 2:4.

Mellor, A. C. 1994. "Resource Costs of Capitation Maintenance Care in Britain." *Community Dental Health* 11:188–91.

Miljöförbundet. 1993. *EG, EES och Miljön* Göteborg: Miljöförbundet.

Miller, Irwin. 1996. *American Health Care Blues: Blue Cross, HMOs, and Pragmatic Reform Since 1960*. New Brunswick, N.J.: Transaction.

Miller, S. M., ed. 1963. *Max Weber: Selections from His Work*. New York: Crowell.

Milner, Henry. 1989. *Sweden: Social Democracy in Practice*. New York: Oxford University Press.

Milton, A. 1991. *En Ny Primärvård: Idékiss från Läkarförbundet*. Stockholm: Läkarförbundet.
Ministry of Finance. 1992. *The Swedish Budget 1992–1993: Budget Statement and Summary*. Stockholm: Allmänna Förlaget.
Misgeld, Klaus, Karl Molin, and Klas Åmark, eds. 1992. *Creating Social Democracy: A Century of the Social Democratic Labor Party in Sweden*. Translated by Jan Teeland, University Park: Pennsylvania State University Press.
Mollstedt, Bengt. 1992. "The Future of Regional Policy in Health and Medical Care." Paper presented at Emory University, Atlanta, 22 May.
———. 1993. Personal communication, 2 January, in Stockholm.
Monekosso, G. L. 1993. "Meeting the Challenges of the African Health Crisis in the Decade of the Nineties." *African J. Medicine and Medical Science* 22, no. 4:7–12.
Montiero, Lois. 1973. "Cost Is No Object: Income and Physician Visits Reconsidered." *J. Health and Social Behavior* 14:99.
Morreim, E. Haavi. 1995. *Balancing Act: The New Medical Ethics of Medicine's New Economics*, Washington, D.C.: Georgetown University Press.
Moses, Jonathon W. 1992. "The Effect of European Integration on the Institutions of Social Democracy." Paper presented at the annual meeting of the Society for the Advancement of Scandinavian Studies, Minneapolis, 1 May.
Murray, C. J., J. Kruser, and W. Whang. 1994. "Cost-Effectiveness Analysis and Policy Choices: Investing in Health Systems." *Bulletin of the World Health Organization* 72:663–74.
Myrdal, Gunnar. 1982. *Hur styrs landet?* Stockholm: Rabén och Sjögren.
Møgedal, Sigrun, S. H. Steen, and G. Mpelumbe. 1995. "Health Sector Reform and Organizational Issues at the Local Level: Lessons from Selected African Countries." *J. International Development* 7:349–67.
Navarro, V. 1989. "The Jackson National Health Program." *International J. Health Services* 19:19–44.
Naylor, C. D. 1987. "Privatization of South African Health Services—Are the Underlying Assumptions Correct?" *South African Medical J.* 72:673–78.
———. 1988. "Private Medicine and the Privatization of Health Care in South Africa." *Social Science and Medicine* 27:1153–70.
Nej till EG. 1992. *Kritiska Europa Fakta*, Nr 18, November.
———. 1993. *15 skäl att säga nej till EES*. Göteborg: Folkrörelsen Nej till EG.
———. n.d. "EG och demokratin." In *Faktablad EG: Demokratin*. Göteborg: Nej till EG.
———. n.d. *Kritiska Europa Fakta: EES special No. 2.*
———. n.d. "Medlemskap i EG Syftande till neutralitet i krig." In *Faktablad EG: Neutraliteten*. Göteborg: Nej till EG.
OECD. 1987. *Financing and Delivering Health Care: A Comparative Analysis of OECD Countries*. Paris: OECD.
Ogbu, O. and M. Gallagher. 1992. "Public Expenditures and Health Care in Africa." *Social Science and Medicine* 34:615–24.
Olby, Britta. 1991. "Omsorg i hemmiljö: Aspekter på omsorgskvalitet ur skilda perspektiv." *Vård* 3:14–25.
Olsson, Sven. 1993. *Social Policy and Welfare State in Sweden*. Lund: Arkiv.

O'Neill, D., and M. Pearson. 1995. "Appropriateness of Hospital Use in the United Kingdom: A Review of Activity in the Field." *International J. Quality of Health Care* 7:239–44.

Ording, Jan. 1991. "Människor utanför arbetsmarknaden föga uppmärksammade." In *Den sociala dimensionen in Europasamarbetet: Rapport från ett seminarium in februari 1991.* Stockholm: Utrikesdepartment, 52–54.

Owens, Colodia. 1995. *Managed Care Organizations: Practical Implications for Medical Practices and Other Providers.* New York: McGraw-Hill.

Parsons, Talcott. 1951. *The Social System.* Glencoe, Ill.: Free Press.

———. 1964. *Social Structure and Personality,* Glencoe, Ill.: Free Press.

———. 1968. "Professions." *International Encyclopedia of the Social Sciences* 12:536.

———. 1975. "The Sick Role and the Role of the Physician Reconsidered." *Milbank Memorial Fund Quarterly* 53:257–78. Reprinted in *Action Theory and the Human Condition.* Edited by T. Parsons. New York: Free Press 17–34.

Picciotto, Sol. 1991. "The Internationalization of the State." *Capital and Class* 43:43–63.

Pierce, R. V. 1895. *The People's Common Sense Medical Adviser in Plain English: or Medicine Simplified.* Buffalo, N.Y.: World's Dispensary Printing Office and Bindery.

Pitelis, Christos. 1991. "Beyond the Nation State: The Transnational Firm and the Nation State." *Capital and Class* 43:131–52.

Press, Irwin. 1984. "The Predisposition to File Claims: The Patients' Perspective," *Law, Medicine and Health Care* 12, no. 2:53–66.

R&D Tema. 1993. "Så Föddes EES." In *Sverige och EES.* Stockholm: Från Riksdag och Departmentet.

Regeringens propositionen (government proposal). 1981/82:97. *Hälso- och sjukvårdslag, m.m.,*

———. 1983/84:190. *Om vissa ersättningar till sjukvårdshuvudmännen.*

———. 1992/93:160. *Proposition om Husläkare.*

Regeringens skrivelse. 1990/91:71. *Överenkommelse mellan Regering och Landstingsförbundet angående vårdgaranti för 1992.*

Relman, Howard. 1980. "The New Medical–Industrial Complex." *New England J. Medicine* 303:963–70.

———. 1983. "Investor-Owned Hospitals and Health Care Costs." *New England J. Medicine,* 309:370–72.

Richmond, C. 1996. "NHS Waiting Lists Have Been a Boone for Private Medicine in the U.K." *Canadian Medical Association J.* 154:378–81.

Riksdag. 1992. *Riksdagen har sagt ja till EES.* Stockholm: Riksdag.

Rosenthal, Marilyn. 1988. *Dealing with Medical Malpractice: The British and Swedish Experience.* Durham, N.C.: Duke University Press.

———. 1989. "Physician Surplus and the Growth of Private Practice: The Case of Sweden." *Scandinavian Studies* 61:169–84.

Rosero-Bixby, L. 1991. "Socioeconomic Development, Health Interventions and Mortality Decline in Costa Rica." *Scandinavian J. Med Suppl* 46:33–42.

Roy, M. J. 1993. "The German Health Care System: Model or Mirage?" *Southern Medical J.,* 86:1389–94.

Ruggie, Mary. 1996. *Realignments in the Welfare State: Health Policy in the United States, Britain and Canada*. New York: Columbia University Press.
SAF (*Svenska Arbetsgivareföreningen*). 1975. *Om Demokrati på Arbetsplatsen ur SAFs Remissvar*. Stockholm: SAF.
———. 1991. *Rätt man in Europa är ofta en kvinna: Om jämställdhet i Sverige och EG*. Stockholm: SAF.
———. 1992. *EG på 10 minuter*. Stockholm: SAF.
Saltman, Richard. 1992. *Patient Choice and Patient Empowerment: A Conceptual Analysis* (Occasional Paper #40). Stockholm: Studieförbundet Näringsliv och Samhälle.
Saltman, Richard, and Casten von Otter. 1987. "Revitalizing Public Health Care Systems: A Proposal for Public Competition in Sweden." *Health Policy* 7:21–40.
———. 1989. "Public Competition versus Mixed Markets: An Analytical Comparison." *Health Policy* 11:43–55.
———. 1992. *Planned Markets and Public Competition: Strategic Reform in Northern European Health Systems* London: Open University Press.
SAP (Social Democratic Party). 1993. *Konsument eller Mänslig Resurs? 10 Fristånde inlägg i debatten om förnyelsen av den offentliga sektorn*. Stockholm: SAP.
Sassen, Saskia. 1993. *The Global City: New York, London, Tokyo*. Princeton, N.J.: Princeton University Press.
Saward, Edward. 1970. Interviewed by author.
Scarpaci, J. L. 1987. "HMO Production and the Privatization of Health Care in Chile." *J. Health Politics, Policy and Law* 12:551–67.
Schein, Harry. 1990. *"Makten."* Stockholm: Bonniers.
Schreter, Robert, Steven Sharfstein, Carol Schreter, eds. 1994. *Allies and Adversaries: The Impact of Managed Care on Mental Health Services*. Washington, D.C.: American Psychiatric Press.
Schyman, Gudrun. 1992. "Vad händer med välfärden." In *EG/EU —Till Vilket Pris?* edited by W. Agrell. Stockholm: Lts Förlag, 77–91.
Selwyn, B. J., and M. Ruiz de Chavez. 1985. "Coverage and Patterns of Ambulatory Medical Care Use in Talpan, Mexico City." *Social Science and Medicine* 21:77–86.
SFS (Government Printing Office). 1962:242. *Sjukvårdslagen*.
———. 1990:1402. *Lag om övertagande av vissa sjukhem och andra vårdinrättningar.*
———. 1990:1403. *Lag om ändring i socialtjänsten (1980:620).*
———. 1990:1404. *Lag om kommunernas betalninganswar för viss hälso- och sjukvård.*
———. 1990:1405, *Lag on ändring i lagen (1985:569) om införande av lagen (1985:568) om särskilda omsorger om psykiskt utvecklingsstörda m fl.*
Shactman, David. 1995. *Market Consolidation, Antitrust, and Public Policy in the Health Care Industry: Agenda for Future Research*. Princeton, N.J.: Robert Wood Johnson Foundation.
Sharpe, Virginia, and Alan Faden. 1996. "Appropriateness in Patient Care: A New Conceptual Framework." *Milbank Quarterly* 74:115–38.
Sherrill, R. 1995. "The Madness of the Market: Dangerous to your Health." *Nation*, 260:45.
Shi, L. 1993. "Health Care in China: A Rural–Urban Comparison After the Socioeconomic Reform." *Bulletin of the World Health Organization* 71:723–36.

SHSTF. 1990. *Vården Spränger Ramarna*. Stockholm: Kommunals press—och informationsenhet.

———. n.d. "SHSTFs Medlemmar och Husläkarna—Synpunkter och Förslag," Stockholm: Vårdörbundet SHSTF (mimio).

SIAR. 1990. *Människor i samspel: Struktur för sjukvården i Dalarna under 90-talet*. Lund: SIAR (Project L-417).

Sigeman, Tore. 1991. "EG-rättens förhållande till nationell rätt: Arbetsrättsliga aspekter." In *Den sociala dimensionen in Europasamarbetet: Rapport från ett seminarium in februari 1991*. Stockholm: Utrikesdepartment, 29–34.

Simpson, Richard L. 1971. "Imperative Control, Associationalism, and the Moral Order." In *Institutions and Exchange: The Sociologies of Talcott Parsons and George Homans*. edited by H. Turk and R. Simpson. Indianapolis: Bobbs-Merrill.

Soberón, G., J. Frenk, and J. Sepulveda. 1986. "The Health Care Reform in Mexico: Before and After the 1985 Earthquakes." *American J. Public Health* 76:673–80.

Socialdemokratiska Riksdagsgruppen. 1993. *Strategi för välfärdens överlevnad och utveckling: Sociademokraternas välfärdspolitiska motion I januari 1993*. Stockholm: Riksdag.

Socialstyrelsen. 1991. *God vård i rätt tid—1992 års vårdgaranti: Allmänna råd från Socialstyrelsen* (Ds 1991:11).

———. 1992a. *Husläkare—för kontinuitet och trygghet i vården* (Ds 1992:41).

———. 1992b. *Sammanställning av remissytranden över departmentspromemoria med Förslag om husläkarsystem*, (Ds 1992:113).

———. 1993a. *Ädelreformen: Arsrapport 1993* (Socialstyrelsen Följer Upp och Utvärderar, 1993:8).

———. 1993b. *Vårdgaranti 1992: Uppföljning och utvärdering* (1993:11).

Socialutskottet. 1992/93. *Socialutskottets betankande Husläkare m.m.* (SoU22).

SOU (Statens Offentliga Utredningen). 1948:14. *Den Öppna Läkarvården i Riket*, Stockholm: Inrekesdepartmentet.

———. 1978:74. *Husläkare: en enklare och tryggare sjukvård.*

———. 1979:78. *Mål och Medel för hälso- och sjukvården.*

———. 1987:21. *Äldreomsog i utveckling.*

———. 1990:14. *Långtidsutredningen 1990*, Stockholm: Finansdepartmentet.

———. 1993:16. *Nya Villkor för Ekonomi och Politik—Ekonomikommisionens Förslag.*

———. 1993:38. *Hälso— och Sjukvården I Framtiden: Tre Modeller: Rapport från expertgruppen till HSU 200.*

———. 1993:52. *Ersättning vid arbetslöshet: Betänkande från utredning om en ny arbetslöshetsförsäkring.*

———. 1994:115. *Sjukvårdsreformer I andra länder.*

———. 1995:104. *Skattereformen 1990–1991: en utvärdering: betänkande av Kommittén för utvärding av skattereformen (KUSK).*

———. 1996:113. *En allmän och aktiv försäkring vid sjukdom och rehabilitaring.*

———. 1996:158. *Sverige och EU.*

———. 1996:163. *Behov och resurser I vården—en analys.*

———. 1996:175. *Styrning och samverkan.*

———. 1997:50. *Riksbankens ställning.*

———. 1997:85. *Förmån efter inkomst.*

———. 1997:116. *Barnets bästa I främsta rummet.*
———. 1997:118. *Delade städer—underlagsrapport från storstadskommittén.*
———. 1997:119. *En tydligare roll för hälso- och sjukvården I folkhälsoarbetet.*
———. 1997:131. *Lag om premiepension.*
———. 1997:154. *Patienten har rätt.*
———. 1998:2. *Tänder hela livet—nytt ersättningssystem för vuxentandvård.*
———. 1998:72. *Kommunala finansförbund.*
———. 1998:78. *Regelförenkling för framtiden, småföretagardelegations rapport.*
———. 1998:93. *Kapitalförsjörjning till småföretag.*
———. 1998:106. *Unga I hälsoförsäkring.*

Spasoff, R. A. 1995. "Health Department Administration of the Canadian Health Care Program," *J. Public Health Policy* 16:141–51.

Spencer, Herbert. 1858. *Essays: Scientific, Political and Speculative.* New York: Appleton.

SPRI. 1993. "Systemskifte med Stockholmodellen." *SPRI Informerar* 3:8–9.

Starr, Paul. 1982. *The Social Transformation of American Medicine.* New York: Basic.

Statistiska Centralbyrån (SCB). 1988. *Nationalräkenskaperna* Stockholm: SCB.

———. 1991. *The Cost and Financing of the Social Services in Sweden in 1991.* Stockholm: Statistics Sweden.

———. 1993. *Statistiska Årsbok '93 för Sverige.* Stockholm: SCB.

Stebbins, K. R. 1986. "Curative Medicine, Preventive Medicine and Health Status: The Influence of Politics on Health Status in a Rural Mexican Village." *Social Science and Medicine* 23:139–48.

Stevens, Rosemary. 1966. *Medical Practice in Modern England.* New Haven: Yale University Press.

———. 1971. *American Medicine and the Public Interest.* New Haven: Yale University Press.

Stigler, George. 1968. "Competition." *International Encyclopedia of the Social Sciences.* 3:181–86.

Strender, Börje. 1974. *Appropå Nya Arbetsformer.* Stockholm: Svenska Arbetsgivareföreningen.

Ståhl, Ingemar. 1993. "Den Reglerade Arbetsmarknaden." *Ekonomikommissionen,* Bilaga 23, Bilagadel 2, 337–59.

Sullivan, P. 1995. "Private Health Care Dominates Meeting as General Council Calls for National Debate on Issue." *Canadian Medical Association J.* 153:801–3.

Sumner, William Graham. 1883. *What Social Classes Owe to Each Other.* New York: Harper and Row. Reprint, 1961, Caldwell, Idaho: Caxton.

Svenska Fredskommittén. 1993. *Fred och Solidaritet.* No. 1: *Skulle du skicka ditt barn till en EU-armé?* Stockholm: Svenska Fredskommittén.

Svensson, Ronny. 1992. "Kommer EG att tredubbla arbetslösheten i Sverige?" In *EG/EU—Till Vilket Pris?* edited by W. Agrell. Stockholm: Lts Förlag, 57–76.

Swartz, D. 1993. "The Politics of Reform: Public Health Insurance in Canada." *International J. Health Services* 23:219–38.

Söderlund, N. 1994. "Product Definition for Healthcare Contracting: An Overview of Approaches to Measuring Hospital Output with Reference to the UK Internal Market." *J. Epidemiology and Community Health* 48:244–31.

Tajimi, K., Y. Shimada, S. Nishimura, and C. A. Sirio. 1994. "Cost Containment: The Pacific: Japan." *New Horizons* 2:404–12.

Tambour, M. 1997. "The Impact of Health Care Policy Initiatives on Productivity." *Health Economics* 6:57–70.

Terbörn, Göran. A. Kjellberg, S. Marklund, and U. Öhlund. 1978. "Sweden Before and After Social Democracy: A First Overview." *Acta Sociologica* Supplement, 21:3758.

Thibaud, Ewa. 1993. "EG-anpassning i otakt: Opinionen steget efter regeringens närmande till Europa." *Dagens Nyheter*, 14 November, p. A13.

Thorgren, Gunilla. 1992. "Kvinnornas ställning på arbetsmarknaden." In *EG/EU—Till Vilket Pris?* edited by W. Agrell. Stockholm: Lts Förlag, 92–100.

Thorslund, Mats. 1992. "Vad påverkar vårdbehov och vårdpotential?" In *Fler vårdbehovande: Familjens roll och samhällets ansvar*, edited by M. Thorslund. Helsingfors.

Thorslund, Mats, and Marti G. Parker. 1992. "Care of the Elderly in the Changing Swedish Welfare State." Paper presented at the British Society of Gerontology, University of Kent, Canterbury.

Tibblin, Gösta. 1979. Interview with the author, Göteborg.

Tierney, A. J., S. Sladden, J. Andersson, M. King, I. Lapsley, S. Llewellyn. 1994. "Measuring the Costs and Quality of Palliative Care: A Discussion Paper." *Palliative Medicine* 8:273–81.

Toguchi, T. 1995. "The Role of Nurses in Restructuring the Japanese Health System for the Benefits of Consumers." *J. American Academy of Nurse Practice* 7:431–34.

Toon, P. D. 1994. "Justice for Gatekeepers." *Lancet* 343:585–87.

Traska, Maria. 1995. *Managed Care Strategies: An Annual Report on the Latest Practices and Policies in the New Managed Care Environment.* New York: Faulkner and Gray's Healthcare Information Center.

Twaddle, Andrew C. 1976. "Discussion by Andrew Twaddle." In *The Doctor–Patient Relationship in the Changing Health Scene*, edited by E. Gallagher. Washington, D.C.: DHEW NIH (publication no. 78-183) 255–58.

———. 1979. *Sickness Behavior and the Sick Role*. Boston: G. K. Hall.

———. 1980. "Sickness and the Sickness Career: Some Implications." In *The Relevance of Social Science for Medicine*, edited by L. Eisenberg and A. Klineman. Dordrech, Holland: D. Reidel.

———. 1982. "From Medical Sociology to the Sociology of Health: Some Changing Concerns in the Sociological Study of Sickness and Treatment." In *Sociology: The State of the Art*, edited by T. Bottomore, M. Sokolowska, and S. Nowak. London and Beverly Hills: Sage, 323–57.

———. 1986. "Swedish Physicians' Perspectives on Work and the Medical Care System: I. The Case of District General Practitioners." *Social Science and Medicine* 25:763–71.

———. 1987. "Swedish Physicans' Perspectives on Work and the Medical Care System: II. The Case of Child and Maternal Health Physicians." *Social Science and Medicine* 25:515–24.

———. 1988. "Swedish Physicans' Perspectives on Work and the Medical Care System: III. Private Physicians on the Public System." *Social Science and Medicine* 27:761–68.

———. 1989. "Scandinavian Medical Care and the Crisis in Western Medicine." *Scandinavian Studies* 61:115–27.

———. 1992. "Reforming Swedish Medical Care." Paper tabled at the 12th International Conference on Social Science and Medicine, September, in Peebles, Scotland.

———. 1994a. "Recent Changes in the Swedish Medical Care System." Paper presented at the Annual Meeting of the Society for the Advancement of Scandinavian Studies, May, in Pullman, Wash.

———. 1994b. *Restructuring Medical Care: Swedish Opinion Leaders on the Medical Care Crisis (If there Is One).* Linköping: Tema H, Universitet i Linköping.

———. 1997. "EU or Not EU? The Swedish Debate on Entering the European Union 1993–1994." *Scandinavian Studies* 69:189–211.

Twaddle, Andrew C., and Richard Hessler. 1977. *A Sociology of Health*. St. Louis: Mosby.

———. 1986. "Power and Change: The Case of the Swedish Commission of Inquiry on Health and Sickness Care." *J. Health Politics, Policy and Law* 11:19–40.

———. 1987. *A Sociology of Health*. New York: MacMillan.

Twaddle, Andrew C., and Lennart Nordenfelt. 1994. *Disease, Illness and Sickness.* Studies in Health and Society, Linköping, Tema: Universitet i Linköping.

Twaddle, Andrew C., and John Stoeckle. 1971. *A Model of the Development of Western Medicine*. Boston: Massachusetts General Hospital (mimeo).

Uddhammar, Emil. 1993. *Partierna och den Stora Staten: En Analys av Statsteorier och Svensk Politik under 1900-talet*. Stockholm: City University Press.

Ugalde, A. 1984. "Where There Is a Doctor: Strategies to Increase Productivity at Lower Costs: The Economics of Rural Health Care in the Dominican Republic." *Social Science and Medicine* 19:441–50.

Ulvskog, Marita. 1992. "EES—en medelväg." In *EG/EU—Till Vilket Pris?* edited by W. Agrell. Stockholm: Lts Förlag, 150–58.

Urwitz, Gabriel, and Staffan Viotti. 1993. "Det Financiella Systemet—Dagens Problem och Synpunkter på Framtiden." *Ekonomikommissionen* Bilaga 25, Bilagadel 2, 393–412.

U.S. General Accounting Office. 1993. *1993 German Health Reforms: New Cost Control Initiatives: Report to the Chairman, Committee on Governmental Affairs.* Washington, D.C.: U.S. Senate (microfilm).

U.S. Congress. Senate. 1991. *Cutting Health Care Costs, Experiences in France, Germany and Japan: Joint Hearing before the Committee on Governmental Affairs and the Special Committee on Aging.* 102nd Cong., 1st sess. 19 November.

Utrikesdepartmentet. 1990. "Offentlig Upphandling i Ett Nytt Europa." In *Fakta Europa* Stockholm: Utrikesdepartmentor.

———. 1991. "Arbetsmiljön och EG." In *Fakta Europa*, Stockholm: Utrikesdepartmentor.

———. 1992. *Avtalet om Europiska Ekonomiska Samarbetsområdet: EES-Avtalet, Februari 1992*. Stockholm: Utrikesdepartmentor.

———. 1993. *EG inför folkomröstningen, Europa Information.* Stockholm: Sekretariat för Europainformation UD.

Vall-Spinosa, A. 1991. "Lessons from London: The British Are Reforming their National Health Service." *American J. Public Health* 81:1566–70.

Virdesten, Per. 1991. "Arbetsrätten i EG." In *Den sociala dimensionen in Europasamarbetet: Rapport från ett seminarium in februari 1991*. Stockholm: Utrikesdepartment, 27–28.

Viveros-Long, A. 1986. "Changes in Health Financing: The Chilean Experience." *Social Science and Medicine* 22:379–85.

von Otter, Casten, and Richard Saltman. 1990. *Valfrihet som Styrmedel*. Stockholm: Arbetslivscentrum.

Vågerö. D. 1994. "Equity and Efficiency in Health Reform: A European View." *Social Science and Medicine* 39:1204–10.

Wardwell, Walter. 1952. "A Marginal Professional Role: The Chiropractor." *Social Forces* 30:339–48.

———. 1980. "The Future of Chiropractic." *New England J. Medicine*. 302:688–90.

———. 1992. *Chiropractic: History and Evolution of a Profession*, St. Louis: Mosby Year Book.

Weber, Max. 1947. *The Theory of Social and Economic Organization*. Glencoe, Ill.: The Free Press.

Wedge, J. H. 1994. "The Impact of Health Care Reform on Orthopaedic Surgery in the United States and Canada." *Clinical Orthopedics* 308:271–80.

Westerberg, Bengt, and Sture Nordh. 1993. *Välfärdsstatens Vägval och Villkor*. Stockholm: Brombergs.

Westergaard, Kaj. 1991. "De nordiska traditionerna och den sociala dimensionen i EG." in *Den sociala dimensionen in Europasamarbetet: Rapport från ett seminarium in februari 1991*. Stockholm: Utrikesdepartment, 42–43.

Wibe, Sören. 1992. "EG och en ekonomiska tillväxten." In *Eg/Eu—Till Vilket Pris?* edited by W. Agrell. Stockholm: Lts Förlag, 32–56.

Wickbom, Ulf. 1989. *Blågula Rosor: Nedslag i Svensk Samtidshistoria 1969–1989*. Stockholm: LTs Förlag.

Williams, Michael. 1992. "Flyktningpolitiken—skydd för eller mot flyktningar?" In *Eg/Eu—Till Vilket Pris?* edited by W. Agrell. Stockholm: Lts Förlag, 138–49.

Wilsford, D. 1995. "States Facing Interests: Struggles over Health Care Policy in Advanced, Industrial Democracies." *J. Health Politics, Policy and Law* 20:571–613.

Yang, P. L., V. Lin, and J. Lawson. 1991. "Health Policy Reform in the People's Republic of China." *International J. Health Services* 21:481–91.

Zetterberg, Hans. 1979. *Hälsovården vid sprängpunkten*. Vällingby: Svenska Institut för Opinionsundersökningar, AB.

Zheng, X., and S. Hiller. 1995. "The Reforms of the Chinese Health Care System: County Level Changes: The Jiangxi Study." *Social Science and Medicine* 41:1057–64.

Zola, Irving. 1975. "Medicine as a System of Social Control." In *A Sociology of Medical Practice*, edited by C. Cox and A. Mead. London: Collier-MacMillan, Ltd.

Åsbrink, Erik. 1990. *Århundradets Skattereform: En Populärsammanfattning*. Stockholm: Allmänna Förlaget.

"Ädel var en viktig reform: Helheten är ett framsteg men vårdkompetensen på sjukhemmen behöver uppmarksammas." *Dagens Nyheter*, 1 October, 1993. p. A2.

Äldredelegationen. 1987. *Ansvaret för äldreomsorgen* (Ds 1987:27). Stockholm: Socialdepartmentet.

Name Index

The Swedish letters Å and Ö follow the English alphabet.

Subject Index

ABOUT THE AUTHOR

Andrew C. Twaddle is Professor of Sociology at the University of Missouri, Columbia.

ISBN 0-86569-289-0
90000>
EAN
9 780865 692893
HARDCOVER BAR CODE